Pocket Guide to

CLINICAL
MICROBIOLOGY

3RD EDITION

3RD EDITION

Pocket Guide to

CLINICAL MICROBIOLOGY

Patrick R. Murray, Ph.D., ABMM
Senior Scientist and Chief,
Clinical Microbiology Service
NIH Clinical Center
Bethesda, Maryland

Yvonne R. Shea, M.S.
Supervisor, Mycology and
Mycobacteriology Laboratories
Clinical Microbiology Service
NIH Clinical Center
Bethesda, Maryland

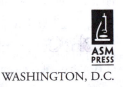

ASM
PRESS

WASHINGTON, D.C.

Address editorial correspondence to ASM Press, 1752 N St. NW, Washington, DC 20036-2904, USA

Send orders to ASM Press, P.O. Box 605,
Herndon, VA 20172, USA
Phone: 800-546-2416; 703-661-1593
Fax: 703-661-1501
E-mail: books@asmusa.org
Online: www.asmpress.org

Library of Congress Cataloging-in-Publication Data

Murray, Patrick R.
  Pocket guide to clinical microbiology / Patrick R. Murray,
Yvonne R. Shea—3rd ed.
     p. ; cm.
  Includes bibliographical references and index.
  ISBN 1-55581-288-0 (softcover)
  1. Medical microbiology—Handbooks, manuals, etc. I. Title:
Clinical microbiology. II. Shea, Yvonne R. III. Title.
  [DNLM: 1. Microbiology—Handbooks. 2. Antibiosis—
Handbooks. 3. Microbial Sensitivity Tests—Handbooks.
4. Microbiological Techniques—Handbooks. QW 39 M983p 2004]

QR46.M92 2004

616.9′041—dc22

2003070890

10 9 8 7 6 5 4 3 2 1

The role of Patrick R. Murray and Yvonne R. Shea in preparation of this book was carried out in their private capacity and does not reflect official support or endorsement by the National Institutes of Health or Department of Health and Human Services.

*To Melissa and David for their
patient support and loving understanding
while we labored with this project*

Contents

SECTION 5
Viral Diagnosis   233

SECTION 6
Fungal Diagnosis   255

SECTION 8
Vaccines, Susceptibility Testing Methods, and Susceptibility Patterns   **345**

Preface

Writing is an art of organizing and refining information. The challenge for authors is to identify what is important and express it in a coherent, logical manner. By its nature, a pocket guide is a condensation of many disparate facts. This makes the challenge more daunting — what information should be included and excluded, and how can it be logically presented without creating a book that expands beyond the limits of a lab coat pocket? This is the third edition of the *Pocket Guide to Clinical Microbiology*. The genesis of this series sprang from the observation that our clinical colleagues were never far removed from an assortment of pocket-sized reference texts that they used to confirm clinical diagnoses and treatment options. Like our colleagues, clinical microbiologists must constantly make decisions — about the choice of diagnostic tests such as culture, detection of microbial antigens or serologic responses, and genome-based approaches; how to collect, transport, and process specimens; and what methods should be used to identify an isolated organism and determine its susceptibility to a spectrum of antimicrobial agents. A number of good reference texts exist that can guide the clinical microbiologist (refer to the Bibliography of this pocket guide), but these volumes are hardly pocket-size. Hence, the first edition of this text was born. As with most projects of this nature, each subsequent edition is a refinement of the previous. In this third edition, both the content and the organization have been modified. Some of these changes are transparent, others are obvious. The most obvious change is the addition of a second author, Yvonne R. Shea, who has assumed responsibilities for the mycology and mycobacteriology sections of the *Pocket Guide*. Another obvious change is that we have reorganized the diagnostic sections. In the previous two editions, specimen processing, organism isolation and identification, and immunodiagnostic testing were in separate sections. In this edition we have combined this information into separate diagnostic sections for bacteria, viruses, fungi, and parasites. We hope the readers will find this more useful. We have also carefully updated the information presented in this text, using as our guide the published literature and available reference texts, particularly the eighth edition of the *Manual of Clinical Microbiology* and other ASM publications. Obviously, not all information can be incorporated into this pocket guide. Rather, we hope the readers will use this text as the beginning and not the end. It should serve as a quick reference. The users of this pocket guide should refer to the available reference books for a more expansive coverage of the topics presented here. For your additional convenience, the *Pocket Guide* is now available via ASM Press in PDA format.

As with any project of this nature, there are many people who should be thanked. We have been fortunate to work with many excellent clinical microbiologists at Washington University, the University of Maryland, and the National Institutes of Health Clinical Center, as well as colleagues in many national and international laboratories. Special thanks go to colleagues from the editorial board of the *Manual of Clinical Microbiology* (Ellen Jo Baron, Jim Jorgensen, Mike Pfaller, and Bob Yolken) and Davise Larone, who graciously allowed us to borrow heavily from her text, *Medically Important Fungi, a Guide to Identification*. We also thank once more the staff at ASM Press, particularly Susan Birch and Jeff Holtmeier. Without their efforts, encouragement, and patience, this pocket guide would never have been possible. Finally, we thank all those who have offered suggestions for improving the *Pocket Guide to Clinical Microbiology*. We hope this effort will not fall short of their expectations.

Patrick R. Murray
Yvonne R. Shea

Taxonomic Classification of Medically Important Microorganisms

In the previous editions of this pocket guide, the first section was devoted to a taxonomic listing of common (and some uncommon) organisms associated with humans. Unfortunately, lists of this sort are becoming increasingly complex with the rapid proliferation of new species of organisms. In large part this is a direct result of the use of more sophisticated phenotypic tests and genomic analyses (e.g., sequencing of housekeeping and rRNA genes). We have attempted to provide the current taxonomic classification of microbes. However, because any listing of organisms will rapidly become outdated, it seems appropriate to provide electronic references for the latest classification of organisms.

It should be appreciated that despite appearances, changes in nomenclature are regulated by a system of rules with oversight governed by the International Code of Biological Nomenclature (www.biosis.org.uk/zrdocs/codes/codes.htm). The International Code of Nomenclature of Bacteria governs bacterial taxonomy, and all bacteria named after 1980 must be validly published in the *International Journal of Systematic and Evolutionary Microbiology*. A current listing of bacteria can be found at http://www.bacterio.net, http://www.bacterio.cict.fr/, and http://www.dsmz.de/bactnom/bactname.htm. The International Committee on Taxonomy of Viruses (ICTV) governs viral taxonomy, and all currently recognized viruses can be found at www.ncbi.nlm.nih.gov/ICTVdb/. The International Code of Botanical Nomenclature governs fungal classification, and additional information can be found at www.bgbm.org/iapt/nomenclature/code/.

Taxonomic Classification of Bacteria

Eubacteria have been subdivided into at least 11 divisions, including 5 with medically important organisms.

1. Division: Proteobacteria
   Subdivision: Alpha subclass
      Subgroup 1
         Genus. *Brevundimonas*
      Subgroup 2
         Family. *Bartonellaceae*
         Genus. *Bartonella*
         Family. *Rickettsiaceae*
         Genus. *Rickettsia*
         Genus. *Orientia*

Family. *Anaplasmataceae*
  Genus. *Ehrlichia*
  Genus. *Anaplasma*
  Genus. *Neorickettsia*
  Genus. *Wolbachia*
Family. *Brucellaceae*
  Genus. *Brucella*
  Genus. *Ochrobactrum*

Subdivision: Beta subclass
Subgroup 1
  Genus. *Burkholderia*
Subgroup 2
Family. *Neisseriaceae*
  Genus. *Eikenella*
  Genus. *Kingella*
  Genus. *Neisseria*
  Genus. *Simonsiella*
Family. *Alcaligenaceae*
  Genus. *Alcaligenes*
  Genus. *Acromobacter*
  Genus. *Bordetella*
Uncertain classification
  Genus. *Chromobacterium*
Subgroup 3
Family. *Comamonadaceae*
  Genus. *Acidovorax*
  Genus. *Comamonas*

Subdivision: Delta subclass
  Genus. *Desulfovibrio*

Subdivision: Gamma subclass
Subgroup 1
Family. *Legionellaceae*
  Genus. *Legionella*
Family. *Francisellaceae*
  Genus. *Francisella*
Uncertain classification
  Genus. *Coxiella*
Subgroup 2
Family. *Enterobacteriaceae*
  Genus. *Cedecea*
  Genus. *Citrobacter*

Genus. *Edwardsiella*
Genus. *Enterobacter*
Genus. *Escherichia*
Genus. *Ewingella*
Genus. *Hafnia*
Genus. *Klebsiella*
Genus. *Kluyvera*
Genus. *Leclercia*
Genus. *Moellerella*
Genus. *Morganella*
Genus. *Pantoea*
Genus. *Plesiomonas*
Genus. *Proteus*
Genus. *Providencia*
Genus. *Salmonella*
Genus. *Serratia*
Genus. *Shigella*
Genus. *Tatumella*
Genus. *Yersinia*
Family. *Vibrionaceae*
Genus. *Listonella*
Genus. *Shewanella*
Genus. *Vibrio*
Family. *Pasteurellaceae*
Genus. *Actinobacillus*
Genus. *Haemophilus*
Genus. *Mannheimia*
Genus. *Pasteurella*
Family. *Aeromonadaceae*
Genus. *Aeromonas*

Subgroup 3
Family. *Pseudomonadaceae*
Genus. *Pseudomonas*
Family. *Moraxellaceae*
Genus. *Acinetobacter*
Genus. *Branhamella*
Genus. *Moraxella*
Uncertain classification
Genus. *Stenotrophomonas*

Subgroup 4
Family. *Cardiobacteriaceae*
Genus. *Cardiobacterium*
Genus. *Suttonella*

Subdivision: Epsilon subclass
  Family. *Campylobacteraceae*
    Genus. *Arcobacter*
    Genus. *Campylobacter*
  Uncertain classification
    Genus. *Helicobacter*
    Genus. *Wolinella*

Division: "Gram-positive" bacteria
Subdivision 1: Gram-negative anaerobes
  Family. *Veillonellaceae*
    Genus. *Acidaminococcus*
    Genus. *Megasphaera*
    Genus. *Veillonella*
  Uncertain classification
    Genus. *Selenomonas*
Subdivision 2: *Heliobacterium*
Subdivision 3: Bacteria with low G+C mol%
  Order. *Bacillales*
  Family. *Bacillaceae*
    Genus. *Aneurinibacillus*
    Genus. *Bacillus*
        B. subtilis group
        B. cereus group (includes *B. anthracis*)
        B. sphaericus group
    Genus. *Brevibacillus*
    Genus. *Gemella*
    Genus. *Listeria*
    Genus. *Paenibacillus*
    Genus. *Planococcus*
    Genus. *Staphylococcus*
    Genus. *Virgibacillus*
  Family. *Streptococcaceae*
    Genus. *Enterococcus*
    Genus. *Lactococcus*
    Genus. *Streptococcus*
  Family. *Lactobacillaceae*
    Genus. *Lactobacillus*
    Genus. *Leuconostoc*
    Genus. *Pediococcus*
  Family. *Peptococcaceae*
    Genus. *Anaerococcus*

Genus: *Coprococcus*
Genus. *Finegoldia*
Genus: *Peptococcus*
Genus. *Micromonas*
Genus. *Peptoniphilus*
Genus: *Ruminococcus*
Genus: *Sarcina*
Uncertain affiliation
Genus. *Aerococcus*
Genus. *Kurthia*
Order. *Clostriadiales*
Family. *Clostridiaceae* I
Genus. *Clostridium* (e.g., *C. perfringens*,
C. butyricum)
Family. *Clostridiaceae* II
Genus. *Clostridium* (e.g., *C. difficile*)
Genus. *Eubacterium*
Genus. *Peptostreptococcus*
Family. *Clostridiaceae* III
Genus. *Clostridium* (e.g., *C. sphenoides*)
Family. *Clostridiaceae* IV
Genus. *Clostridium* (e.g., *C. innocuum*,
C. ramosum)
Genus. *Erysipelothrix*
Genus. *Lactobacillus* (e.g., *L. catenaforme*)
Order. *Mycoplasmatales*
Family. *Mycoplasmataceae*
Genus. *Mycoplasma*
Genus. *Ureaplasma*
Order. *Acholeplasmatales*
Family. *Acholeplasmataceae*
Genus. *Acholeplasma*

Subdivision 4: Bacteria with high G+C mol%
Order. *Actinomycetales*
Suborder. *Actinomycineae*
Family. *Actinomycetaceae*
Genus. *Actinomyces*
Genus. *Arcanobacterium*
Genus. *Mobiluncus*
Suborder. *Corynebacterineae*
Family. *Corynebacteriaceae* (coryneform
bacteria)
Genus. *Corynebacterium*

Family. *Dietziaceae*
 Genus. *Dietzia*
Family. *Mycobacteriaceae*
 Genus. *Mycobacterium*
Family. *Nocardiaceae*
 Genus. *Nocardia*
 Genus. *Rhodococcus*
Family. *Tsukamurellaceae*
 Genus. *Tsukamurella*
Suborder. *Micrococcineae*
Family. *Brevibacteriaceae*
 Genus. *Brevibacterium*
Family. *Cellulomonadaceae*
 Genus. *Cellulomonas*
 Genus. *Oerskovia*
 Genus. *Tropheryma*
Family. *Dermatophilaceae*
 Genus. *Dermatophilus*
Family. *Micrococcaceae*
 Genus. *Arthrobacter*
 Genus. *Micrococcus*
 Genus. *Rothia* (*Stomatococcus*)
Suborder. *Micromonosporineae*
Family. *Micromonosporaceae*
 Genus. *Micromonospora*
Suborder. *Propionibacterinaeae*
Family. *Nocardioidaceae*
 Genus. *Nocardioides*
Family. *Propionibacteriaceae*
 Genus. *Luteococcus*
 Genus. *Propionibacterium*
Suborder. *Pseudonocardinaeae*
Family. *Pseudonocardiaceae*
 Genus. *Amycolata*
 Genus. *Amycolatopsis*
 Genus. *Saccharomonospora*
 Genus. *Saccharopolyspora*
Suborder. *Streptomycineae*
Family. *Streptomycetaceae*
 Genus. *Streptomyces*
Suborder. *Streptosporangineae*
Family. *Nocardiospsaceae*
 Genus. *Nocardiopsis*

Family. *Thermomonosporaceae*
Genus. *Actinomadura*
Genus. *Thermomonospora*
Order. *Bifidobacteriales*
Family. *Bifidobacteriaceae*
Genus. *Bifidobacterium*
Genus. *Gardnerella*
Unclassified *Bifidobacteriales*
Family. *Turicella*
Genus. *Turicella*

3. Division: Spirochaetes

Order. *Spirochaetales*
Family. *Spirochaetaceae*
Genus. *Borrelia*
Genus. *Cristispira*
Genus. *Serpulina*
Genus. *Spirochaeta*
Genus. *Treponema*
Family. *Leptospiraceae*
Genus. *Leptonema*
Genus. *Leptospira*

4. Division: Aerobic and anaerobic bacilli in RNA superfamily V
Subgroup 1

Family. *Bacteroidaceae*
Genus. *Bacteroides*
Genus. *Bilophila*
Genus. *Porphyromonas*
Genus. *Prevotella*
Uncertain classification
Genus. *Fusobacterium*
Genus. *Leptotrichia*
Subgroup 2

Family. *Flavobacteriaceae*
Genus. *Capnocytophaga*
Genus. *Flavobacterium*
Uncertain classification
Genus. *Cytophaga*
Genus. *Flexibacter*

5. Division: Chlamydiae

    Order. *Chlamydiales*

        Family. *Chlamydiaceae*

            Genus. *Chlamydia*

            Genus. *Chlamydophila*

Taxonomic Classification of Human Viruses

Single-stranded, nonenveloped DNA viruses

    Family. *Parvoviridae*

        Genus. *Erythrovirus*: B19 virus

        Genus. *Dependovirus*: Adeno-associated viruses

Double-stranded, nonenveloped DNA viruses

    Family. *Polyomaviridae*

        Genus. *Polyomavirus*: Simian virus 40 (SV40), JC polyomavirus, BK polyomavirus

    Family. *Papillomaviridae*

        Genus. *Papillomavirus*: Human papillomavirus

    Family. *Adenoviridae*

        Genus. *Mastadenovirus*: Human adenoviruses (types 1 through 51)

Double-stranded, enveloped DNA viruses

    Family. *Poxviridae*

        Genus. *Orthopoxvirus*: Vaccinia virus, smallpox virus, cowpox virus, monkeypox virus

        Genus. *Molluscipoxvirus*: Molluscum contagiosum virus

        Genus. *Parapoxvirus*: Orf virus

        Genus. *Suipoxvirus*: Swinepox virus

    Family. *Hepadnaviridae*

        Genus. *Orthohepadnavirus*: Hepatitis B virus

    Family. *Herpesviridae*

        Genus. *Simplexvirus*: Human herpesvirus 1 (herpes simplex virus type 1; HHV-1), human herpesvirus 2 (herpes simplex virus type 2; HHV-2)

        Genus. *Varicellovirus*: Human herpesvirus 3 (varicella-zoster virus [VZV]; HHV-3)

        Genus. *Lymphocryptovirus*: Human herpesvirus 4 (Epstein-Barr virus [EBV]; HHV-4)

        Genus. *Cytomegalovirus*: Human herpesvirus 5 (CMV; HHV-5)

Genus. *Roseolovirus*: Human herpesvirus 6 (roseola virus; HHV-6), human herpesvirus 7 (HHV-7)

Genus. *Rhadinovirus*: Human herpesvirus 8 (HHV-8)

Single-stranded, positive-sense, nonenveloped RNA viruses

Family. *Picornaviridae*

Genus. *Human enterovirus A*: Human coxsackievirus A (types 2, 3, 5, 7, 8, 10, 12, 14, and 26), enterovirus 71

Genus. *Human enterovirus B*: Human coxsackievirus A (type 9), human coxsackievirus B (types 1 through 6)

Genus. *Human enterovirus C*: Human coxsackievirus A (types 1, 11, 13, 15, 17 through 22, and 24)

Genus. *Human enterovirus D*: Human enterovirus (types 68 and 70)

Genus. *Poliovirus*: Human poliovirus (types 1 through 3)

Genus. *Human rhinovirus A*: Human rhinovirus (types 1, 2, 7, 9, 11, 15, 16, 21, 29, 36, 39, 49, 50, 59, 62, 65, 85, and 89)

Genus. *Human rhinovirus B*: Human rhinovirus (types 3, 14, and 72)

Genus. *Aphthovirus*: Foot-and-mouth disease virus

Genus. *Hepatovirus*: Human hepatitis A virus (HHAV)

Family. *Caliciviridae*

Genus. *Norovirus*: Norwalk virus

Genus. *Sapovirus*: Sapporo virus

Family. *Astroviridae*

Genus. *Astrovirus*: Human astrovirus (types 1 through 8)

Single-stranded, positive-sense, enveloped RNA viruses

Family. *Coronaviridae*

Genus. *Coronavirus*: Human coronavirus

Genus. *Torovirus*: Human torovirus

Family. *Togaviridae*

Genus. *Alphavirus*: Sindbis virus, Eastern equine encephalitis (EEE) virus, Western equine encephalitis (WEE) virus, Venezuelan equine encephalitis (VEE) virus, many other viruses

Genus. *Rubivirus*: Rubella virus

Family. *Flaviviridae*

Genus. *Flavivirus*: Yellow fever virus, West Nile virus, St. Louis encephalitis (SLE) virus, Japanese encephalitis (JE) virus, Dengue virus (types 1 through 4), many other viruses

Genus. *Hepacivirus*: Hepatitis C virus (HCV; types 1 through 6)

Single-stranded, negative-sense, enveloped RNA viruses

Family. *Rhabdoviridae*

Genus. *Vesiculovirus*: Vesicular stomatitis virus

Genus. *Lyssavirus*. Rabies virus

Family. *Filoviridae*

Genus. "Marburg-like viruses": Marburg virus

Genus. "Ebola-like viruses": Ebola virus

Family. *Orthomyxoviridae*

Genus. *Influenzavirus A*: Influenza A virus

Genus. *Influenzavirus B*: Influenza B virus

Genus. *Influenzavirus C*: Influenza C virus

Family. *Paramyxoviridae*

Genus. *Respirovirus*: Sendai virus, Human parainfluenza virus (types 1 and 3)

Genus. *Rubulavirus*: Mumps virus, Human parainfluenza virus (types 2 and 4)

Genus. *Morbillivirus*: Measles virus, Rinderpest virus

Genus. *Henipavirus*: Hendravirus, Nipahvirus

Genus. *Avulavirus*: Newcastle disease virus

Genus. *Pneumovirus*: Human respiratory syncytial virus (RSV), human metapneumovirus

Family. *Bunyaviridae*

Genus. *Orthobunyavirus*: Bunyamwera virus, California encephalitis virus, La Crosse virus, many other viruses

Genus. *Hantavirus*: Hantaan virus, Sin Nombre virus, other viruses

Genus. *Nairovirus*: Crimean-Congo hemorrhagic fever virus (CCFV), other viruses

Genus. *Phlebovirus*: Rift Valley fever virus, other viruses

Family. *Arenaviridae*

Genus. *Arenavirus*: Lymphocytic choriomeningitis (LCM) virus, Lassa virus, Junin virus, Machupo virus, Sabia virus, other viruses

Double-stranded, enveloped RNA viruses

Family. *Retroviridae*

Genus. *Deltaretrovirus*: Human T-lymphotropic virus type 1 (HTLV-1), human T-lymphotropic virus type 2 (HTLV-2)

Genus. *Lentivirus*: Human immunodeficiency virus
type 1 (HIV-1), human immunodeficiency virus
type 2 (HIV-2)
Family. *Reoviridae*
Genus. *Rotavirus*: Rotavirus (types A through G)
Genus. *Coltivirus*: Colorado tick fever virus
Genus. *Orthoreovirus*: Human reovirus

Mammalian prions

Agents of spongiform encephalopathies: scrapie, transmis
sible mink encephalopathy, chronic wasting disease
bovine spongiform encephalopathy, kuru, Creutzfeld
Jakob disease, Gerestmann-Straussler-Scheinker syr
drome, fatal familial insomnia

Taxonomic Classification of Fungi

The taxonomic classification of fungal organisms is comple
because fungi can be classified by different methods. The cor
rect phylogenic taxonomy for fungi is represented in this chap
ter. Fungi, or the kingdom Eumycota, are divided into fou
divisions: Chytridomycota, Zygomycota, Ascomycota, an
Basidiomycota. No fungi with clinical significance have bee
attributed to the Chytridomycota. The Protozoa and Chromist
kingdoms are included because some members may possess
fungus-like appearance and are clinically relevant. The tele
omorph (sexual state) name, when known, is listed on the le
side of the slanted line; the anamorph and synamorph (asexua
states) names are listed on the right of the slanted line.

The syn(anamorph) state of fungi is most frequently seen i
the laboratory, and therefore fungi are sometimes grouped int
an artificial classification (or form group) called the Deutero
mycetes. This group is subdivided into the yeasts (Blastomy
cetes), conidia produced in fruiting bodies (Coelomycetes), an
moulds with septate hyphae (Hyphomycetes). The hyphomy
cetes are further differentiated into groups based on hyph
pigmentation: Moniliaceae (lacking melanin) and Dematiacea
(possessing melanin). Deuteromycete terminology is used whe
considering fungal identification later in this book.

Kingdom: Protozoa
Division. Mesomycetozoa
Genus. *Rhinosporidium*/——

Kingdom: Chromista
Division. Oomycota
    Genus. *Pythium*/—

Kingdom: Eumycota
Division. Zygomycota (lower fungi)
    Order. Mucorales
        Genus. *Absidia*/—
        Genus. *Apophysomyces*/—
        Genus. *Cokeromyces*/—
        Genus. *Cunninghamella*/—
        Genus. *Mucor*/—
        Genus. *Rhizomucor*/—
        Genus. *Rhizopus*/—
        Genus. *Syncephalastrum*/—
        Genus. *Saksenaea*/—
    Order. Mortierrellales
        Genus. *Mortierella*/—
    Order. Entomophthorales
        Genus. *Basidiobolus*/—
        Genus. *Conidiobolus*/—
Division. Ascomycota (higher fungi)
Class. Archiascomycetes
    Order. Pneumocystidales
        Genus. *Pneumocystis jiroveci (carinii)*/—
Class Hemiascomycetes (Endomycetes)
    Order. Saccharomycetales
        Genus. *Issatchenkia orientalis/Candida krusei*
        Genus. *Saccharomyces cerevisiae*/—
        Genus. *Stephanoascus ciferrii/Candida ciferrii*
        Genus. *Pichia guilliermondii/Candida guillermondii*
        Genus. *Hansenula anomala/Candida pelliculosa*
        Genus. *Clavispora lusitaniae/Candida lusitaniae*
        Genus. *Galactomyces geotrichum/Geotrichum candidum*
        Genus. *Dipodascus capitatus/Geotrichum capitatum*
        Genus. *Kluyveromyces marxianus/Candida kefyr*
        Genus. *Yarrowia lipolytica/Candida lipolytica*
    Order. Saccharomycetales (mitosporic)
        Genus. —/*Candida albicans*
        Genus. —/*Candida glabrata*

Genus. —/*Candida inconspicua*
Genus. —/*Candida parapsilosis*
Genus. —/*Candida tropicalis*
Class. Euascomycetes
Order. Onygenales
Genus. —/*Epidermophyton*
Genus. *Arthroderma/Microsporum, Trichophyton*
Genus. *Ajellomyces/Blastomyces*
Genus. *Ajellomyces/Emmonsia*
Genus. *Ajellomyces/Histoplasma*
Genus. —/*Paracoccidioides*
Genus. *Aphanoascus/Chrysosporium*
Genus. *Nanizziopsis/Chrysosporium*
Genus. *Uncinocarpus/Chrysosporium*
Order. Eurotiales
Genus. *Eremomyces/Arthrographis*
Genus. *Eurotium/Aspergillus*
Genus. *Neosartorya/Aspergillus*
Genus. *Fennellia/Aspergillus*
Genus. *Emericella/Aspergillus*
Genus. —/*Paecilomyces*
Genus. —/*Penicillium*
Order. Chaetothyriales
Genus. —/*Cladophialophora*
Genus. —/*Exophiala*
Genus. —/*Fonsecaea*
Genus. —/*Philophora*
Genus. —/*Ramichloridium*
Order. Claviciptales
Genus. —/*Beauvaria*
Genus. —/*Paecilomyces*
Order. Microascales
Genus. *Microascus/Scopulariopsis*
Genus. *Petriella/Scedosporium, Graphium*
Genus. *Pseudallescheria/Scedosporium*
Genus. *Pseudallescheria/Graphium*
Order. Ophiostomatales
Genus. —/*Sporothrix*
Order. Dothideales
Genus. *Discosphaerina/Aureobasidium*
Genus. *Sydowia/Hormonema*
Genus. —/*Hotaea*
Genus. —/*Nattrassia*

Genus. —/*Cladosporium*
Genus. —/*Madurella*
Order. Pleosporales
Genus. *Cochliobolus/Bipolaris, Curvularia*
Genus. —/*Dreschlera*
Genus. *Setosphaeria/Exserohilum*
Genus. —/*Phoma*
Genus. —/*Ulocladium*
Order. Sordarilaes
Genus. *Chaetomium*
Genus. —/*Acrophialophora*
Genus. —/*Phaeoacremonium*
Genus. —/*Phialemonium*
Genus. —/*Oidiodendron*
Genus. —/*Nigrospora*
Genus. —/*Geomyces*
Order. Leotiales
Genus. —/*Ochroconis (Dactylaria)*
Order. Hypocreales
Genus. *Neocosmospora/Acremonium*
Genus. *Nectria/Cylindrocarpon*
Genus. *Cosmospora/Fusarium*
Genus. *Gibberella/Fusarium*
Genus. *Nectria/Fusarium*
Genus. *Hypocrea/Trichoderma*
Division. Basidiomycota
Class. Urediniomycetes
Order. Sporidiales
Genus. *Rhodosporidium/Rhodotorula*
Genus. *Sporidiobolus/Sporobolomyces*
Class. Hymenomycetes
Order. Tremellales
Genus. *Filobasidella/Cryptococcus*
Genus. —/*Malassezia*
Genus. —/*Trichosporon*
Order. Stereales
Genus. *Schizophyllum/—*

Microbial Taxonomy

Taxonomic Classification of Parasites[a]

Kingdom. Protozoa
Subkingdom 1. Archezoa
Phylum. Metamonada (intestinal flagellates)

Class. Trepomonadea
    Order. Diplomonadida
        Genus. *Giardia lamblia*
    Order. Enteromonadida
        Genus. *Enteromonas hominis*
Class. Retortamonadea
    Order. Retortamonadida
        Genus. *Chilomastix mesnili, Retortamonas intestinalis*

Phylum. Parabasalia
    Class. Trichomonadea (intestinal and related flagellates)
        Order. Trichomonadida
            Genus. *Dientamoeba fragilis, Trichomonas vaginalis, T. tenax, Pentatrichomonas hominis*

Subkingdom 2. Neozoa
Infrakingdom 1. Discicristata
    Phylum. Percolozoa
        Class. Heterolobosea (flagellated amoebae)
            Order. Schizopyrenida
                Genus. *Naegleria fowleri*
    Phylum. Euglenozoa
        Class. Kinetoplastea (kinetoplastid flagellates)
            Order. Trypanosomatida
                Genus. *Leishmania donovani, L. infantum (= L. chagasi), L. major, L. tropica, L. braziliensis, L. mexicana, Trypanosoma cruzi, T. brucei gambiense, T. brucei rhodesiense, T. rangeli*

Infrakingdom 2. Sarcomastigota
    Phylum. Amoebozoa
    Subphylum. Lobosa
        Class. Amoebaea
            Order. Acanthopodida
                Genus. *Acanthamoeba* spp., *Balamuthia mandrillaris*
    Subphylum. Conosa
        Class. Entamoebidea
            Order. Euamoebida
                Genus. *Entamoeba histolytica, E. coli, E. dispar, E hartmanni, E. gingivalis, E.*

    chattoni (= *E. polecki*), *Endolimax*
    nana, Iodamoeba buetschlii

Infrakingdom 3. Alveolata
    Phylum. Sporozoa (sporozoans)
        Class. Coccidea
            Order. Eimeriida
                Genus. *Cryptosporidium parvum, Toxo-*
                      plasma gondii, Cyclospora cayetanensis,
                      Isospora belli, Sarcocystis hominis
            Order. Piroplasmida
                Genus. *Babesia microti, B. divergens,*
                      B. gibsoni
            Order. Haemosporida
                Genus. *Plasmodium falciparum, P.*
                      malariae, P. ovale, P. vivax
    Phylum. Ciliophora (ciliates)
        Class. Litostomatea
            Order. Vestibulifera
                Genus. *Balantidium coli*

Kingdom. Chromista
  Subkingdom. Chromobiota
    Phylum. Bigyra
        Class. Blastocystea
            Genus. *Blastocystis hominis*
Incertae Cedis
    Phylum. Microspora (microsporidians)
        Class. Microsporea
                Genus. *Encephalitozoon cuniculi, E. hellem,*
                      E. intestinalis, Enterocytozoon bieneusi,
                      Nosema ocularum, Brachiola connori, B.
                      vesicularum, Microsporidium ceylonen-
                      sis, M. africanum, Vittaforma corneae,
                      Trachipleistophora hominis,
                      T. anthropophtheca

Kingdom. Animalia
  Subkingdom 1. Radiata
  Subkingdom 2. Myxozoa
  Subkingdom 3. Bilateria
  Infrakingdom 1. Ecdysozoa
    Phylum. Nemathelminthes (Infraphylum Nematoda.
    Roundworms)

Class. Adenophorea (Asphasmidea)
Superfamily. Trichinelloidea
Family. Trichinellidae
Genus. *Trichinella spiralis*
Family. Trichuridae
Genus. *Trichuris trichiura*
Class. Secernentea (Phasmidea)
Superfamily. Ancylostomatoidea
Family. Ancylostomatidae
Genus. *Ancylostoma duodenale, Necator americanus*
Superfamily. Ascaridoidea
Family. Ascarididae
Genus. *Ascaris lumbrioides, Toxocara canis, T. cati*
Family. Anisakidae
Genus. *Anisakis simplex*
Superfamily. Dracunculoidea
Family. Dracunculidae
Genus. *Dracunculus medinensis*
Superfamily. Filarioidea
Family. Onchocercidae
Genus. *Brugia malayi, Loa loa, Wuchereria bancrofti, Onchocerca volvulus, Brugia timori, Dirofilaria immitis, Mansonella ozzardi, M. perstans*
Superfamily. Oxyuroidea
Family. Oxyuridae
Genus. *Enterobius vermicularis*
Superfamily. Rhabditoidea
Family. Strongyloididae
Genus. *Strongyloides stercoralis*

Infrakingdom 2. Platyzoa
Phylum. Platyhelminthes
Class. Digenea (Trematoda, flukes)
Order. Strigeida
Family. Schistosomatidae
Genus. *Schistosoma haematobium, S. japonicum, S. mansoni, S. mekongi, S. intercalatum*
Order. Echinostomatida
Family. Fasciolidae

Genus. *Fasciola hepatica, Fasciolopsis buski*

Order. Plagiorchiida

    Family. Heterophyidae

        Genus. *Heterophyes heterophyes*

    Family. Opisthorchiidae

        Genus. *Opisthorchis (Clonorchis) sinensis, O. felineus, O. viverrini*

    Family. Paragonimidae

        Genus. *Paragonimus westermani*

Class. Cestoidea (Cestoda, tapeworms)

    Order. Pseudophyllidea

        Family. Diphyllobothriidae

            Genus. *Diphyllobothrium latum*

    Order. Cyclophyllidea

        Family. Dipylidiidae

            Genus. *Dipylidium caninum*

        Family. Hymenolepididae

            Genus. *Hymenolepis (Rodentolepsis) nana, Hymenolepis diminuta*

        Family. Taeniidae

            Genus. *Taenia saginata, T. solium, Echinococcus granulosus, Echinococcus multilocularis*

---

[a]Adapted from P. R. Murray, E. J. Baron, J. H. Jorgensen, M. A. Pfaller, and R. H. Yolken (ed.), *Manual of Clinical Microbiology*, 8th ed., ASM Press, Washington, D.C., 2003.

Indigenous and Pathogenic Microbes of Humans

Humans are exposed to microbes at birth, which leads to one of three outcomes: transient colonization, persistent colonization, or pathogenic interaction. The majority of organisms are unable to become established on the skin or mucosal surfaces and are considered an insignificant finding when recovered in clinical specimens. Examples include the moulds and many of the nonfermentative gram-negative bacilli that can be isolated in soil, vegetation, water, and food products. These organisms are unable to compete with the normal microbial population of the body or cannot survive on the skin surface.

Other organisms are able to establish long-term residency on or in the human body. The successes of these interactions are influenced by complex microbial and host factors (e.g., favorable environment [pH, atmosphere, moisture, available nutrients], ability to adhere to surfaces, resistance to bacteriocins, antibiotics, and phagocytic cells). These microbes generally exist in a symbiotic relationship with their human host and produce disease only when they invade normally sterile body sites such as tissues and body fluids. Table 2.1 is a listing of the organisms most commonly recovered from the body surfaces of healthy individuals. This table is intended to serve as an interpretive guideline for cultured specimens. It should be remembered that many organisms cannot be detected when present in a mixed population (typical of many body sites). Additionally, as the taxonomic classification of microbes is updated and more sophisticated identification systems are introduced, our understanding of the prevalence of organisms at specific body sites can change. The quantitative and qualitative presence of specific microbes will also vary with the individual host, including dramatic changes in the indigenous flora in hospitalized patients. Thus, only qualitative data (presence or absence of the organisms) are presented. Data for viruses are not listed because replication of viruses generally is associated with host tissue destruction or an immunologic response (although this can range from a clinically asymptomatic infection to host death).

Most diseases in humans are caused by infections with endogenous bacteria and yeasts or exposure to opportunistic moulds, parasites, and viruses. However, some interactions between microbes and humans commonly lead to disease. The most common microbes responsible for human disease are summarized in this section.

Selected pathogens are monitored routinely, with all clinical laboratories required to report specific organisms or diseases to their State Public Health Department. This group of organisms and the diseases associated with them are reported weekly in *Morbidity and Mortality Weekly Report*. Data for 2002 are summarized in this section.

Unfortunately, with the anthrax attack in 2001, bioterrorism has become a renewed concern of all. The Department of Health and Human Services (HHS) and the U.S. Department of Agriculture (USDA) have published a list of Select Agents and Toxins. This list is presented in this section and can be found on the CDC website (www.cdc.gov/od/sap/docs/salist.pdf).

Arthropods, parasites in their own right, can also serve as vectors for human disease. A listing of the most common arthropod vectors and their associated diseases is included in Table 2.2. Tables 2.3 and 2.4 are listings of fungi and parasites isolated from humans and their geographic distribution. For additional information about indigenous and pathogenic microbes, please consult the reference texts listed in the Bibliography.

Microbes of Humans

Microbes of Humans

Table 2.1 Human indigenous flora[a]

Organism	Prevalence of carriage in[b]:			
	Resp tract	GI tract	GU tract	Skin, ear, and eye
Abiotrophia defectiva	+	0	0	0
Acholeplasma laidlawii	+	0	0	0
Acidaminococcus fermentans	+	+	0	0
Acinetobacter spp.	+	+	+	+
Actinobacillus spp.	+	0	+	0
Actinomyces spp.	+	+	+	0
Aerococcus christensenii	0	0	+	0
Aerococcus viridans	0	0	0	+
Aerococcus urinae	0	0	+	0
Aeromonas spp.	0	+	0	0
Alloiococcus otitis	0	0	0	+
Anaerococcus hydrogenalis	0	+	+	+
Anaerococcus lactolyticus	0	+	+	0
Anaerococcus prevotii	0	+	+	0
Anaerorhabdus furcosus	0	0	0	0
Arcanobacterium spp.	+	+	0	+
Bacillus spp.	0	+	0	+
Bacteroides caccae	0	+	0	0
Bacteroides distasonis	0	+	0	0
Bacteroides eggerthii	0	+	0	0
Bacteroides fragilis	0	+	+	0
Bacteroides merdae	0	+	0	0

Organism				
Bacteroides ovatus	0	+	0	0
Bacteroides splanchnicus	0	+	0	0
Bacteroides thetaiotaomicron	0	+	0	0
Bacteroides vulgatus	0	+	0	0
Bifidobacterium adolescentis	0	+	+	0
Bifidobacterium bifidum	0	+	+	0
Bifidobacterium breve	0	+	+	0
Bifidobacterium catenulatum	+	+	+	0
Bifidobacterium dentium	0	+	+	0
Bifidobacterium longum	+	+	+	0
Bilophila wadsworthia	0	0	+	0
Blastocystis hominis	0	0	0	0
Blastoschizomyces capitatus	0	0	0	+
Brevibacterium casei	0	0	0	+
Brevibacterium epidermidis	+	0	0	+
Burkholderia cepacia complex	0	+	0	+
Butyrivibrio fibrisolvens	+	+	0	0
Campylobacter concisus	+	+	0	0
Campylobacter curvus	+	+	0	0
Campylobacter gracilis	0	+	0	0
Campylobacter jejuni	+	+	0	0
Campylobacter rectus	0	+	0	0
Campylobacter showae	+	0	0	0
Campylobacter sputorum	+	+	0	0
Candida albicans	+	+	+	+

(continued)

Microbes of Humans

Microbes of Humans

Table 2.1 Human indigenous flora[a] *(continued)*

Organism	Prevalence of carriage in[b]:			
	Resp tract	GI tract	GU tract	Skin, ear, and eye
Candida glabrata	+	+	+	+
Candida guilliermondii	+	+	+	+
Candida kefyr	+	+	+	+
Candida krusei	+	+	+	+
Candida lusitaniae	+	+	+	+
Candida parapsilosis	+	+	+	+
Candida tropicalis	+	+	+	+
Capnocytophaga gingivalis	+	0	0	0
Capnocytophaga granulosum	+	0	0	0
Capnocytophaga haemolytica	+	0	0	0
Capnocytophaga ochracea	+	+	+	0
Cardiobacterium hominis	+	0	0	0
Centipeda periodontii	0	+	0	0
Chilomastix mesnilii	0	+	0	0
Citrobacter freundii	0	+	0	0
Citrobacter koseri	0	+	0	0
Clostridium spp.	0	+	0	+
Corynebacterium accolens	+	0	0	+
Corynebacterium afermentans	+	0	0	+
Corynebacterium amycolatum	0	0	0	+
Corynebacterium auris	0	0	0	+
Corynebacterium diphtheriae	+	0	0	+

Organism				
Corynebacterium duram	+	0	0	0
Corynebacterium glucuronolyticum	0	0	+	0
Corynebacterium jeikeium	0	0	0	+
Corynebacterium macginleyi	+	0	0	+
Corynebacterium matruchotii	0	0	0	0
Corynebacterium minutissimum	+	0	0	+
Corynebacterium propinquum	+	0	0	0
Corynebacterium pseudodiphtheriticum	0	0	0	0
Corynebacterium riegelii	0	0	0	0
Corynebacterium simulans	+	0	+	+
Corynebacterium striatum	+	0	0	+
Corynebacterium ulcerans	0	0	0	0
Corynebacterium urealyticum	+	0	0	+
Cryptococcus albidus	0	0	+	0
Dermabacter hominis	+	0	0	+
Dermacoccus nishinomiyaensis	0	0	0	+
Desulfomonas pigra	0	+	0	0
Dysgonomonas spp.	+	+	0	0
Eikenella corrodens	0	+	0	0
Endolimax nana	0	+	0	0
Entamoeba coli	+	+	0	0
Entamoeba gingivalis	0	0	0	0
Entamoeba hartmanni	+	+	0	0
Entamoeba polecki	0	+	0	0
Enterobacter aerogenes	0	+	0	0

Microbes of Humans

(continued)

Table 2.1 Human indigenous flora[a] *(continued)*

Organism	Prevalence of carriage in[b]:			
	Resp tract	GI tract	GU tract	Skin, ear, and eye
Enterobacter cloacae	0	+	0	0
Enterobacter gergoviae	0	+	0	0
Enterobacter sakazakii	0	+	0	0
Enterobacter taylorae	0	+	0	0
Enterococcus spp.	0	+	0	0
Epidermophyton floccosum	0	0	0	+
Escherichia coli	0	+	+	0
Escherichia fergusonii	0	+	0	0
Escherichia hermanii	0	+	0	0
Escherichia vulneris	0	+	0	0
Eubacterium spp.	+	+	0	0
Ewingella americana	+	0	0	+
Finegoldia magnus	0	+	+	+
Fusobacterium alocis	+	0	+	0
Fusobacterium gonidiaformans	0	+	+	0
Fusobacterium mortiferum	0	+	0	0
Fusobacterium naviforme	0	+	+	0
Fusobacterium necrophorum	+	+	0	0
Fusobacterium nucleatum	+	0	0	0
Fusobacterium russii	0	+	0	0
Fusobacterium sulci	+	0	0	0
Fusobacterium varium	0	+	0	0

Gardnerella vaginalis	0	+	+	0
Gemella haemolysans	+	0	0	0
Gemella morbillorum	+	+	0	0
Geotrichum spp.	+	+	+	+
Granulicatella spp.	+	0	0	0
Haemophilus spp.	0	0	0	0
Hafnia alvei	0	+	0	0
Helcococcus kunzii	0	0	0	+
Helicobacter spp.	0	+	0	0
Kingella spp.	+	0	0	0
Klebsiella spp.	0	+	0	0
Kocuria spp.	0	0	0	+
Kytococcus sedantarius	+	0	+	+
Lactobacillus acidophilus	+	+	+	0
Lactobacillus breve	+	0	0	0
Lactobacillus casei	0	0	0	0
Lactobacillus cellobiosus	+	+	+	0
Lactobacillus fermentum	0	+	+	0
Lactobacillus reuteri	0	0	0	0
Lactobacillus salivarius	0	0	0	0
Lactococcus spp.	+	+	+	0
Leclercia adecarboxylata	+	+	0	0
Leminorella spp.	0	0	0	0
Leptotrichia buccalis	+	+	+	0
Leuconostoc spp.	0	+	+	0

(continued)

Microbes of Humans

Table 2.1 Human indigenous flora[a] (continued)

	Prevalence of carriage in[b]:			
Organism	Resp tract	GI tract	GU tract	Skin, ear, and eye
Listeria monocytogenes	0	+	0	0
Malassezia spp.	0	0	0	+
Megasphaera elsdenii	0	+	0	0
Micrococcus luteus	+	0	0	+
Micrococcus lylae	+	0	0	+
Micromonas micros	+	0	0	0
Microsporum spp.	0	0	0	+
Mitsuokella multiacidus	0	+	0	0
Mobiluncus curtisii	0	+	+	0
Mobiluncus mulieris	0	+	+	0
Moellerella wisconsensis	0	+	0	0
Moraxella catarrhalis	+	0	0	0
Morganella morganii	0	+	+	0
Mycoplasma buccale	+	0	+	0
Mycoplasma faucium	+	0	+	0
Mycoplasma fermentans	+	0	0	0
Mycoplasma genitalium	+	0	+	0
Mycoplasma hominis	+	0	+	0
Mycoplasma lipophilum	+	0	0	0
Mycoplasma orale	+	0	0	0
Mycoplasma penetrans	0	0	+	0
Mycoplasma pneumoniae	+	0	0	0

Mycoplasma primatum	o	o	+	o
Mycoplasma salivarium	+	o	o	o
Mycoplasma spermatophilum	o	o	+	o
Neisseria cinerea	+	o	o	o
Neisseria flavescens	+	o	o	o
Neisseria lactamica	+	o	o	o
Neisseria meningitidis	+	o	o	o
Neisseria mucosa	+	o	o	o
Neisseria polysaccharea	+	o	o	o
Neisseria sicca	o	o	o	o
Neisseria subflava	o	o	+	o
Oligella ureolytica	o	o	+	o
Oligella urethralis	+	+	+	o
Pantoea agglomerans	o	o	o	o
Pasteurella bettyae	o	o	+	+
Pasteurella multocida	+	+	o	+
Pentatrichomonas hominis	o	o	+	o
Peptococcus niger	o	+	o	o
Peptoniphilus asaccharolyticus	o	o	+	o
Peptoniphilus lacrimalis	+	+	+	+
Peptostreptococcus anaerobius	+	o	o	o
Peptostreptococcus productus	o	+	o	o
Peptostreptococcus vaginalis	o	o	o	o
Porphyromonas asaccharolytica	o	+	+	+
Porphyromonas catoniae	+	o	+	o

Microbes of Humans

(continued)

Microbes of Humans

Table 2.1 Human indigenous flora[a] *(continued)*

Organism	Resp tract	GI tract	GU tract	Skin, ear, and eye
		Prevalence of carriage in[b]:		
Porphyromonas endodontalis	+	0	0	0
Porphyromonas gingivalis	+	0	0	0
Prevotella bivia	0	0	+	0
Prevotella buccae	+	0	0	0
Prevotella buccalis	+	0	+	0
Prevotella corporis	+	0	0	0
Prevotella dentalis	+	0	0	0
Prevotella denticola	+	0	0	0
Prevotella disiens	0	0	+	0
Prevotella enoeca	+	0	0	0
Prevotella heparinolytica	+	0	0	0
Prevotella intermedia	+	0	0	0
Prevotella loescheii	+	0	+	0
Prevotella melaninogenica	+	0	+	0
Prevotella nigrescens	+	0	0	0
Prevotella oralis	+	0	+	0
Prevotella oris	+	0	0	0
Prevotella oulorum	+	0	0	0
Prevotella tannerae	+	0	0	0
Prevotella veroralis	+	0	+	0
Prevotella zoogleoformans	+	0	0	0
Propionibacterium acnes	0	0	0	+

Propionibacterium avidum	o	o	o	+
Propionibacterium granulosum	+	o	o	+
Propionibacterium propionicum	o	o	o	o
Propionferax innocuum	o	+	+	+
Proteus mirabilis	o	+	+	o
Proteus penneri	o	+	+	o
Proteus vulgaris	o	+	o	o
Providencia rettgeri	o	+	o	o
Providencia stuartii	o	o	o	o
Pseudomonas aeruginosa	+	o	o	o
Retortamonas intestinalis	o	+	o	o
Rothia dentocariosa	+	+	o	o
Rothia mucilaginosa	o	o	o	o
Ruminococcus productus	+	+	+	o
Saccharomyces spp.	+	+	o	o
Selenomonas spp.	o	o	o	o
Serratia liquefaciens	o	+	o	+
Serratia marcescens	o	+	o	+
Serratia odorifera	+	+	+	+
Staphylococcus aureus	o	o	o	+
Staphylococcus auricularis	o	o	o	+
Staphylococcus capitis	o	o	o	+
Staphylococcus caprae	o	o	o	+
Staphylococcus cohnii	o	o	o	+
Staphylococcus epidermidis	+	o	+	+

(continued)

Microbes of Humans

Microbes of Humans

Table 2.1 Human indigenous flora[a] *(continued)*

Organism	Prevalence of carriage in[b]:			
	Resp tract	GI tract	GU tract	Skin, ear, and eye
Staphylococcus haemolyticus	0	0	0	+
Staphylococcus hominis	0	0	0	+
Staphylococcus lugdunensis	0	0	0	+
Staphylococcus pasteuri	0	0	0	+
Staphylococcus saccharolyticus	0	0	0	+
Staphylococcus saprophyticus	0	0	+	+
Staphylococcus simulans	0	0	0	+
Staphylococcus xylosus	0	0	0	+
Staphylococcus warneri	0	0	0	+
Streptococcus agalactiae	0	+	+	0
Streptococcus anginosus	+	+	+	0
Streptococcus bovis	+	+	+	0
Streptococcus constellatus	+	+	0	0
Streptococcus cricetus	+	0	0	0
Streptococcus crista	+	0	0	0
Streptococcus equisimilis	+	0	0	0
Streptococcus gordonii	+	0	0	0
Streptococcus intermedius	+	+	+	0
Streptococcus mitis	+	0	0	0
Streptococcus mutans	+	0	0	0
Streptococcus oralis	+	0	0	0
Streptococcus parasanguis	+	0	0	0

Streptococcus pneumoniae	+	0	0	0
Streptococcus pyogenes	+	0	0	+
Streptococcus salivarius	+	0	0	0
Streptococcus sanguis	+	0	0	0
Streptococcus sobrinus	+	0	0	0
Streptococcus vestibularis	+	0	0	0
Succinivibrio dextrinosolvens	0	+	0	0
Tissierella praeacuta	0	0	0	0
Treponema denticola	+	+	0	0
Treponema maltophilum	+	0	0	0
Treponema minutum	0	0	+	0
Treponema phagedenis	0	0	+	0
Treponema refringens	0	0	+	0
Treponema socranskii	+	0	0	0
Treponema vincentii	+	0	0	0
Trichomonas tenax	+	0	0	0
Trichophyton spp.	0	0	0	+
Trichosporon spp.	+	+	+	+
Turicella otitidis	0	0	0	+
Ureaplasma urealyticum	+	+	+	0
Veillonella spp.	+	+	0	0
Weeksella virosa	0	0	+	0

[a] Adapted from P. R. Murray, Human microbiota, p. 295–306, *in* L. Collier, A. Balows, and M. Sussman (ed.), *Topley & Wilson's Microbiology and Microbial Infections*, 9th ed., Arnold, London, 1998.

[b] Resp, respiratory tract including nasopharynx and oropharynx; GI, gastrointestinal tract; GU, genitourinary tract; +, commonly present; 0, not typically isolated in healthy individuals.

Microbes of Humans

BONE AND JOINT INFECTIONS

Arthritis
    Bacteria
        Neisseria gonorrhoeae
        Staphylococcus aureus
        Borrelia burgdorferi
        Brucella spp.
        Pseudomonas aeruginosa
        Pasteurella multocida
        Eikenella corrodens
        Streptobacillus moniliformis
        Mycoplasma hominis
        Ureaplasma urealyticum
        Mycobacterium marinum (and other
            Mycobacterium spp.)
    Viruses
        Rubella virus
        Hepatitis B virus
        Mumps virus
        Lymphocytic choriomeningitis virus
        Parvovirus B19
        Human immunodeficiency virus
    Fungi
        Sporothrix schenckii
        Candida spp.
        Coccidioides immitis

Osteomyelitis
    Bacteria
        Staphylococcus aureus (and other
            Staphylococcus spp.)
        Streptococcus, beta-hemolytic groups
        Streptococcus pneumoniae
        Escherichia coli
        Salmonella spp. (and other
            Enterobacteriaceae)
        Pseudomonas aeruginosa
        Mycobacterium tuberculosis (and other
            Mycobacterium spp.)
    Fungi
        Candida spp.

Aspergillus spp.
Cryptococcus neoformans
Blastomyces dermatitidis
Coccidioides immitis

CARDIOVASCULAR INFECTIONS

Endocarditis

Bacteria

Staphylococcus aureus (and other
   Staphylococcus spp.)
Streptococcus, viridans group (primarily *S. mitis*,
   S. oralis, *S. sanguis*, and *S. mutans*)
Streptococcus bovis
Streptococcus pneumoniae
Abiotrophia defectiva
Granulicatella adiacens
Rothia mucilaginosa
Enterococcus spp. (primarily *E. faecalis* and
   E. faecium)
Haemophilus spp. (primarily *H. aphrophilus*)
Actinobacillus actinomycetemcomitans
Cardiobacterium hominis
Eikenella corrodens
Kingella kingae
Salmonella spp.
Serratia spp. (and other enteric
   gram-negative rods)
Pseudomonas aeruginosa
Brucella spp.
Bartonella spp. (primarily *B. henselae*)
Corynebacterium spp. (primarily in damaged or
   prosthetic valves)
Erysipelothrix rhusiopathiae
Coxiella burnetii
Chlamydophila psittaci

Fungi

Candida spp. (*C. parapsilosis*, *C. albicans*, *C. tropicalis*,
   and others)
Aspergillus spp.

Myocarditis

Bacteria

Corynebacterium diphtheriae

Microbes of Humans

Clostridium perfringens
Streptococcus pyogenes
Borrelia burgdorferi
Neisseria meningitidis
Staphylococcus aureus
Salmonella spp.
Mycoplasma pneumoniae
Chlamydophila spp. (*C. pneumoniae* and
    C. psittaci)
Rickettsia rickettsii
Orientia tsutsugamushi
Viruses
    Coxsackievirus groups A and B
    Echoviruses
    Poliovirus
    Mumps virus
    Rubeola virus
    Influenza A and B viruses
    Herpesvirus group
    Adenoviruses
    Flaviviruses
    Arenaviruses
Fungi
    Aspergillus spp.
    Candida spp.
    Cryptococcus neoformans
Parasites
    Trypanosoma spp.
    Trichinella spiralis
    Toxoplasma gondii
Pericarditis
Bacteria
    Streptococcus pneumoniae
    Staphylococcus aureus
    Neisseria spp. (primarily *N. meningitidis* and
        N. gonorrhoeae)
    Mycoplasma pneumoniae
    Mycobacterium tuberculosis (and other
        Mycobacterium spp.)
Viruses
    Coxsackievirus groups A and B
    Echovirus
    Adenovirus

Mumps virus
Influenza A and B viruses
Herpesvirus group

Fungi

Histoplasma capsulatum
Coccidioides immitis
Blastomyces dermatitidis
Cryptococcus neoformans
Candida spp.
Aspergillus spp.

Parasites

Toxoplasma gondii
Entamoeba histolytica
Schistosoma spp.

Sepsis

Bacteria

Staphylococcus aureus (and other
Staphylococcus spp.)
Escherichia coli
Enterococcus spp. (primarily *E. faecalis* and *E. faecium*)
Klebsiella spp.
Streptococcus pneumoniae
Pseudomonas aeruginosa
Enterobacter spp.
Streptococcus, beta-hemolytic (primarily groups A, B, C,
and F)
Proteus mirabilis
Streptococcus, viridans group
Acinetobacter spp.
Serratia spp.
Citrobacter spp.
Stenotrophomonas maltophilia
Salmonella spp.
Haemophilus spp.
Morganella morganii
Mycobacterium avium complex
Mycobacterium tuberculosis

Fungi

Candida albicans
Candida glabrata
Candida parapsilosis
Candida tropicalis

Microbes of Humans

Candida krusei
Cryptococcus neoformans
Trichosporon spp.
Malassezia spp.
Histoplasma capsulatum
Fusarium spp.

Transfusion-associated sepsis
  Bacteria
    Yersinia enterocolitica
    Staphylococcus, coagulase-negative spp.
    Pseudomonas fluorescens/putida
    Salmonella spp.
    Serratia marcescens (and other
      Enterobacteriaceae)
    Campylobacter jejuni
    Treponema pallidum
    Bacillus cereus
    Borrelia spp.
  Viruses
    Hepatitis viruses (primarily types A, B, C, and D)
    Cytomegalovirus
    Epstein-Barr virus
    Human immunodeficiency virus
    Human T-cell leukemia virus
    Parvovirus B19
    Colorado tick fever virus
  Parasites
    Plasmodium spp.
    Babesia microti
    Toxoplasma gondii
    Trypanosoma cruzi
    Leishmania spp.

Suppurative thrombophlebitis
  Bacteria
    Staphylococcus aureus
    Klebsiella (and other *Enterobacteriaceae*)
    Pseudomonas aeruginosa
    Enterococcus spp. (primarily *E. faecalis* and
      E. faecium)
    Bacteroides fragilis group
    Campylobacter fetus

Fungi
    Candida spp.
    Malassezia spp.

CENTRAL NERVOUS SYSTEM INFECTIONS

Acute meningitis

Bacteria
    Escherichia coli
    Streptococcus agalactiae (group B)
    Streptococcus pneumoniae
    Neisseria meningitidis
    Listeria monocytogenes
    Haemophilus influenzae
    Other gram-negative rods (e.g., *Klebsiella* and
        Pseudomonas spp.)
    Staphylococcus aureus (and other
        Staphylococcus spp.)
    Propionibacterium acnes
    Nocardia spp.
    Treponema pallidum
    Borrelia burgdorferi
    Leptospira spp.
    Mycobacterium tuberculosis
    Mycobacterium avium complex (and other
        Mycobacterium spp.)
    Rickettsia spp.
    Orientia tsutsugamushi
    Ehrlichia spp.

Viruses
    Enteroviruses (echovirus and coxsackievirus groups A
        and B)
    Orbivirus (Colorado tick fever virus)
    Mumps virus
    Measles virus
    Adenovirus
    Herpes simplex virus
    Human immunodeficiency virus

Fungi
    Cryptococcus neoformans
    Histoplasma capsulatum
    Coccidioides immitis

Candida spp.
Scedosporium spp.
Parasites
   Naegleria fowleri
   Acanthamoeba spp.
   Angiostrongylus cantonensis

Chronic meningitis
Bacteria
   Brucella spp.
   Borrelia burgdorferi
   Treponema pallidum
   Mycobacterium tuberculosis (and other
      Mycobacterium spp.)
   Actinomyces spp.
   Nocardia spp.
Fungi
   Candida spp.
   Coccidioides immitis
   Histoplasma capsulatum
   Cryptococcus neoformans
   Sporothrix schenckii
Parasites
   Acanthamoeba spp.
   Angiostrongylus cantonensis

Encephalitis
Bacteria
   Listeria monocytogenes
   Treponema pallidum
   Leptospira spp.
   Actinomyces spp.
   Nocardia spp.
   Borrelia spp. (associated with Lyme disease and
      relapsing fever)
   Rickettsia rickettsii
   Coxiella burnetii
   Mycoplasma pneumoniae
   Mycobacterium tuberculosis
Viruses
   Enteroviruses (poliovirus, coxsackievirus, echovirus,
      and hepatitis A virus)
   Herpesvirus group
   Alphaviruses (Eastern, Western, and Venezuelan equine
      encephalitis viruses)

Flaviviruses (St. Louis encephalitis virus, West Nile
  virus, Japanese encephalitis virus, and
  Dengue virus)
Bunyaviruses (La Crosse virus and Rift
  Valley virus)
Arenaviruses (lymphocytic choriomeningitis virus,
  Machupo virus, Lassa virus, and Junin virus)
Filoviruses (Ebola virus and Marburg virus)
Rabies virus
Human immunodeficiency virus
Mumps virus
Measles virus
Rubella virus
Adenovirus

Fungi
  Cryptococcus neoformans
  Histoplasma capsulatum

Parasites
  Naegleria fowleri
  Acanthamoeba spp.
  Toxoplasma gondii
  Plasmodium falciparum
  Trypanosoma spp.

Brain abscess
Bacteria
  Staphylococcus aureus
  Enterobacteriaceae (*Proteus*, *Escherichia*,
    Klebsiella, and other spp.)
  Pseudomonas aeruginosa
  Streptococcus, viridans group (*S. anginosus* group)
  Bacteroides spp. (and other anaerobic
    gram-negative rods)
  Peptostreptococcus spp. (and other anaerobic
    gram-positive cocci)
  Actinomyces spp.
  Clostridium spp.
  Listeria monocytogenes
  Nocardia spp.
  Rhodococcus equi
  Mycobacterium tuberculosis
Fungi
  Cryptococcus neoformans

Microbes of Humans

   Candida spp.
   Coccidioides immitis
   Aspergillus spp.
   Zygomycetes
   Cladiophialophora spp.
   Scedosporium spp.
   Exophiala spp.
  Parasites
   Acanthamoeba spp.
   Toxoplasma gondii

EAR INFECTIONS
Otitis externa
 Bacteria
  Pseudomonas aeruginosa
  Staphylococcus aureus
  Streptococcus pyogenes
 Fungi
  Aspergillus spp. (primarily *A. fumigatus* and
   A. niger)
  Candida albicans
  Pseudallescheria boydii
  Malassezia spp.
Otitis media
 Bacteria
  Streptococcus pneumoniae
  Haemophilus influenzae
  Moraxella catarrhalis
  Staphylococcus aureus
  Streptococcus pyogenes
  Mixed anaerobes
 Viruses
  Respiratory syncytial virus
  Influenza virus
  Enterovirus
  Rhinovirus

EYE INFECTIONS
Conjunctivitis
 Bacteria
  Streptococcus pneumoniae
  Streptococcus agalactiae

    Streptococcus, viridans group
    Staphylococcus aureus
    Moraxella catarrhalis
    Haemophilus aegyptius
    Neisseria gonorrhoeae
    Pseudomonas aeruginosa
    Corynebacterium diphtheriae
    Francisella tularensis
    Borrelia burgdorferi
    Bartonella henselae
    Chlamydia trachomatis
Viruses
    Adenovirus
    Herpesvirus group
    Papillomavirus
    Rubella virus
    Influenza virus
    Measles virus
Fungi
    Candida spp.
    Sporothrix schenckii
Parasites
    Onchocera volvulus
    Loa loa
    Wuchereria bancrofti
    Leishmania donovani
    Microsporidia (most commonly
      Encephalitozoon spp.)
    Toxocara canis

Microbes of Humans

Endophthalmitis
Bacteria
    Staphylococcus aureus (and other
      Staphylococcus spp.)
    Pseudomonas aeruginosa
    Propionibacterium spp.
    Corynebacterium spp.
    Bacillus cereus (and other *Bacillus* spp.)
    Rapidly growing mycobacteria (primarily *M. chelonae*
      and *M. abscessus*)
Viruses
    Herpesvirus group
    Rubella virus
    Measles virus

Fungi
Candida albicans (and other *Candida* spp.)
Aspergillus spp.
Histoplasma capsulatum
Opportunistic fungi
Parasites
Toxoplasma gondii
Toxocara spp.
Cysticercus cellulosae

Keratitis
Bacteria
Staphylococcus aureus (and other *Staphylococcus* spp.)
Streptococcus pneumoniae
Streptococcus pyogenes
Enterococcus faecalis
Pseudomonas aeruginosa
Proteus mirabilis (and other enteric gram-negative rods)
Bacillus spp. (primarily *B. cereus*)
Clostridium perfringens
Neisseria gonorrhoeae
Viruses
Herpesvirus group
Adenovirus
Measles virus
Fungi
Fusarium spp.
Aspergillus spp.
Candida spp.
Parasites
Onchocerca volvulus
Acanthamoeba spp.
Leishmania braziliensis
Trypanosoma spp.
Microsporidia (primarily *Nosema* and *Encephalitozoon* spp.)

GASTROINTESTINAL INFECTIONS
Esophagitis
Viruses
Cytomegalovirus

Herpes simplex virus
Human immunodeficiency virus
Fungi
Candida albicans (and other *Candida* spp.)

Noninflammatory diarrhea
Bacteria
Escherichia coli
Staphylococcus aureus
Bacillus cereus
Clostridium perfringens
Vibrio spp. (primarily *V. cholerae* and
V. parahaemolyticus)
Viruses
Rotaviruses
Caliciviruses
Adenoviruses
Astroviruses
Coronaviruses

Inflammatory diarrhea
Bacteria
Escherichia coli
Salmonella spp.
Shigella spp.
Campylobacter spp.
Clostridium difficile
Yersinia enterocolitica
Vibrio parahaemolyticus
Plesiomonas shigelloides
Edwardsiella tarda
Aeromonas spp.
Viruses
Adenoviruses
Cytomegalovirus
Fungi
Zygomycetes
Parasites
Giardia lamblia
Entamoeba histolytica
Balantidium coli
Cryptosporidium parvum

> *Isospora belli*
> Microsporidia
> *Cyclospora cayetanensis*
> *Diphyllobothrium latum*
> *Trichinella spiralis*
> *Strongyloides stercoralis*
> *Schistosoma* spp. (primarily *S. mansoni* and
>   *S. japonicum*)

GENITAL INFECTIONS

Cervicitis
Bacteria
> *Neisseria gonorrhoeae*
> *Neisseria meningitidis*
> *Chlamydia trachomatis*
> *Actinomyces* spp.

Viruses
> Herpes simplex virus
> Cytomegalovirus
> Adenovirus
> Measles virus
> Papillomavirus

Genital ulcers and skin nodules
Bacteria
> *Treponema pallidum*
> *Haemophilus ducreyi*
> *Chlamydia trachomatis*
> *Klebsiella granulomatis*
> *Mycobacterium ulcerans*
> *Mycobacterium tuberculosis*

Viruses
> Herpes simplex virus
> Molluscipoxviruses

Fungi
> *Histoplasma capsulatum*

Urethritis
Bacteria
> *Neisseria gonorrhoeae*
> *Chlamydia trachomatis*
> *Ureaplasma urealyticum*

Vaginitis
Bacteria
Mobiluncus spp.
Gardnerella vaginalis
Mycoplasma hominis

GRANULOMATOUS INFECTIONS
Bacteria
Brucella spp.
Francisella tularensis
Listeria monocytogenes
Burkholderia pseudomallei
Actinomyces spp.
Bartonella henselae
Tropheryma whippelii
Mycobacterium spp.
Chlamydia trachomatis
Coxiella burnetii
Treponema pallidum
Nocardia spp.

Viruses
Cytomegalovirus
Measles virus
Mumps virus
Epstein-Barr virus

Fungi
Cryptococcus neoformans
Candida spp.
Sporothrix schenckii
Histoplasma capsulatum
Paracoccidioides brasiliensis
Coccidioides immitis
Blastomyces dermatitidis
Aspergillus spp.
Phialophora spp.
Exophiala spp.
Fonsecaea spp.
Penicillium marneffei
Pseudallescheria boydii

Parasites
Leishmania spp.
Toxoplasma gondii

Schistosoma spp.
Toxocara spp.

INTRA-ABDOMINAL INFECTIONS
Peritonitis
Bacteria
Escherichia coli
Klebsiella pneumoniae (and other enteric
gram-negative rods)
Pseudomonas aeruginosa
Streptococcus pneumoniae
Staphylococcus aureus
Enterococcus spp.
Bacteroides fragilis group (and other
Bacteroides spp.)
Fusobacterium spp.
Clostridium spp.
Peptostreptococcus spp. (and other anaerobic
gram-positive cocci)
Neisseria gonorrhoeae
Chlamydia trachomatis
Mycobacterium tuberculosis
Fungi
Candida albicans
Parasites
Strongyloides stercoralis

Dialysis-associated peritonitis
Bacteria
Staphylococcus aureus (and other
Staphylococcus spp.)
Streptococcus spp.
Corynebacterium spp.
Propionibacterium spp.
Escherichia coli (and other *Enterobacteriaceae*)
Pseudomonas aeruginosa
Acinetobacter spp.
Fungi
Candida albicans
Candida parapsilosis (and other *Candida* spp.)

Aspergillus spp.
Fusarium spp.
Exophiala spp.

Visceral abscesses
Bacteria
Escherichia coli (and other *Enterobacteriaceae*)
Enterococcus spp.
Staphylococcus aureus
Bacteroides fragilis group
Fusobacterium spp.
Actinomyces spp.
Mixed aerobes and anaerobes
Yersinia enterocolitica
Mycobacterium tuberculosis
Mycobacterium avium complex (and other *Mycobacterium* spp.)
Fungi
Candida albicans (and other *Candida* spp.)
Parasites
Entamoeba histolytica (primarily hepatic abscesses)
Echinococcus (hepatic abscesses)

RESPIRATORY TRACT INFECTIONS
Cold
Bacteria
Streptococcus pyogenes
Viruses
Rhinovirus
Coronavirus
Parainfluenza virus
Respiratory syncytial virus
Influenza virus
Adenovirus
Metapneumovirus

Pharyngitis
Bacteria
Streptococcus pyogenes
Streptococcus dysgalactiae (groups C and G)

Microbes of Humans

    Archanobacterium haemolyticum
    Chlamydophila pneumoniae
    Neisseria gonorrhoeae
    Corynebacterium diphtheriae
    Corynebacterium ulcerans
    Mycoplasma pneumoniae
    Yersinia enterocolitica
    Treponema pallidum
Viruses
    Respiratory syncytial virus
    Rhinovirus
    Coronavirus
    Adenovirus
    Herpes simplex virus
    Parainfluenza virus
    Influenza virus
    Coxsackievirus A
    Epstein-Barr virus
    Cytomegalovirus
    Human immunodeficiency virus

Laryngitis
Bacteria
    Mycoplasma pneumoniae
    Chlamydophila pneumoniae
    Streptococcus pyogenes
Viruses
    Rhinovirus
    Influenza virus
    Parainfluenza virus
    Adenovirus
    Coronavirus

Laryngotracheobronchitis (croup)
Bacteria
    Mycoplasma pneumoniae
Viruses
    Parainfluenza virus
    Influenza A and B viruses
    Respiratory syncytial virus
    Adenovirus
    Rhinovirus
    Enterovirus

Sinusitis

Bacteria

Streptococcus pneumoniae
Haemophilus influenzae
Moraxella catarrhalis
Streptococcus, viridans group
Mixed anaerobes
Staphylococcus aureus
Streptococcus pyogenes
Chlamydophila pneumoniae
Pseudomonas aeruginosa (and other
    gram-negative rods)

Viruses

Rhinovirus
Influenza virus
Parainfluenza virus
Adenovirus

Fungi

Aspergillus spp. (allergic sinusitis)
Hyphomycetes (allergic sinusitis)
Zygomycetes (invasive disease)

Bronchitis

Bacteria

Mycoplasma pneumoniae
Chlamydophila pneumoniae
Bordetella pertussis
Moraxella catarrhalis
Haemophilus influenzae

Viruses

Rhinovirus
Coronavirus
Parainfluenza virus
Influenza virus
Respiratory syncytial virus
Adenovirus

Empyema

Bacteria

Staphylococcus aureus
Streptococcus pneumoniae
Streptococcus pyogenes

Microbes of Humans

      Bacteroides fragilis
      Klebsiella pneumoniae (and other gram-negative rods)
      Actinomyces spp.
      Nocardia spp.
      Mycobacterium tuberculosis (and other
        Mycobacterium spp.)
  Fungi
      Aspergillus spp.

Community-acquired pneumonia
  Bacteria
      Streptococcus pneumoniae
      Staphylococcus aureus
      Klebsiella pneumoniae
      Haemophilus influenzae
      Moraxella catarrhalis
      Neisseria meningitidis
      Mycoplasma pneumoniae
      Chlamydia trachomatis
      Chlamydophila spp. (primarily *C. pneumoniae* and
        C. psittaci)
      Pseudomonas aeruginosa
      Legionella spp.
      Bacteroides fragilis (and other anaerobes in
        mixed infections)
      Nocardia spp.
      Rhodococcus equi
      Mycobacterium tuberculosis (and other
        Mycobacterium spp.)
      Coxiella burnetii
      Many other bacteria
  Viruses
      Respiratory syncytial virus
      Parainfluenza virus
      Influenza virus
      Adenovirus
      Rhinovirus
      Enteroviruses
      Herpesviruses
      Measles virus
  Fungi
      Pneumocystis jiroveci (carinii)
      Cryptococcus neoformans

    Histoplasma capsulatum
    Blastomyces dermatitidis
    Coccidioides immitis
    Paracoccidioides brasiliensis
    Zygomycetes (primarily *Rhizopus* and *Mucor* spp.)
Parasites
    Ascaris lumbricoides
    Strongyloides stercoralis
    Toxoplasma gondii
    Paragonimus westermani

Hospital-acquired pneumonia

Bacteria
    Streptococcus pneumoniae
    Staphylococcus aureus
    Haemophilus influenzae
    Klebsiella pneumoniae
    Enterobacter spp.
    Escherichia coli
    Serratia marcescens
    Stenotrophomonas maltophilia
    Acinetobacter spp.
    Moraxella catarrhalis
    Proteus mirabilis
    Citrobacter spp.
    Enterococcus spp.
Viruses
    Cytomegalovirus
    Respiratory syncytial virus
Fungi
    Aspergillus fumigatus
    Zygomycetes (primarily *Rhizopus* and *Mucor* spp.)
Parasites
    Toxoplasma gondii

SKIN AND SOFT TISSUE INFECTIONS

Primary pyodermas

Bacteria
    Staphylococcus aureus

Streptococcus pyogenes
Pseudomonas aeruginosa
Bacillus anthracis
Treponema pallidum
Haemophilus ducreyi
Francisella tularensis
Corynebacterium diphtheriae
Mycobacterium spp. (primarily *M. ulcerans* and
  M. marinum)
Fungi
  Candida spp.
  Sporothrix schenckii

Gangrenous cellulitis
Bacteria
  Streptococcus pyogenes
  Pseudomonas aeruginosa
  Clostridium spp. (primarily *C. perfringens*, *C. septicum*,
    and *C. novyi*)
  Mixed aerobes and anaerobes (e.g., *E. coli*,
    Bacteroides spp., and *Peptostreptococcus* spp.)
Fungi
  Aspergillus spp.
  Zygomycetes (primarily *Rhizopus*, *Absidia*, and
    Mucor spp.)

Nodular lesions
Bacteria
  Staphylococcus aureus
  Nocardia spp.
  Mycobacterium marinum
  Bartonella spp.
Fungi
  Candida spp.
  Sporothrix schenckii
Parasites
  Leishmania spp.

Secondary skin infections
Bacteria
  Staphylococcus aureus

    Streptococcus pyogenes
    Pseudomonas aeruginosa
    Enterobacter spp. (and other *Enterobacteriaceae*)
    Anaerobic gram-positive cocci
    Pasteurella spp. (primarily *P. multocida* and *P. canis*)
Fungi
    Candida spp.
    Aspergillus spp.

Disseminated infections with cutaneous manifestations

Bacteria
    Staphylococcus aureus
    Streptococcus pyogenes
    Neisseria spp. (primarily *N. meningitidis* and
       N. gonorrhoeae)
    Pseudomonas aeruginosa
    Salmonella enterica serovar Typhi
    Listeria monocytogenes
    Leptospira interrogans
    Streptobacillus moniliformis
    Burkholderia spp. (primarily *B. pseudomallei* and
       B. mallei)
    Bartonella spp.
    Mycobacterium tuberculosis (and other
       Mycobacterium spp.)
    Nocardia spp.
Fungi
    Candida spp.
    Blastomyces dermatitidis
    Aspergillus spp.
    Coccidioides immitis
    Fusarium spp.

URINARY TRACT INFECTIONS

Cystitis and pyelonephritis

Bacteria
    Escherichia coli
    Enterococcus spp. (primarily *E. faecalis*
       and *E. faecium*)

Proteus mirabilis
Klebsiella spp.
Pseudomonas aeruginosa
Enterobacter spp.
Staphylococcus aureus
Staphylococcus saprophyticus (and other
    Staphylococcus spp.)
Streptococcus agalactiae (group B)
Aerococcus urinae
Mycobacterium tuberculosis
Viruses
  Adenovirus
  Cytomegalovirus
  BK virus
Fungi
  Candida glabrata
  Candida albicans (and other *Candida* spp.)
Parasites
  Schistosoma haematobium

Renal calculi
Bacteria
  Proteus spp.
  Morganella morganii
  Klebsiella pneumoniae
  Corynebacterium urealyticum
  Staphylococcus saprophyticus
  Ureaplasma urealyticum

Prostatitis
Bacteria
  Escherichia coli
  Klebsiella spp.
  Proteus mirabilis
  Enterobacter spp.
  Enterococcus spp.
  Neisseria gonorrhoeae
  Mycobacterium spp.
Fungi
  Candida spp.
  Cryptococcus neoformans

Microbes of Humans

Summary of Notifiable Infectious Diseases: United States, 2002[a]

Microbes of Humans

Bacterial

Anthrax (*Bacillus anthracis*) (2)

Botulism, food-borne (*Clostridium botulinum*) (28)

Botulism, infant (69)

Botulism, other (21)

Brucellosis (*Brucella* spp.) (125)

Chancroid (*Haemophilus ducreyi*) (67)

Chlamydia (*Chlamydia trachomatis*) (834,555)

Cholera (*Vibrio cholerae*) (2)

Diphtheria (*Corynebacterium diphtheriae*) (1)

Ehrlichiosis, human granulocytic (*Anaplasma phagocytophilum*) (511)

Ehrlichiosis, human monocytic (*Ehrlichia chaffeensis*) (216)

Escherichia coli O157:H7 (3,840)

Gonorrhea (*Neisseria gonorrhoeae*) (351,852)

Haemophilus influenzae, invasive (1,743)

Hansen disease, leprosy (*Mycobacterium leprae*) (96)

Legionellosis (*Legionella* spp.) (1,321)

Listeriosis (*Listeria monocytogenes*) (665)

Lyme disease (*Borrelia burgdorferi*) (23,763)

Meningococcal disease (*Neisseria meningitidis*) (1,814)

Pertussis (*Bordetella pertussis*) (9,771)

Plague (*Yersinia pestis*) (2)

Psittacosis (*Chlamydophila psittaci*) (18)

Q fever (*Coxiella burnetii*) (61)

Rocky Mountain spotted fever (*Rickettsia rickettsii*) (1,104)

Salmonellosis (*Salmonella* spp.) (44,264)

Shigellosis (*Shigella* spp.) (23,541)

Streptococcal disease, invasive (*Streptococcus pyogenes*) (4,720)

Streptococcal toxic shock (*S. pyogenes*) (118)

Streptococcus pneumoniae, drug resistant, invasive (2,546)

Streptococcus pneumoniae, <5 years, invasive (513)

Syphilis, all stages (*Treponema pallidum*) (32,871)

Syphilis, primary and secondary (6,852)

Syphilis, congenital (412)

Tetanus (*Clostridium tetani*) (25)

(continued)

Toxic shock syndrome (*Staphylococcus aureus*) (109)

Tuberculosis (*Mycobacterium tuberculosis*) (15,075)

Tularemia (*Francisella tularensis*) (90)

Typhoid fever (*Salmonella enterica* serovar Typhi) (321)

Hepatitis A (8,795)
Hepatitis B (7,996)
Hepatitis C (1,835)
Measles (44)
Mumps (270)
Rabies, animal (7,609)
Rabies, human (3)
Rubella (18)
Rubella (congenital) (1)
Varicella (22,841)
Yellow fever (1)

Viral

AIDS (human immunodeficiency virus) (42,745)

AIDS, pediatric infection (163)

Encephalitis, California (164)

Encephalitis, Eastern equine (10)

Encephalitis, Powassan (1)

Encephalitis, St. Louis (28)

Encephalitis, West Nile (2,840)

Hantavirus pulmonary syndrome (19)

Fungal

Coccidioidomycosis (*Coccidioides immitis*) (4,968)

Parasitic

Cryptosporidiosis (*Cryptosporidium parvum*) (3,016)

Cyclosporiasis (*Cyclospora cayetanensis*) (156)

Giardiasis (*Giardia lamblia*) (21,206)

Malaria (*Plasmodium* spp.) (1,430)

Trichinosis (*Trichinella spiralis*) (14)

[a] Data from *Morb. Mortal. Wkly. Rep.* **S2**(31):741–750, 2003. Numbers in parentheses represent the number of cases reported in 2002.

Microbes of Humans

HHS and USDA Select Agents and Toxins

HHS Nonoverlap select agents and toxins
>Crimean-Congo hemorrhagic fever virus
>*Coccidioides posadasii*
>Ebola viruses
>Cercopithecine herpesvirus 1 (herpes B virus)
>Lassa fever virus
>Marburg virus
>Monkeypox virus
>*Rickettsia prowazekii*
>*Rickettsia rickettsii*

>South American hemorrhagic fever viruses
>>Junin virus
>>Machupo virus
>>Sabia virus
>>Flexal virus
>>Guanarito virus

>Tick-borne encephalitis complex viruses (flaviviruses)
>>Central European tick-borne encephalitis virus
>>Far Eastern tick-borne encephalitis virus
>>Russian spring and summer encephalitis virus
>>Kyasanur forest disease virus
>>Omsk hemorrhagic fever virus

>Variola major virus (smallpox virus)
>Variola minor virus (Alastrim)
>*Yersinia pestis*
>Abrin
>Conotoxins
>Diacetoxyscirpenol
>Ricin
>Saxitoxin
>Shiga-like ribosome-inactivating proteins
>Tetrodotoxin

High-consequence livestock pathogens and toxins/select agents (overlap agents)
>*Bacillus anthracis*
>*Brucella abortus*

(continued)

Microbes of Humans

Brucella melitensis
Brucella suis
Burkholderia mallei
Burkholderia pseudomallei
Botulinum neurotoxin-producing *Clostridium* spp.
Coccidioides immitis
Coxiella burnetii
Eastern equine encephalitis virus
Hendra virus
Francisella tularensis
Nipah virus
Rift Valley fever virus
Venezuelan equine encephalitis virus
Botulinum neurotoxin
Clostridium perfringens epsilon toxin
Shiga toxin
Staphylococcal enterotoxin
T-2 toxin

USDA high-consequence livestock pathogens and toxins (nonoverlap agents and toxins)

Akabane virus
African swine fever virus
African horse sickness virus
Avian influenza virus (highly pathogenic)
Blue tongue virus (exotic)
Bovine spongiform encephalopathy agent
Camel pox virus
Classical swine fever virus
Cowdria ruminantium (heartwater)
Foot and mouth disease virus
Goat pox virus
Lumpy skin disease virus
Japanese encephalitis virus
Malignant catarrhal fever virus (exotic)
Menangle virus
Mycoplasma capricolum/M.F38/*M. mycoides capri*
Mycoplasma mycoides mycoides
Newcastle disease virus (VVND)
Peste Des Petits Ruminants virus
Rinderpest virus
Sheep pox virus

(continued)

Swine vesicular disease virus
Vesicular stomatitis virus (exotic)

Listed plant pathogens

Liberobacter africanus
Liberobacter asiaticus
Peronosclerospora philippinensis
Phakospora pachyrhizi
Plum pox virus
Ralstonia solanacearum race 3, biovar 2
Schlerophthora rayssiae var. *zeae*
Synchytrium endobioticum
Xanthomonas oryzae
Xylella fastidiosa (citrus variegated chlorosis strain)

Microbes of Humans

Table 2.2 Arthropod vectors of medically important diseases[a]

Arthropod	Etiologic agent	Disease
Crustacea		
Decapods	*Paragonimus* spp.	Paragonimiasis
Copepods	*Diphyllobothrium* spp.	Diphyllobothriasis
	Dracunculus medinensis	Guinea worm disease
	Gnathostoma spinigerum	Gnathostomiasis
Insecta		
Anopleura		
Pediculus	*Rickettsia prowazekii*	Epidemic typhus
	Bartonella quintana	Trench fever
	Borrelia recurrentis	Epidemic relapsing fever
Siphonaptera		
Xenopsylla, Nosophyllus	*Yersinia pestis*	Plague
	Rickettsia typhi	Murine typhus
	Hymenolepis diminuta	Rat tapeworm
Pulex, Oropsylla	*Yersinia pestis*	Plague
Ctenocephalides	*Dipylidium caninum*	Dog tapeworm disease
Hemiptera		
Panstrongylus, Rhodnius, Triatoma	*Trypanosoma cruzi*	Chagas' disease

Diptera

Aedes	*Wuchereria, Brugia*	Filariasis
	Flaviviruses	Dengue, yellow fever
	Other arboviruses	Encephalitis
Anopheles	*Plasmodium* spp.	Malaria
	Wuchereria, Brugia	Filariasis
	Arboviruses	Encephalitis
Culex	*Wuchereria*	Filariasis
	Arboviruses	Encephalitis
Culicoides	*Mansonella* spp.	Filariasis
Glossina	*Trypanosoma brucei*	African sleeping sickness
Chrysops	*Loa loa*	Loiasis
	Francisella tularensis	Tularemia
Simulium	*Onchocerca volvulus*	Onchocerciasis
	Mansonella ozzardi	Filariasis
Phlebotomus, Lutzomyia	*Leishmania* spp.	Leishmaniasis
	Bartonella bacilliformis	Bartonellosis
	Phlebovirus	Sandfly fever

Arachnida

Acari (ticks)

Ixodes	*Borrelia burgdorferi*	Lyme disease
	Anaplasma phagocytophilum	Anaplasmosis
	Rickettsia conorii	Boutonneuse fever
	Babesia spp.	Babesiosis

(continued)

Microbes of Humans

Table 2.2 Arthropod vectors of medically important diseases[a] *(continued)*

Arthropod	Etiologic agent	Disease
Dermacentor	*Rickettsia rickettsii*	Rocky Mountain spotted fever
	Francisella tularensis	Tularemia
	Coltivirus	Colorado tick fever
	Flavivirus	Omsk hemorrhagic fever
Amblyomma	*Rickettsia rickettsii*	Rocky Mountain spotted fever
	Francisella tularensis	Tularemia
	Ehrlichia chaffeensis	Human monocytic ehrlichiosis
Hyalomma	Nairovirus	Crimean-Congo hemorrhagic fever
Rhipicephalus	*Rickettsia conorii*	Boutonneuse fever
	Rickettsia rickettsii	Rocky Mountain spotted fever
Ornithodoros	*Borrelia* spp.	Relapsing fever
Acari (mites)		
Leptotrombidium	*Orientia tsutsugamushi*	Scrub typhus
Liponyssoides	*Rickettsia akari*	Rickettsialpox

[a] Adapted from P. R. Murray, E. J. Baron, J. H. Jorgensen, M. A. Pfaller, and R. H. Yolken (ed.), *Manual of Clinical Microbiology*, 8th ed., ASM Press, Washington, D.C., 2003.

Table 2.3 Fungal pathogens and geographic distribution

Fungi	Human body sites	Geographic distribution
Yeasts		
Candida spp.	Opportunistic pathogen involving any part of body	Worldwide
Cryptococcus neoformans	Opportunistic pathogen primarily involving lungs and central nervous system; other body sites can be infected	Worldwide
Cryptococcus, other spp.	Opportunistic pathogen rarely implicated in disease	Worldwide
Blastoschizomyces capitatus	Opportunistic pathogen uncommonly implicated in systemic infections	Worldwide
Geotrichum candidum	Opportunistic pathogen uncommonly implicated in systemic infections	Worldwide
Hansenula spp.	Opportunistic pathogen uncommonly implicated in systemic infections	Worldwide
Malassezia spp.	Opportunistic pathogen involving skin surface (tinea versicolor, atopic dermatitis, folliculitis) and systemic disease (associated with lipid therapy)	Worldwide
Rhodotorula spp.	Opportunistic pathogen uncommonly implicated in systemic infections	Worldwide

(continued)

Microbes of Humans

Microbes of Humans

Table 2.3 Fungal pathogens and geographic distribution *(continued)*

Fungi	Human body sites	Geographic distribution
Trichosporon spp.	Opportunistic pathogen involving capital, axillary or crural hairs (white piedra); systemic infections in immunocompromised patients	Worldwide
Pneumocystis (carinii) jiroveci	Opportunistic pathogen primarily involving respiratory tract	Worldwide
Dimorphic fungi		
Blastomyces dermatitidis	Blastomycosis is primarily a pulmonary infection with dissemination to skin (cutaneous and subcutaneous lesions), genitourinary tract, bone, and central nervous system	Ohio and Mississippi River valleys, as well as Missouri and Arkansas River basins; southern Canada, South America, and portions of Africa
Coccidioides immitis, *Coccidioides posadasii*	Coccidioidomycosis is primarily a pulmonary infection with dissemination to skin, bone, joints, lymph nodes, adrenal glands, and central nervous system	Southwestern United States, northwestern Mexico, Argentina, and other dry areas of Central and South America
Histoplasma capsulatum	Histoplasmosis is primarily a pulmonary infection with dissemination to central nervous system, adrenal glands, mucocutaneous surfaces, and other tissues	Temperate, tropical, and subtropical regions throughout the world, particularly Ohio, Missouri, and Mississippi River valleys, southern portions of Central and South America, and areas in Central and South America
H. capsulatum var. *duboisii*	African histoplasmosis; pulmonary infection less common with more frequent involvement of skin and bones	Central Africa (between 20°N and 20°S)

Paracoccidioides brasiliensis	Paracoccidioidomycosis (South American blastomycosis) is primarily a pulmonary infection with dissemination commonly to nose and mouth, less commonly to lymph nodes, spleen, liver, gastrointestinal tract, and adrenal glands	Central and South America
Penicillium marneffei	Disseminated infection involving bone, skin, lung, lymph nodes, genitourinary and gastrointestinal tracts, central nervous system, and other tissues	Mountainous provinces of northern Thailand, Laos, Myanmar, and southeastern China
Sporothrix schenckii	Sporotrichosis involving skin and subcutaneous tissues with dissemination commonly via lymphatics to lymph nodes and, less commonly, to other internal organs	Worldwide, primarily in soil and decaying plant material
Cutaneous fungi		
Epidermophyton floccosum	Infection of nails and skin, particularly of the groin and feet	Worldwide; anthropophilic
Microsporum audouinii	Infection of scalp in children; rarely infects adults	Worldwide but primarily in Africa (Nigeria), eastern Europe, and Haiti; rarely in North America or western Europe; anthropophilic
Microsporum canis	Infection of scalp in children, infection of beard and glabrous skin in all ages	Worldwide; zoophilic (dogs, cats)
Microsporum ferrugineum	Infection of scalp	Africa, East Asia, eastern Europe; anthropophilic
Microsporum gypseum	Infection of scalp and glabrous skin	Worldwide; geophilic

(continued)

Microbes of Humans

Table 2.3 Fungal pathogens and geographic distribution *(continued)*

Fungi	Human body sites	Geographic distribution
Microsporum persicolor	Infection of scalp, glabrous skin, and feet	Worldwide; zoophilic (small rodents)
Phaeoannellomyces (Exophiala) werneckii	Infection (tinea nigra) of palms of hands, occasionally, the dorsa of the feet	Tropical areas of Central and South America, Africa, and Asia; southeastern United States
Piedraia hortae	Infection (black piedra) of scalp hair; less commonly beard, axillary, or pubic hairs	Tropical regions of Africa, Asia, and Central and South America
Trichophyton concentricum	Infection of glabrous skin	Southwestern Pacific islands, Southeast Asia, Central and South America; anthropophilic
Trichophyton megninii	Infection of glabrous skin, scalp, and beard	Europe (particularly Portugal, Spain, and Sardinia), African nation of Burundi; rare in Western Hemisphere; anthropophilic
Trichophyton mentagrophytes	Infection of all body surfaces including nails, hair, and (particularly) feet	Worldwide; anthropophilic or zoophilic (primarily small mammals)
Trichophyton rubrum	Infection of skin and nails (most common pathogenic dermatophyte)	Worldwide; anthropophilic
Trichophyton schoenleinii	Infection of scalp (favus) and occasionally nails and skin	Primarily in Eurasia and Africa; anthropophilic
Trichophyton soudanense	Infection of scalp and hair	Central and West Africa; anthropophilic
Trichophyton tonsurans	Infection of scalp (most common pathogen), as well as skin and nails	Worldwide, particularly in the United States and Latin America; anthropophilic
Trichophyton verrucosum	Infection of scalp, beard, nails, and other skin surfaces	Worldwide distribution; zoophilic (cattle, horses)

Trichophyton violaceum	Infection of scalp, as well as glabrous skin, nails, and soles of feet	North Africa, Middle East, Europe, South America, and Mexico; anthropophilic
Zygomycosis		
Apophysomyces elegans	Rare cause of traumatic zygomycosis	Worldwide
Absidia corymbifera	Pulmonary infections, as well as infections of the skin, meninges, and kidneys	Worldwide
Basidiobolus ranarum	Subcutaneous zygomycosis of limbs, chest, back, or buttocks	Worldwide
Conidiobolus coronatus	Subcutaneous zygomycosis of nasal mucosa, with spread into adjacent tissues	Worldwide, primarily in tropical and subtropical areas
Cunninghamella bertholletiae	Rare cause of pulmonary or disseminated zygomycosis	Primarily in Mediterranean or subtropical areas
Mucor spp.	Uncommon cause of disseminated zygomycosis	Worldwide
Rhizomucor pusillus	Pulmonary, disseminated, or cutaneous zygomycosis	Worldwide
Rhizopus spp.	Primary cause of invasive zygomycosis, particularly involving spread from nasopharynx to brain	Worldwide
Saksenaea vasiformis	Occasional cause of rhinocerebral zygomycosis, as well as involvement of bone, skin, and subcutaneous tissues	Worldwide

(continued)

Microbes of Humans

Table 2.3 Fungal pathogens and geographic distribution *(continued)*

Fungi	Human body sites	Geographic distribution
Eumycotic mycetoma		
Acremonium spp. (*A. falciforme*, *A. kiliense*, *A. recifei*)	Mycetoma (*A. falciforme* is the second most common cause in the United States)	India, Thailand, United States, Africa, Romania, Venezuela, Brazil
Curvularia spp. (*C. geniculata*, *C. lunata*)	Mycetoma (*C. geniculata* in dogs)	United States (*C. geniculata*); Senegal (*C. lunata*)
Exophiala jeanselmei	Mycetoma; subcutaneous phaeohyphomycosis; peritonitis	United States, Europe, India, Malaya, Thailand, Argentina
Leptosphaeria spp. (*L. senegalensis*, *L. tompkinsii*)	Mycetoma	Northern tropical West Africa (especially Senegal and Mauritania), India
Madurella spp. (*M. grisea*, *M. mycetomatis*)	Mycetoma	Venezuela, Argentina, Paraguay, Chile, Brazil, British West Indies, India, Zaire (*M. grisea*); Venezuela, Argentina, Romania, India, Sudan, Senegal, Somalia (*M. mycetomatis*)
Neotestudina rosatii	Mycetoma	Australia, Cameroon, Guinea, Senegal, Somalia
Pseudallescheria boydii	Mycetoma (most common cause in United States)	United States, Mexico, Venezuela, Argentina, Uruguay, India, Romania
Pyrenochaeta romeroi	Mycetoma	Somalia, Senegal, India, South America

Moniliaceous fungi

Aspergillus spp.	*A. fumigatus*, *A. flavus*, and *A. niger* are the most common pathogens; capable of colonization, invasive disease, toxicoses, or allergy	Worldwide
Fusarium spp.	*F. solani*, *F. oxysporum*, and *F. moniliforme* are the most common pathogens; cause eye infection and, less commonly, systemic infection, sinusitis, skin and nail infection, and mycetoma	Worldwide
Paecilomyces spp.	*P. varioti* and *P. lilacinus* are the most common pathogens; cause keratitis and, less commonly, endocarditis, sinusitis, nephritis, pulmonary infection, and skin and soft tissue infection	Worldwide
Penicillium spp.	With the exception of *P. marneffei*, most isolates are contaminants	Worldwide
Scopulariopsis spp.	*S. brevicaulis* is the most common pathogen, as well as a frequent lab contaminant; infection of toenails and (less commonly) fingernails	Worldwide

Dematiaceous fungi

Alternaria spp.	Phaeohyphomycosis of bone, skin, ears, eyes, sinuses, and urinary tract (this genus and other dematiaceous fungi are frequently isolated as lab contaminants)	Worldwide

(continued)

Microbes of Humans

Table 2.3 Fungal pathogens and geographic distribution *(continued)*

Fungi	Human body sites	Geographic distribution
Aureobasidium pullulans	Phaeohyphomycosis of nail, skin, subcutaneous, and deep tissues	Worldwide
Bipolaris spp.	*B. australiensis, B. hawaiiensis,* and *B. spicifera* are associated with infection of meninges, eye, sinuses, respiratory tract, and subcutaneous tissues	Worldwide
Chaetomium spp.	Phaeohyphomycosis of skin, nails, and deep tissues	Worldwide
Cladophialophora spp.	Chromoblastomycosis (*C. carrionii* is the most common cause in Africa, Australia, and Madagascar)	Worldwide
Cladosporium spp.	Cutaneous, subcutaneous, and eye infections	Worldwide
Curvularia spp.	Common cause of fungal sinusitis and keratitis; less commonly associated with other infections	Worldwide
Dactylaria spp.	Opportunistic pathogen	Worldwide
Exserohilum spp.	*E. longirostratum, E. mcginnisii,* and *E. rostratum* are associated with phaeohyphomycosis of skin, subcutaneous tissue, and sinuses	Worldwide
Fonsecaea spp.	*F. compacta* is the most common cause of chromoblastomycosis; *F. pedrosoi* is a rare cause	Worldwide

Lasiodiplodia theobromae	keratitis; rare cause of subcutaneous infection	Worldwide
Lecythophora spp.	*L. hoffmannii* and *L. mutabilis* cause subcutaneous phaeohyphomycosis, endocarditis, and peritonitis	Worldwide
Scytalidium spp. (a pycnidial form, *Nattrassia mangiferae*)	Phaeohyphomycosis of skin and nail	Worldwide
Phialemonium spp.	*P. curvatum* and *P. obovatum* cause infection of subcutaneous tissues, endocarditis, and peritonitis	Worldwide
Phialophora spp.	*P. verrucosa* is the leading cause of chromoblastomycosis in North America; phaeohyphomycosis, endocarditis, keratitis, osteomyelitis, and opportunistic infections	Worldwide
Phoma spp.	Phaeohyphomycosis involving skin and subcutaneous tissues, lung, cornea, and sinuses	Worldwide
Rhinocladiella spp.	*R. aquaspersa* is a rare cause of chromoblastomycosis	Brazil, Mexico
Exophiala dermatitidis	Phaeohyphomycosis of skin and subcutaneous tissues	Worldwide

Table 2.4 Parasitic pathogens and geographic distribution

Parasites	Human body sites[a]	Geographic distribution
Protozoa: amoebae		
Acanthamoeba spp.	Brain, skin, eye, lung	Worldwide
Balamuthia mandrillaris	Brain, CSF	Worldwide
Blastocystis hominis	Small and large intestine	Worldwide
Endolimax nana	Lumen of colon and cecum	Worldwide
Entamoeba histolytica/dispar	Lumen of colon and cecum; extraintestinal sites include liver, lung, brain, skin	Worldwide
Entamoeba hartmanni	Lumen of colon and cecum	Worldwide
Entamoeba gingivalis	Mouth	Worldwide
Entamoeba coli	Lumen of colon and cecum	Worldwide
Entamoeba polecki	Lumen of colon and cecum	Worldwide
Iodamoeba butschlii	Lumen of colon and cecum	Worldwide
Naegleria fowleri	Brain, CSF	Worldwide
Protozoa: flagellates		
Chilomastix mesnili	Primarily large intestine	Worldwide
Dientamoeba fragilis	Colon	Worldwide
Giardia lamblia	Small intestine	Worldwide

Leishmania chagasi, L. donovani, L. infantium	Visceral leishmaniasis: amastigotes in bone marrow or aspirates from spleen, lymph nodes, or liver	*L. chagasi* in Central and South America; *L. donovani* in China, India, Middle East, Africa; *L. infantum* in North Africa, Southwest Asia, Mediterranean, Europe, Central and South America
Leishmania tropica, L. braziliensis, L. major, other *Leishmania* spp.	Cutaneous leishmaniasis: amastigotes in cutaneous lesions	Many species worldwide
Pentatrichomonas (Trichomonas) hominis	Cecum	Worldwide
Trichomonas tenex	Mouth	Worldwide
Trichomonas vaginalis	Vagina, urethra, prostate, epididymis	Worldwide
Trypanosoma brucei gambiense	Trypomastigotes in blood, CSF, brain, lymph nodes, and spleen	West Central Africa south of Sahara Desert
Trypanosoma brucei rhodesiense	As with *T. b. gambiense*	East Central Africa south of Sahara Desert
Trypanosoma cruzi	Trypomastigotes in blood; amastigotes and epimastigotes in pseudocysts in cardiac and smooth muscle, glial cells, and phagocytes	Western Hemisphere from southern United States south to Argentina
Protozoa: ciliates		
Balantidium coli	Colon	Widespread in temperate and warm climates

(continued)

Microbes of Humans

Microbes of Humans

Table 2.4 Parasitic pathogens and geographic distribution (*continued*)

Parasites	Human body sites[a]	Geographic distribution
Protozoa: apicomplexans		
Babesia spp.	Parasite of erythrocytes	*B. microti* in North America and Europe; other species (e.g., *B. divergens, B. equi*) with worldwide distribution in tropics and subtropics
Cryptosporidium parvum	Intracellular parasite of intestinal epithelial cells; also in respiratory tract and biliary system	Worldwide
Cyclospora cayetanensis	Intracellular parasite of jejunum enterocytes	North, Central, and South America; Caribbean, Africa, Southeast Asia, Eastern and Western Europe, Australia
Isospora belli	Intracellular parasite of duodenum and jejunum	Worldwide
Plasmodium falciparum	Ring forms and gametocytes infect erythrocytes of all ages; trophozoites and schizonts not typically seen in peripheral blood; no persistent exoerythrocytic stage	Widely distributed in tropics and subtropics, particularly Africa and Asia; chloroquine-resistant strains reported in all areas except Central America and the Caribbean
Plasmodium malariae	Trophozoites, schizonts, and gametocytes parasitize mature erythrocytes; no persistent exoerythrocytic stage, but low-level parasitemia can persist for years	Present in tropics and subtropics (e.g., tropical Africa, India, Myanmar, Sri Lanka, Malaysia, Indonesia) but less common than other plasmodia
Plasmodium ovale	Trophozoites, schizonts, and gametocytes parasitize reticulocytes; hypnozoites persist in hepatic parenchymal cells	Present in tropical Africa (particularly in West Africa), New Guinea, Philippines; also reported in Southeast Asia

Plasmodium vivax	Trophozoites, schizonts, and gametocytes in erythrocytes, with preference for reticulocytes; hypnozoites persist in hepatic parenchymal cells	Worldwide; predominant species in temperate areas; less commonly in tropics such as West Africa; chloroquine-resistant strains reported in Indonesia, Papua New Guinea, Myanmar, and Guyana
Sarcocystis spp.	Intracellular parasite of intestinal epithelium; cysts in skeletal and cardiac muscle	Worldwide
Toxoplasma gondii	Cysts in skeletal muscle, myocardium, brain; tachyzoites in blood, CSF, ocular fluid, bronchoalveolar lavage fluid	Worldwide
Protozoa: microsporidia		
Encephalitozoon spp.	Parasite of intestinal enterocytes and macrophages of lamina propria; kidney, liver, and bronchial epithelium; uroepithelium; cells of cornea and respiratory tract	Worldwide
Enterocytozoon bieneusi	Primarily in epithelium of the small intestine and biliary tree; also in respiratory epithelium, liver, and pancreas	Worldwide
Nosema spp.	Eye	Worldwide
Pleistophora spp.	Muscle	Unknown
Trachipleistophora spp.	Eye, muscle, sinuses	Unknown
Vittaforma spp.	Eye	Unknown

(continued)

Microbes of Humans

Table 2.4 Parasitic pathogens and geographic distribution (*continued*)

Parasites	Human body sites[a]	Geographic distribution
Nematodes		
Ancylostoma duodenale	Adults: small intestine; eggs: feces	Southern Europe, northern Africa, China, India, Japan
Angiostrongylus cantonensis	Larvae and young adults in CSF	Thailand, Tahiti, Taiwan, Indonesia, Hawaii; less commonly in Cuba, Central America, and Louisiana
Angiostrongylus costricensis	Adults: terminal ileus, cecum, colon, regional lymph nodes, mesenteric arteries; larvae and eggs in surrounding tissue	Central and South America
Anisakis spp.	Larvae: wall of stomach or intestine; occasionally in extraintestinal sites	Worldwide where uncooked fish is consumed
Ascaris lumbricoides	Adults: small intestine; larvae: small intestine, liver, lungs; eggs: feces	Worldwide (particularly in warm, moist regions)
Brugia malayi	Adults: lymphatic system; microfilaria: blood	Southeast Asia, Philippines, Korea, southern China, India
Brugia timori	Adults: lymphatic system; microfilaria: blood	Lesser Sunda Islands of eastern Indonesian archipelago
Capillaria hepatica	Adults: liver	Worldwide

Capillaria philippinensis	Adults: intestine; eggs: feces; larvae: occasionally found in feces	Philippines, Thailand, Japan, Taiwan, Egypt, Iran, Colombia
Dirofilaria immitis	Larvae in pulmonary nodules	Worldwide in tropical, subtropical, and warm temperate regions; southern coastal and southeastern United States
Dracunculus medinensis	Adults in cutaneous lesions	Worldwide
Enterobius vermicularis	Adults: cecum, appendix, colon, rectum; eggs: deposited in perianal area	Worldwide
Eustrongyloides spp.	Adults: abdominal cavity, intestines	Worldwide where uncooked fish is consumed (rare)
Gnathostoma spp.	Larvae: tissues	China, Philippines, Thailand, Japan
Loa loa	Adults: subcutaneous tissue; microfilaria: blood	Equatorial rain forests of Central and West Africa south of Sahara Desert
Mansonella ozzardi	Adults: subcutaneous tissue; microfilaria: blood	Central America (e.g., Mexico, Panama) and northern part of South America, West Indies
Mansonella perstans	Adults: abdominal cavity, mesenteries, peritoneal tissues; microfilaria: blood	West and Central Africa south of Sahara Desert, South America, some Caribbean islands
Mansonella streptocerca	Adults: subcutaneous tissues; microfilaria: skin snips	Rain forests of Central and West Africa (e.g., Zaire, Ghana, Nigeria, Cameroon)

(continued)

Microbes of Humans

Microbes of Humans

Table 2.4 Parasitic pathogens and geographic distribution *(continued)*

Parasites	Human body sites[a]	Geographic distribution
Necator americanus	Adults: small intestine; eggs: feces	Western Hemisphere, Central and South Africa, southern Asia, India, Melanesia, Polynesia
Onchocerca volvulus	Adults: subcutaneous nodules; microfilaria: skin snips; occasionally blood or urine	West and Central Africa south of Sahara Desert; Yeman, Central America (southern Mexico, Guatemala), South America (Venezuela, Colombia, Ecuador, Brazil)
Strongyloides stercoralis	Adults: small intestine; larvae: feces	Worldwide (particularly in warm, moist regions)
Toxocara spp.	Visceral larva migrans; larvae found in various tissues including liver, eye, and central nervous system	Worldwide (particularly in warm, moist regions)
Trichinella spiralis	Adults: intestines; larvae: encyst in muscle tissue	Worldwide (primarily in Europe and North America; less commonly in tropical countries)
Trichostrongylus spp.	Adults: small intestine; eggs: feces	Worldwide (associated with herbivorous animals)
Trichuris trichiura	Adults: large intestine, cecum, appendix; eggs: feces	Worldwide (particularly in warm, moist regions)
Wuchereria bancrofti	Adults: lymphatic system; microfilaria: blood	Widespread in tropics and subtropics (India, Bangladesh, China, Indonesia, Malaysia, Papua New Guinea, Philippines, Sri Lanka, Thailand, Vietnam, South Pacific islands, Africa, Egypt, Costa Rica, Brazil, West Indies)

Trematodes

Clonorchis sinensis	Adults: bile ducts; eggs: feces
Dicrocoelium dendriticum	Adults: bile ducts; eggs: feces
Echinostoma hortense	Adults: small intestine; eggs: feces
Fasciola hepatica	Adults: bile ducts; eggs: feces
Fasciolopsis buski	Adults: small intestine; eggs: feces
Gastrodiscoides hominis	Adults: cecum, colon; eggs: feces
Heterophyes heterophyes	Adults: small intestine; eggs: feces
Metagonimus yokogawai	Adults: small intestine; eggs: feces
Metorchis conjunctus	Adults: bile ducts; eggs: feces
Nanophyetus salmincola	Adults: small intestine; eggs: feces
Neodiplostomum seoulense	Adults: small intestine; eggs: feces
Opisthorchis spp.	Adults: bile ducts; eggs: feces
Paragonimus westermani	Adults: lung parenchyma; occasionally in abdominal wall, connective tissues, and organs; subcutaneous tissues; brain; eggs: feces or sputum

Clonorchis sinensis	China, Taiwan, Japan, Korea, Vietnam
Dicrocoelium dendriticum	Europe, former USSR, northern Africa, northern Asia, Far East, Western Hemisphere
Echinostoma hortense	Southeast Asia
Fasciola hepatica	Worldwide (particularly in sheep-raising countries)
Fasciolopsis buski	China, Taiwan, Thailand, Indonesia, India, Bangladesh, Cambodia, Myanmar, Vietnam
Gastrodiscoides hominis	India, Southeast Asia, former USSR
Heterophyes heterophyes	Nile River delta, Turkey, East and Southeast Asia
Metagonimus yokogawai	China, Japan, Southeast Asia, Balkan states
Metorchis conjunctus	Canada
Nanophyetus salmincola	Northwest North America
Neodiplostomum seoulense	Southeast Asia
Opisthorchis spp.	*O. viverrini*: Thailand, Laos; *O. felineus*: Eastern Europe, former USSR
Paragonimus westermani	China, Japan, Korea; other species in Latin America, Southeast Asia, Africa

(continued)

Microbes of Humans

Microbes of Humans

Table 2.4 Parasitic pathogens and geographic distribution *(continued)*

Parasites	Human body sites[a]	Geographic distribution
Phaneropsolus bonnei	Adults: small intestine; eggs: feces	Southeast Asia
Prosthodendrium molenkampi	Adults: small intestine; eggs: feces	Southeast Asia
Pygidiopsis summa	Adults: small intestine; eggs: feces	Southeast Asia
Schistosoma haematobium	Adults: venous plexuses of bladder and rectum; eggs: biopsy of bladder wall or rectum, feces	Africa, Madagascar, Arabian peninsula, Iraq, Iran, Syria, Lebanon, Turkey, India
Schistosoma japonicum	Adults: venous plexuses of small intestine; eggs: feces, rectal biopsy	China, Philippines, Indonesia, Thailand
Schistosoma mansoni	Adults: venous plexuses of colon and lower ileum; hepatic portal system; eggs: feces, rectal biopsy	Africa, Madagascar, Arabian peninsula, Caribbean islands, including Puerto Rico, South America (Brazil, Suriname, Venezuela)
Schistosoma mekongi	Adults: venous plexuses of small intestine; eggs: feces, rectal biopsy	Laos, Cambodia, Thailand
Cestodes		
Diphyllobothrium latum	Adults: small intestine; eggs and proglottids: feces	Fish tapeworm in cold lakes of northern Europe, Baltic countries, North America, Japan; other species found in Alaska, Peru, and Japan
Dipylidium caninum	Adults: small intestine; eggs and proglottids: feces	Worldwide (dog tapeworm)

Echinococcus granulosus	Unilocular hydatid disease; larvae form cysts in any tissue including liver, lung, and brain	Sheep-raising countries (e.g., Australia, New Zealand, southern Africa, southern South America); parts of Europe, North America, and the Orient
Echinococcus multilocularis	Multilocular hydatid disease; larvae form cysts in any tissue, particularly liver	Northern Europe, Japan, China, India, North America (Alaska, Canada, northern midwestern United States)
Echinococcus vogeli	Polycystic hydatid disease; larvae form cysts primarily in liver	Latin America
Hymenolepis diminuta	Adults: small intestine; eggs: feces	Worldwide (rat tapeworm)
Hymenolepis nana	Adults: small intestine; eggs: feces	Worldwide (dwarf tapeworm)
Spirometra mansoni	Larvae migrate to brain	China, Japan, Korea, Vietnam
Spirometra mansonoides	Larvae migrate in subcutaneous tissues	United States
Taenia multiceps	Larva form cysts in subcutaneous tissues, muscle, eye, and central nervous system	Sheep-raising countries
Taenia saginata	Adults: small intestine; eggs and proglottids: feces	Worldwide (beef tapeworm)
Taenia solium	Adults: small intestine; eggs and proglottids: feces; larvae (*Cysticercus cellulosae*) form cysts in various tissues including brain and muscle	Worldwide (pork tapeworm), particularly in middle European countries, Mexico, Latin America, India, China

[a] CSF, cerebrospinal fluid.

Microbes of Humans

Specimen Collection and Transport

The most important aspects of microbiological testing are collection of the right specimen and transport of the specimen to the testing site in a manner that ensures the reliability of the diagnostic procedure (e.g., culture, microscopy, and antigen or antibody tests). The following guidelines can be used for most commonly submitted specimens. For further information, please consult the ASM *Manual of Clinical Microbiology*, 8th ed., and Miller's *A Guide to Specimen Management in Clinical Microbiology*, 2nd ed.

As a general guideline for all specimens, the following considerations should be kept in mind.

1. Appropriate safety precautions must be used for the collection and transport of all specimens. Specimens should always be considered infectious. Therefore, gloves should always be worn when handling specimens and all procedures should be performed behind barrier protection, preferably in a biosafety cabinet.

2. Many infections are caused by members of the patient's indigenous microbial population. For this reason, it is important to avoid contamination of the specimen with these organisms.

3. Specimens should be collected from the areas where organisms are present and replicating. Although it seems obvious, this principle is often ignored. For example, pus typically contains relatively few viable organisms. A more appropriate specimen would be scrapings or a biopsy specimen from the wall of an abscess. Likewise, the material collected from the surface of a wound is often not representative of the organisms present deep in the wound. Finally, the diagnosis of a lower respiratory tract infection requires collection of material from that site (e.g., sputum) and not from the mouth (e.g., saliva).

4. The quantity of specimen collected must be sufficient to ensure that all requested tests (cultures, microscopy, antigen tests, nucleic acid probes, and amplification tests) can be performed properly. If only a limited amount of specimen can be collected, tests should be performed selectively. If too many tests are attempted, no test will be performed adequately.

5. As a general rule, swabs collect an inadequate quantity of specimen, are easily contaminated, and are subject to drying with subsequent loss of most organisms.

6. Transport of specimens should maintain the viability of the etiologic agent (if culture is performed) and prevent overgrowth with contaminating organisms.

7. Specimens should always be transported in a leakproof container inserted in a leakproof plastic bag with a separate compartment for the requisition. Use of plastic bags allows the specimen to be examined before the bag is opened. Every effort should be made to collect a second specimen if the original specimen is received in a leaking container. However, if an additional specimen cannot be collected, the laboratory should attempt to process the specimen if it can be done safely.

8. For off-site delivery specimen transport guidelines, refer to the International Air Transport Association (IATA) Dangerous Goods Regulations (http://www.IATA.org/dangerousgoods/index), the U.S. Department of Transportation (http://hazmat.dot.gov/rules.htm), and the International Civil Aviation Organization (ICAO) regulations. The IATA and ICAO have established two categories of specimens: diagnostic and infectious substances. Each specimen type requires specific packaging and handling procedures. When preparing a specimen for transport, always check the specimen transport guidelines of the receiving laboratory.

Collection and Transport

Collection and Transport

Table 3.1 Bacteriology: collection and transport guidelines [a,b]

Specimen type	Collection guidelines	Transport device and/or minimum vol	Transport time and temp	Comments
Abscess				
General	Remove surface exudate by wiping with sterile saline or 70% alcohol			Tissue or fluid is always superior to a swab specimen. If swabs must be used, collect 2, 1 for culture and 1 for Gram staining. Preserve swab material by placing in Stuart's or Amies medium.
Open	Aspirate if possible or pass a swab deep into the lesion to firmly sample the lesion's "fresh border"	Swab transport system	≤2 h, RT	Samples of the base of the lesion and abscess wall are most productive.
Closed	Aspirate abscess material with needle and syringe; aseptically transfer *all* material into anaerobic transport device	Anaerobic transport system, ≥1 ml	≤2 h, RT	Contamination with surface material will introduce colonizing bacteria not involved in the infectious process.
Bite wound	See Abscess			Do not culture animal bite wounds ≤12 h old (agents are usually not recovered) unless signs of infection are present.

Blood	Disinfect culture bottle; apply 70% isopropyl alcohol or phenolic to rubber stoppers and wait 1 min	Blood culture bottles for bacteria; adult, ≥20 ml/set (higher vol most productive)	≤2 h, RT	Acute febrile episode, antimicrobials to be started or changed immediately: 2 sets from separate sites, all within 10 min (before antimicrobials).
				Nonacute disease, antimicrobials will not be started or changed immediately: 2 or 3 sets from separate sites all within 24 h at intervals no closer than 3 h (before antimicrobials).
				Endocarditis, acute: 3 sets from separate sites, within 1–2 h, before antimicrobials if possible.
				Endocarditis, subacute: 3 sets from separate sites ≥1 h apart, within 24 h. If cultures are negative at 24 h, obtain 2–3 more sets.
	Palpate vein before disinfection of venipuncture site			Fever of unknown origin: 2 or 3 sets from separate sites ≥1 h apart during a 24-h period. If negative at 24–48 h, obtain 2 or 3 more sets.

(continued)

Collection and Transport

Collection and Transport

Table 3.1 Bacteriology: collection and transport guidelines[a,b] (continued)

Specimen type	Collection guidelines	Transport device and/or minimum vol	Transport time and temp	Comments
	Disinfection of venipuncture site: 1. Cleanse site with 70% alcohol 2. Swab concentrically, starting at the center, with an iodine preparation 3. Allow the iodine to dry 4. *Do not palpate vein at this point without sterile glove* 5. Collect blood 6. After venipuncture, remove iodine from the skin with alcohol	Infant and child, 1–20 ml/set depending on weight of patient		Some data indicate that an additional aerobic or fungal bottle is more productive than the anaerobic bottle. Pediatric: Collect immediately; rarely necessary to document continuous bacteremia with hours between cultures. Mycobacteria: Use special culture systems (e.g., Isolator, Bactec 13A, Bactec Myco/F lytic).
Bone marrow aspirate	Prepare puncture site as for surgical incision	Inoculate blood culture bottle or a lysis-centrifugation tube; plated specimen delivered to laboratory immediately	≤24 h, RT, if in culture bottle or tube	Small volumes of bone marrow may be inoculated directly onto culture media. Routine bacterial culture of bone marrow is rarely useful.

Burn	Clean and debride the burn	Tissue is placed into a sterile screw-cap container; aspirate or swab exudate; transport in sterile container or swab transport system	≤24 h, RT	A 3- to 4-mm punch biopsy specimen is optimum when quantitative cultures are ordered. Process for aerobic culture only. Quantitative culture may or may not be valuable. Cultures of surface samples of burns may be misleading.
Catheter i.v.	1. Cleanse the skin around the catheter site with alcohol 2. Aseptically remove catheter and clip 5 cm of distal tip directly into a sterile tube 3. Transport immediately to microbiology laboratory to prevent drying	Sterile screw-cap tube or cup	≤15 min, RT	Acceptable i.v. catheters for semiquantitative culture (Maki method): central, CVP, Hickman, Broviac, peripheral, arterial, umbilical, hyperalimentation, Swan-Ganz.
Foley		Do *not* culture, since growth represents distal urethral flora		Not acceptable for culture.
Cellulitis, aspirate from area of	1. Cleanse site by wiping with sterile saline or 70% alcohol	Sterile tube (syringe transport not recommended)	≤15 min, RT	Yield of potential pathogens in minority of specimens cultured.

(continued)

Collection and Transport

Collection and Transport

Table 3.1 Bacteriology: collection and transport guidelines [a,b] *(continued)*

Specimen type	Collection guidelines	Transport device and/or minimum vol	Transport time and temp	Comments
	2. Aspirate the area of maximum inflammation (commonly the center rather than the leading edge) with a needle and syringe; irrigation with a small amount of sterile saline may be necessary 3. Aspirate saline into syringe, and expel into sterile screw-cap tube			
CSF	1. Disinfect site with iodine preparation 2. Insert a needle with stylet at L3-L4, L4-L5, or L5-S1 interspace 3. Upon reaching the subarachnoid space, remove the stylet and collect 1–2 ml of fluid into each of 3 leakproof tubes	Sterile screw-cap tubes Minimum amount required: bacteria, ≥1 ml; AFB, ≥5 ml	Bacteria: never refrigerate; ≤15 min, RT	Obtain blood for culture also. If only 1 tube of CSF is collected, it should be submitted to microbiology first; otherwise submit tube 2 to microbiology. Aspirate of brain abscess or a biopsy specimen may be necessary to detect anaerobic bacteria or parasites.

Decubitus ulcer	A swab is not the specimen of choice 1. Cleanse surface with sterile saline 2. If a sample biopsy is not available, aspirate inflammatory material from the base of the ulcer	Sterile tube (aerobic) or anaerobic system (for tissue)	≤2 h, RT	Since a swab specimen of a decubitus ulcer provides no clinical information, it should not be submitted. A tissue biopsy sample or needle aspirate is the specimen of choice.
Dental culture: gingival, periodontal, periapical, Vincent's stomatitis	1. Carefully cleanse gingival margin and supragingival tooth surface to remove saliva, debris, and plaque 2. Using a periodontal scaler, carefully remove subgingival lesion material and transfer it to an anaerobic transport system 3. Prepare smear for staining with specimen collected in the same fashion	Anaerobic transport system	≤2 h, RT	Periodontal lesions should be processed only by laboratories equipped to provide specialized techniques for the detection and enumeration of recognized pathogens.

(continued)

Collection and Transport

Collection and Transport

Table 3.1 Bacteriology: collection and transport guidelines ^{a,b} (continued)

Specimen type	Collection guidelines	Transport device and/or minimum vol	Transport time and temp	Comments
Ear				
Inner	Tympanocentesis reserved for complicated, recurrent, or chronic persistent otitis media 1. For intact eardrum, clean ear canal with soap solution and collect fluid via syringe aspiration technique (tympanocentesis) 2. For ruptured eardrum, collect fluid on flexible shaft swab via an auditory speculum	Sterile tube, swab transport medium, or anaerobic system	≤2 h, RT	Results of throat or nasopharyngeal swab cultures are not predictive of agents responsible for otitis media and should not be submitted for that purpose.
Outer	1. Use moistened swab to remove any debris or crust from the ear canal 2. Obtain a sample by firmly rotating the swab in the outer canal	Swab transport	≤2 h, RT	For otitis externa, *vigorous* swabbing is required since surface swabbing may miss streptococcal cellulitis.

Eye			
Conjunctiva	1. Sample each eye with separate swabs (premoistened with sterile saline) by rolling over each conjunctiva 2. Medium may be inoculated at time of collection 3. Smear may be prepared at time of collection; roll swab over 1–2-cm area of slide	Direct culture inoculation: BAP and CHOC; laboratory inoculation: swab transport	Plates: ≤15 min, RT; swabs: ≤2 h, RT	If possible, sample both conjunctiva, even if only one is infected, to determine the indigenous microflora. The uninfected eye can serve as a control with which to compare the agents isolated from the infected eye. If cost prohibits this approach, rely on the Gram stain to assist in interpretation of culture.
Corneal scrapings	1. Specimen collected by ophthalmologist 2. Using sterile spatula, scrape ulcers or lesions, and inoculate scraping directly onto medium 3. Prepare 2 smears by rubbing material from spatula onto 1–2-cm area of slide	Direct culture inoculations: BHI with 10% sheep blood, CHOC, and inhibitory mould agar	≤15 min, RT	If conjunctival specimen is collected, do so before anesthetic application, which may inhibit some bacteria. Corneal scrapings are obtained after anesthesia. Include fungal media.

(continued)

Collection and Transport

Collection and Transport

Table 3.1 Bacteriology: collection and transport guidelines[a,b] *(continued)*

Specimen type	Collection guidelines	Transport device and/or minimum vol	Transport time and temp	Comments
Vitreous fluid aspirates	Prepare eye for needle aspiration of fluid	Sterile screw-cap tube or direct inoculation of small amount of fluid onto media	≤15 min, RT	Include fungal media. Anesthetics may be inhibitory to some etiologic agents.
Feces				
Routine culture	Pass specimen directly into a clean, dry container; transport to microbiology laboratory within 1 h of collection or transfer to Cary-Blair holding medium	Clean, leak-proof, wide-mouth container or use Cary-Blair holding medium (>2 g)	Unpreserved: ≤1 h, RT Holding medium: ≤24 h, RT	Do not perform routine stool cultures for patients whose length of hospital stay is >3 days and the admitting diagnosis was not gastroenteritis, without consultation with physician. Tests for *Clostridium difficile* should be considered for these patients. Swabs for routine pathogens are not recommended except for infants (see Rectal swabs).
C. difficile culture	Pass liquid or soft stool directly into a clean, dry container; soft stool is defined as stool assuming the shape of its container	Sterile, leak-proof, wide-mouth container, >5 ml	≤1 h, RT; 1–24 h, 4°C; ≤24 h, −20°C or colder	Patients should be passing ≥5 liquid or soft stools per 24-h period. Testing of formed or hard stool is not recommended. Freezing at −20°C results in rapid loss of cytotoxin activity.

E. coli O157:H7 and other Shiga-toxin-producing serotypes	Pass liquid or bloody stool into a clean, dry container	Sterile, leak-proof, wide-mouth container, or Cary-Blair holding medium (>2 g)	Unpreserved: ≤1 h, RT Swab transport system: ≤24 h, RT or 4 °C	Bloody or liquid stools collected within 6 days of onset among patients with abdominal cramps have the highest yield. Shiga toxin assay for all EHEC serotypes is better than sorbitol MacConkey culture for O157:H7 only.
Leukocyte detection (not recommended for use with patients who have acute infectious diarrhea)	Pass feces directly into a clean, dry container; transport to microbiology laboratory within 1 h of collection, or transfer to ova and parasite transport system (10% formalin or PVA)	Sterile, leak-proof, wide-mouth container or 10% formalin and/or PVA; >2 ml	Unpreserved: ≤1 h, RT Formalin/PVA: indefinite, RT	This procedure should be discouraged because it provides results of little clinical value. A Gram stain or simple methylene blue stain may be used to visualize leukocytes. Commercial detection methods are also available.
Rectal swab	1. Carefully insert a swab ca. 1 in. beyond the anal sphincter 2. Gently rotate the swab to sample the anal crypts 3. Feces should be visible on the swab for detection of diarrheal pathogens	Swab transport	≤2 h, RT	Reserved for detecting *Neisseria gonorrhoeae*, *Shigella*, *Campylobacter*, and herpes simplex virus and anal carriage of group B *Streptococcus* and other beta-hemolytic streptococci, or for patients unable to pass a specimen.

(continued)

Collection and Transport

Collection and Transport

Table 3.1 Bacteriology: collection and transport guidelines [a,b] (continued)

Specimen type	Collection guidelines	Transport device and/or minimum vol	Transport time and temp	Comments
Fistula	See Abscess			
Fluids: abdominal, amniotic, ascites, bile, joint, paracentesis, pericardial, peritoneal, pleural, synovial, thoracentesis	1. Disinfect overlying skin with iodine preparation 2. Obtain specimen via percutaneous needle aspiration or surgery 3. Always submit as much fluid as possible; *never* submit a swab dipped in fluid	Anaerobic transport system, sterile screw-cap tube, or blood culture bottle for bacteria; transport immediately to laboratory Bacteria, >1 ml	≤15 min, RT	Amniotic and culdocentesis fluids should be transported in an anaerobic system and need not be centrifuged prior to Gram staining. Other fluids are best examined by Gram staining of a cytocentrifuged preparation.
Gangrenous tissue	See Abscess			Discourage sampling of surface or superficial tissue. Tissue biopsy or aspiration should be performed.
Gastric Wash or lavage for mycobacteria	Collect in early morning before patients eat and while they are still in bed. 1. Introduce a nasogastric tube into the stomach 2. Perform lavage with 25–50 ml of chilled, sterile distilled water	Sterile, leak-proof container	≤15 min, RT, or neutralize within 1 h of collection	The specimen must be processed promptly because mycobacteria die rapidly in gastric washings. Neutralize with sodium bicarbonate when holding for >1 h.

	3. Recover sample and place in a leak-proof, sterile container		
Biopsy for *H. pylori*	Collected by gastroenterologist during endoscopy	<1 h, RT	Culture may be needed for antimicrobial testing.
Genital, female			
Amniotic fluid	Aspirate via amniocentesis, or collect during cesarean delivery	≤2 h, RT	Swabbing or aspiration of vaginal secretions is *not* acceptable because of the potential for contamination with the commensal vaginal flora.
Bartholin gland secretions	Anaerobic transport system, ≥1 ml	≤2 h, RT	
	1. Disinfect skin with iodine preparation		
	2. Aspirate fluid from ducts		
Cervical secretions	Swab transport	≤2 h, RT	See the text for collection and transport need for *Chlamydia trachomatis* and *Neisseria gonorrhoeae*.
	1. Visualize the cervix using a speculum without lubricant		
	2. Remove mucus and secretions from the cervical os with swab, and discard the swab		
	3. Firmly yet gently sample the endocervical canal with a new sterile swab		
Cul-de-sac fluid	Anaerobic transport system, >1 ml	≤2 h, RT	
	Submit aspirate or fluid		

(continued)

Collection and Transport

Collection and Transport

Table 3.1 Bacteriology: collection and transport guidelines[a,b] *(continued)*

Specimen type	Collection guidelines	Transport device and/or minimum vol	Transport time and temp	Comments
Endometrial tissue and secretions	1. Collect transcervical aspirate via a telescoping catheter 2. Transfer entire amount to anaerobic transport system	Anaerobic transport system, ≥ 1 ml	≤ 2 h, RT	
Products of conception	1. Submit a portion of tissue in a sterile container 2. If obtained by cesarean delivery, immediately transfer to an anaerobic transport system	Sterile tube or anaerobic transport system	≤ 2 h, RT	Do not process lochia, culture of which may give misleading results.
Urethral secretions	Collect at least 1 h after patient has urinated 1. Remove old exudate from the urethral orifice 2. Collect discharge material on a swab by massaging the urethra; for females, massage the urethra against the pubic symphysis through the vagina	Swab transport	≤ 2 h, RT	If no discharge can be obtained, wash the periurethral area with Betadine soap and rinse with water. Insert a small swab 2–4 cm into the urethra, rotate it, and leave it in place for at least 2 s to facilitate absorption.

Vaginal secretions	1. Wipe away old secretions and discharge 2. Obtain secretions from the mucosal membrane of the vaginal wall with a sterile swab or pipette 3. If a smear is also needed, use a second swab	Swab transport	≤2 h, RT	For intrauterine devices, place entire device into a sterile container and submit at RT. Gram stain, not culture, is recommended for the diagnosis of bacterial vaginosis.
Genital, female or male lesion	1. Clean with sterile saline, and remove lesion's surface with a sterile scalpel blade 2. Allow transudate to accumulate 3. While pressing the base of the lesion, *firmly* rub base with a sterile swab to collect fluid	Swab transport	≤2 h, RT	For dark-field examination to detect *T. pallidum*, touch a glass slide to the transudate, add cover-slip, and transport immediately to the laboratory in a humidified chamber (petri dish with moist gauze). *T. pallidum* cannot be cultured on artificial media.
Genital, male Prostate	1. Cleanse urethral meatus with soap and water 2. Massage prostate through rectum 3. Collect fluid expressed from urethra on a sterile swab	Swab transport or sterile tube for >1 ml of specimen	≤2 h, RT	Pathogens in prostatic secretions may be identified by quantitative culture of urine before and after massage. Ejaculate may also be cultured.

(continued)

Collection and Transport

Collection and Transport

Table 3.1 Bacteriology: collection and transport guidelines[a,b] *(continued)*

Specimen type	Collection guidelines	Transport device and/or minimum vol	Transport time and temp	Comments
Urethra	Insert a small swab 2–4 cm into the urethral lumen, rotate swab, and leave it in place for at least 2 s to facilitate absorption	Swab transport	≤2 h, RT	
Pilonidal cyst	See Abscess			
Respiratory, lower				
Bronchoalveolar lavage, brush or wash, endotracheal aspirate	1. Collect washing or aspirate in a sputum trap 2. Place brush in sterile container with 1 ml of saline	Sterile container, >1 ml	≤2 h, RT	A total of 40–80 ml of fluid is needed for quantitative analysis of BAL fluid. For quantitative analysis of brushings, place brush into 1.0 ml of saline.
Sputum, expectorated	1. Collect specimen under the direct supervision of a nurse or physician 2. Have patient rinse or gargle with water to remove excess oral flora 3. Instruct patient to cough deeply to produce a lower	Sterile container, >1 ml Minimum amount: bacteria, >1 ml	≤2 h, RT	For pediatric patients unable to produce a sputum specimen, a respiratory therapist should collect a specimen via suction. The best specimen should have ≤10 squamous cells/100× field (10× objective and 10× ocular). Mycobacteria: submit an early

			morning specimen on 3 consecutive days.
Sputum, induced	1. Have patient rinse mouth with water after brushing gums and tongue 2. With the aid of a nebulizer, have patients inhale approximately 25 ml of 3–10% sterile saline 3. Collect in a sterile container	Sterile container, >1 ml	≤2 h, RT	Same as above for sputum, expectorated.
Respiratory, upper Oral	1. Remove oral secretions and debris from the surface of the lesion with a swab; discard this swab 2. Using a second swab, vigorously sample the lesion, avoiding any areas of normal tissue	Swab transport or sterile container	≤2 h, RT	Discourage sampling of superficial tissue for bacterial evaluation. Tissue biopsy specimens or needle aspirates are the specimens of choice.

(continued)

Collection and Transport

Collection and Transport

Table 3.1 Bacteriology: collection and transport guidelines[a,b] *(continued)*

Specimen type	Collection guidelines	Transport device and/or minimum vol	Transport time and temp	Comments
Nasal	1. Insert a swab, premoistened with sterile saline, approximately 1–2 cm into the nares 2. Rotate the swab against the nasal mucosa	Swab transport	≤2 h, RT	Anterior nose cultures are reserved for detecting staphylococcal carriers or for nasal lesions.
Nasopharynx	1. Gently insert a small swab (e.g., calcium alginate) into the posterior nasopharynx via the nose 2. Rotate swab slowly for 5 s to absorb secretions	Direct medium inoculation at bedside or examination table, swab transport	Plates: ≤15 min, RT; swabs: ≤2 h, RT	
Throat or pharynx	1. Depress tongue with a tongue depressor 2. Sample the posterior pharynx, tonsils, and inflamed areas with a sterile swab	Swab transport	≤2 h, RT	Throat swab cultures are contra-indicated in patients with epiglottitis. Swabs for *Neisseria gonorrhoeae* should be placed in charcoal-containing transport medium and plated ≤12 h after collection. JEMBEC, Biobags, and the GonoPak are better for transport at RT.

Tissue	Collected during surgery or cutaneous biopsy procedure	Anaerobic transport system or sterile, screw-cap container; add several drops of sterile saline to keep small pieces of tissue moist	≤15 min, RT	Always submit as much tissue as possible. If excess tissue is available, save a portion of surgical tissue at −70°C in case further studies are needed. Never submit a swab that has been rubbed over the surface of a tissue. For quantitative study, a sample of 1 cm³ is appropriate.
Urine				
Female, midstream	1. While holding the labia apart, begin voiding 2. After several milliliters has passed, collect a midstream portion without stopping the flow of urine 3. The midstream portion is used for bacterial culture	Sterile, wide-mouth container, ≥1 ml, or urine transport tube with boric acid preservative	Unpreserved: ≤2 h, RT; preserved: ≤24 h, RT	Chlamydial antigen detection in urine from women is less sensitive than in urine from men. Urine is toxic to cell lines and is therefore not the specimen of choice for chlamydial culture. Cleansing before voiding does not improve urine specimen quality; i.e., midstream urines are equivalent to clean-catch midstream urines. Mycobacteria: collect 3 consecutive early-morning specimens; minimum, 40 ml; 24-h collections are unacceptable.

(continued)

Collection and Transport

Table 3.1 Bacteriology: collection and transport guidelines[a,b] *(continued)*

Specimen type	Collection guidelines	Transport device and/or minimum vol	Transport time and temp	Comments
Male, midstream	1. While holding the foreskin retracted, begin voiding 2. After several milliliters has passed, collect a midstream portion without stopping the flow of urine 3. The midstream portion is used for culture	Sterile, wide-mouth container, ≥1 ml, or urine transport tube with boric acid preservative	Unpreserved: ≤2 h, RT	First part of urine stream is used for probe tests and antigen test for chlamydia. Collect specimen for probe and antigen tests at least 2 h after last urination. Mycobacteria: see above.
Straight catheter	1. Thoroughly cleanse the urethral opening with soap and water 2. Rinse area with wet gauze pads	Sterile, leak-proof container or urine transport tube with boric acid preservative	Unpreserved: ≤2 h, RT; preserved: ≤24 h, RT	Catheterization may introduce members of the urethral flora into the bladder and increase the risk of iatrogenic infection.

	3. Aseptically, insert catheter into the bladder 4. After allowing approximately 15 ml to pass, collect urine to be submitted in a sterile container		
Indwelling catheter	1. Disinfect the catheter collection port with 70% alcohol 2. Use needle and syringe to aseptically collect 5–10 ml of urine 3. Transfer to a sterile tube or container	Sterile leak-proof container or urine transport tube with boric acid preservative	Unpreserved: ≤2 h, RT; preserved: ≤24 h, RT	Patients with indwelling catheters always have bacteria in their bladders. Do not collect urine from these patients unless they are symptomatic.
Wound	See Abscess		

---

[a]Adapted from P. R. Murray, E. J. Baron, J. H. Jorgensen, M. A. Pfaller, and R. H. Yolken (ed.), *Manual of Clinical Microbiology*, 8th ed., ASM Press, Washington, D.C., 2003.

[b]Abbreviations: AFB, acid-fast bacilli; BAL, bronchoalveolar lavage; BAP, blood agar plate; BHI, brain heart infusion; CHOC, chocolate agar; CSF, cerebrospinal fluid; CVP, central venous pressure; i.v., intravenous; PVA, polyvinyl alcohol fixative; RT, room temperature.

Collection and Transport

Collection and Transport

Table 3.2 Specimen collection and transport guidelines for infrequently encountered bacteria[a]

Organism (disease)	Specimen of choice	Transport issues
Anaplasma (human granulocytic ehrlichiosis)	Blood smear, skin biopsy, blood (with heparin or EDTA anticoagulant), CSF,[b] serum	Material for culture sent on ice; keep tissue moist and sterile; hold at 4–20°C until tested or at −70°C for shipment; transport on ice or frozen for PCR test
Bartonella (cat scratch fever)	Blood, tissue, lymph node aspirate	1 wk at 4°C; indefinitely at −70°C
Borrelia burgdorferi (Lyme disease)	Skin biopsy at lesion periphery, blood, CSF	Keep tissue moist and sterile; hand carry to laboratory if possible
Borrelia (relapsing fever)	Blood smear (blood)	Hand carry to laboratory if possible
Brucella (brucellosis)	Blood, bone marrow	Transport at room temperature; pediatric lysis-centrifugation tube is helpful
Klebsiella granulomatis (granuloma inguinale; donovanosis)	Tissue, subsurface scrapings	Transport at room temperature

Organism	Specimen	Transport/Storage
Coxiella (Q fever), *Rickettsia* (spotted fevers; typhus)	Serum, blood, tissue	Blood and tissue are frozen at −70°C until shipped
Ehrlichia (ehrlichiosis)	Blood smear, skin biopsy, blood (with heparin or EDTA anticoagulant), CSF, serum	Material for culture sent on ice; keep tissue moist and sterile; hold at 4–20°C until tested or at −70°C for shipment; transport on ice or frozen for PCR test
Francisella (tularemia)	Lymph node aspirate, scrapings, lesion biopsy, blood, sputum	Rapid transport to laboratory or freeze; ship on dry ice
Leptospira (leptospirosis)	Serum, blood (citrate-containing anticoagulants should not be used), urine (after 1st wk)	Blood,<1 h; urine,<1 h or dilute 1:10 in 1% bovine serum albumin and store at 4–20°C or neutralize with sodium bicarbonate
Streptobacillus (rat bite fever; Haverhill fever)	Blood, aspirates of joint fluid	High-volume bottle preferred

*a*Adapted from P. R. Murray, E. J. Baron, J. H. Jorgensen, M. A. Pfaller, and R. H. Yolken (ed.), *Manual of Clinical Microbiology*, 8th ed., ASM Press, Washington, D.C., 2003.
*b*CSF, cerebrospinal fluid.

Collection and Transport

Table 3.3 Guidelines for collection of specimens for anaerobic culture[a]

Acceptable material (method of collection)	Unacceptable material (method of collection)
Aspirate (by needle and syringe)	Bronchoalveolar lavage washing
Bartholin's gland inflammation or secretions	Cervical secretions
Blood (venipuncture)	Endotracheal secretions (aspirate)
Bone marrow (aspirate)	Lochia secretions
Bronchoscopic secretions (protected specimen brush)	Nasopharyngeal swab
Culdocentesis fluid (aspirate)	Perineal swab
Fallopian tube fluid or tissue (aspirate/biopsy)	Prostatic or seminal fluid
Intrauterine device, for *Actinomyces* spp.	Sputum (expectorated or induced)
Nasal sinus (aspirate)	Stool or rectal swab samples
Placenta tissue (via cesarean delivery)	Tracheostomy secretions
Stool, for *Clostridium difficile*	Urethral secretions
Surgery (aspirate, tissue)	Urine (voided or from catheter)
Transtracheal aspirate	Vaginal or vulvar secretions (swab)
Urine (suprapubic aspirate)	

[a]Adapted from P. R. Murray, E. J. Baron, J. H. Jorgensen, M. A. Pfaller, and R. H. Yolken (ed.), *Manual of Clinical Microbiology*, 8th ed., ASM Press, Washington, D.C., 2003.

Collection and Transport

Virology: General Specimen Guidelines

1. The timing of specimen collection is critical because the duration of viral shedding is influenced by the type of virus, the organ or tissue involved, and the immunocompetence of the patient. For optimal recovery of most viruses, specimens should be collected within 3 to 7 days after onset of symptoms.

2. The method of collection can have a profound effect on detection of viruses. If viral culture is attempted, the viability of the virus must be maintained in appropriate transport medium. If nucleic acid amplification is attempted, the swab composition and anticoagulants can affect the assay.

3. If only a limited amount of material can be collected, the number of tests requested should also be limited.

4. Because viruses are obligate intracellular parasites, wound and skin specimens (e.g., vesicles) should contain cellular material.

5. Specimens should be transported to the laboratory as quickly as possible, particularly for specimens submitted for viral culture. Viability is not required for antigen or nucleic acid amplification tests.

6. Viral transport medium (VTM) should be used to protect specimens from drying. VTM is not required for cerebrospinal fluids, blood, urine, bronchoalveolar lavage specimens, amniotic fluid, and feces.

7. Specimens other than blood should be maintained at 4°C if held for more than 1 h after collection. Freezing should be avoided unless a delay of more than 24 h is anticipated. Recovery of some enveloped viruses (e.g., respiratory syncytial virus, herpes simplex virus, cytomegalovirus, and varicella-zoster virus) is compromised by freezing.

8. A variety of commercial VTM are available. Most contain protein to stabilize the virus, antibiotics to prevent bacterial and fungal growth, and a buffer to control pH. Culturette swabs with Stuart's medium can also be used.

Virology: Specific Specimen Guidelines

Blood

1. An 8–10-ml volume of blood is collected using appropriate aseptic techniques.

2. Anticoagulant tubes (EDTA [purple top], heparin [green top], and acid-citrate-dextrose [yellow top]) are used for detection of viruses in plasma or leukocytes. Heparin inhibits PCR and the infectivity of some viruses.

3. Plasma can be obtained by centrifuging blood collected in tubes with anticoagulants. Plasma partitioning tubes can facilitate separation of plasma from cellular material.

4. Plasma for nucleic acid amplification of RNA viruses should be separated within 4 to 6 h of collection and refrigerated for up to 72 h or frozen at −70°C for longer periods.

5. For serologic testing, acute-phase serum should be collected within the first few days of clinical onset and convalescent-phase serum should be collected 2 to 4 weeks later.

Bone marrow

1. Bone marrow aspirates are collected from the posterior iliac crest, the anterior iliac crest (infants and children), or the sternum or the tibia (infants younger than 18 months).

2. Leukocytes from bone marrow specimens can be cultured for cytomegalovirus (CMV). Varicella-zoster virus (VZV) and human herpesvirus 6 can also be cultured from bone marrow. PCR is used to diagnose parvovirus B19 infections.

CSF

1. Enteroviruses are the most common viruses grown from cerebrospinal fluid (CSF). Herpes simplex virus (HSV) and arboviruses are important causes of sporadic encephalitis but are difficult to culture. These infections are most commonly diagnosed by nucleic acid-based tests. Likewise, CMV, VZV, Epstein-Barr virus (EBV), and JC virus infections are most commonly diagnosed by nucleic acid-based tests.

2. Viral titers are generally low in CSF; therefore, the specimen should not be diluted and tests should be selectively performed.

3. CSF should be collected in a sterile tube without transport medium.

4. CSF for viral culture does not require special processing.

5. CSF for nucleic acid amplification should be processed to remove inhibitors of thermostable polymerases used in PCR.

Respiratory specimens (throat, nasopharyngeal swab, nasopharyngeal aspirate, nasal washings, and bronchoalveolar lavage [BAL] specimens)

1. Influenza viruses, parainfluenza viruses, RSV, adenoviruses, and rhinoviruses are most frequently identified in respiratory specimens. Metapneumoviruses and coronaviruses are also important respiratory pathogens.

2. Nasopharyngeal aspirates are preferred to nasopharyngeal swabs because swabs generally do not collect enough cells.

3. Nasal washes also do not contain a large number of virus-infected cells; however, they are often used when nasal aspiration is contraindicated.

4. Nasopharyngeal aspirates are typically transported in appropriate viral transport medium (VTM). The use of VTM is optional for nasal washes and BAL specimens.

5. All specimens can be used for viral culture. However, nasopharyngeal aspirates and washes are preferred for antigen detection.

6. Mucus in specimens can affect antigen detection by fluorescent-antibody (FA) assay and enzyme immunoassays (EIA). Mucus can inhibit the fixation of cells to slides (FA assay) and can cause nonspecific fluorescence. It can also interfere with penetration of the specimen into EIA membrane devices. Therefore, specimens should be broken up by glass beads or aspiration through a small-bore pipette before processing.

Urine

1. Urine is an important specimen for detection of CMV, enteroviruses, adenoviruses, and BK virus. These days, mumps and rubella viruses are rarely isolated in urine because of the use of vaccines.

2. Urine should be cultured for CMV within 7 days of birth to detect congenital infection.

3. Midstream urine should be collected in a sterile container. VTM is not required.

4. Before urine is cultured, it should be neutralized with 7.5% sodium bicarbonate solution and filtered through a 0.2-μm-pore-size filter to remove contaminating bacteria.

Feces

1. Many viruses responsible for gastroenteritis (e.g., enteric adenovirus, calicivirus, astrovirus, and rotavirus) cannot be cultivated.

2. Enveloped viruses are not normally recovered in feces with the exception of CMV in immunocompromised patients.

3. Fecal specimens (2 to 4 g) are preferred to fecal swabs because an inadequate amount of material is collected on swabs.

Eyes

1. HSV and adenovirus are the most commonly isolated viruses; enterovirus 70 and coxsackievirus A24 may be detected by PCR.

2. Conjunctival swabs are collected from the lower conjunctiva with a flexible, fine-shaft swab moistened with sterile saline and placed in VTM.

3. Scrapings of cornea or conjunctiva should also be placed in VTM.

4. Aqueous and vitreous fluids can inhibit PCR; therefore, the specimen must be diluted or extracted to remove inhibitors.

Tissue

1. Many viruses can be isolated from tissues.

2. Tissues should be transported in VTM.

3. As much tissue as possible should be collected and submitted to the Clinical Microbiology and Surgical Pathology laboratories.

4. Upon receipt in the laboratory, tissues should be ground and centrifuged and the supernatant should be used for processing.

5. Tissue for nucleic acid detection should be minced, treated with proteolytic enzymes, and extracted with chaotropic salts or organic solvents.

Genital specimens

1. HSV-2 and HSV-1 are the most commonly isolated viruses from external genital lesions. HSV-1, HSV-2, and CMV are frequently isolated from the cervix, vagina, and urethra. These viruses can be readily cultured from these sites. Human papillomavirus, an important cause of cervical cancer, can be detected by molecular tests.

2. Genital lesions should be swabbed vigorously to collect cellular material, and the specimen should be transported to the laboratory in VTM.

3. Cervical specimens are collected by inserting a clean swab 1 cm into the cervical canal and rotating it for 5 s. The swab is transported in VTM.

4. To collect urethral specimens, exudates should be expressed and discarded. The patient should not have urinated for at least 1 h prior to specimen collection. A flexible, fine-shafted swab is inserted 4 cm into the urethra, rotated two or three times, removed, and placed in VTM.

Skin

1. Rubella virus, measles virus, adenoviruses, and enteroviruses can cause dermal rashes and be isolated in culture. Parvovirus B19 can cause a rash but is recovered from other sources. HSV, VZV, and enteroviruses can be recovered from vesicular lesions.

2. Fresh dermal lesions (not crusted, healing lesions) should be used for recovery of viruses.

3. Vesicular fluid and cells from the base of the lesion should be collected and transported to the laboratory in VTM.

Table 3.4 Mycology: collection and transport guidelines [a,b]

Specimen type	Collection guidelines	Transport device and/or minimum vol	Time and temp for transport	Comments
Blood Yeasts	Collect as for bacterial cultures; disinfect skin with tincture of iodine; use maximum amount of blood recommended	Automated (BacT/Alert, BACTEC, ESP)	≤2 h, RT	
		Lysis-centrifugation	As above; process in ≤ 16 h	
		Biphasic bottles	≤2 h, RT	
Dimorphic/filamentous fungi	As above	Lysis-centrifugation	As above	
Bone marrow	Prepare site for surgical incision	Lysis-centrifugation	As above	
CSF	Collect as for bacterial culture	Screw-cap tube, ≥2 ml, concentrate	≤15 min, RT or 30°C	Never refrigerate; aspirate or biopsy specimen of brain abscess may be necessary
Ear, external	Firmly rotate swab in outer ear canal	Swab	≤2 h, RT	

(continued)

Collection and Transport

Collection and Transport

Table 3.4 Mycology: collection and transport guidelines [a,b] *(continued)*

Specimen type	Collection guidelines	Transport device and/or minimum vol	Time and temp for transport	Comments
Eye				
Corneal scrapings	Inoculate scrapings directly onto media and slides for staining	Direct inoculation	≤15 min, RT	Inoculate plates in "C" shape
Vitreous fluid	Needle aspiration	Screw-cap tube or direct inoculation	≤15 min, RT	
Hair	With forceps collect 10–12 hairs with shaft intact	Dry container, envelope, Dermapak	≤72 h, RT	Also scrape active borders of lesions if present
Nails	Disinfect with 70% alcohol; clip affected areas; collect debris under nail	Dry container, envelope, Dermapak	≤72 h, RT	For *Candida*, dermatophytes, and agents of dermatomycoses
Prostatic fluid	Bladder emptied followed by prostatic massage	Direct inoculation onto media	≤15 min, RT	Primarily for blastomycosis: occasionally cryptococcosis
Respiratory, lower (BAL, brush, wash, aspirate)	Collect as for bacterial culture	Sterile container, >1 ml	≤2 h, RT	Short survival time for dimorphic pathogens

Respiratory, upper			
Oral	Swab active lesions; saline swish for *Candida*	≤2 h, RT	Selective media useful for yeasts
Nasal sinus	Surgical removal of sinus contents	≤15 min, RT	Maxillary and ethmoid sinuses most common sites
Skin	Disinfect with 70% alcohol; scrape surface of skin at margin of lesion	≤72 h, RT	For dermatophytes and agents of dermatomycoses
Sputum	As for bacterial cultures	≤2 h, RT	Short survival time for thermally dimorphic pathogens
Sterile fluids (pericardial, peritoneal, pleural, synovial)	Collect as for bacterial cultures; concentrate by centrifugation; use sediment for inoculation	≤15 min, RT	May also concentrate small volumes by syringe filtration (0.2 μm)
Subcutaneous granules	Collect from pus, exudate, biopsy, and draining sinus tracts	≤2 h, RT	Fungal grains or granules seen in eumycotic mycetoma
Subcutaneous sites			
Abscess	Aspirate abscess with sterile needle and syringe	≤2 h, RT	Sample base of lesion and abscess wall

Sterile container with >10 ml; may use blood culture bottle for yeasts

Sterile container, 3–5 ml

Clean container or between taped glass slides; Dermapak

Direct inoculation or in sterile moist gauze

Swab or sterile container

Wash granules several times in saline containing antibiotics

Anaerobic transport or direct inoculation; ≥1 ml

Collection and Transport

(continued)

Collection and Transport

Table 3.4 Mycology: collection and transport guidelines [a,b] (continued)

Specimen type	Collection guidelines	Transport device and/or minimum vol	Time and temp for transport	Comments
Open wound	Aspirate or swab deeply	Swab transport system	≤2 h, RT	As above
Tissue biopsy specimen	Surgical collection	Sterile container; add a few drops of sterile saline to keep moist	≤15 min, RT	Punch biopsies may be used for skin lesions
Urine	As for bacterial cultures; early-morning specimen preferred	Sterile wide-mouth container, ≥1 ml	≤2 h, RT	Use midstream collection technique
Vagina	As for bacterial cultures	Swab transport	≤2 h, RT	Primarily for refractory vaginal candidiasis

[a]Adapted from P. R. Murray, E. J. Baron, J. H. Jorgensen, M. A. Pfaller, and R. H. Yolken (ed.), *Manual of Clinical Microbiology*, 8th ed., ASM Press, Washington, D.C., 2003.
[b]Abbreviations: BAL, bronchoalveolar lavage; CSF, cerebrospinal fluid; RT, room temperature.

Table 3.5 Parasitology: specimen guidelines[a]

Body site	Specimen and procedures[b]	Recommended stain(s) and relevant parasites[b]
Blood	Whole or anticoagulated blood. Fresh blood preferred but may not be practical for many laboratories. If anticoagulant is used, EDTA is preferred (purple top).	Giemsa (all blood parasites); hematoxylin-based stain (sheathed microfilariae).
Bone marrow	Aspirate, sterile, collected in EDTA for culture or PCR.	Giemsa (all blood parasites). Sterile specimen required for cultures.
Central nervous system	Spinal fluid, sterile, collected in EDTA for culture or PCR; brain biopsy specimen.	Giemsa (trypanosomes, *Toxoplasma gondii*); Giemsa, trichrome, or Calcofluor (amebae [*Naegleria*—PAM, *Acanthamoeba*, *Balamuthia*—GAE]); Giemsa, acid-fast, PAS, modified trichrome, silver methenamine (microsporidia) (tissue Gram stains also recommended for microsporidia in routine histologic preparations); H&E, PAS, routine histology (larval cestodes: *Taenia solium* cysticerci, *Echinococcus* spp.).
Cutaneous ulcers	Aspirate from below surface, sterile plus air-dried smears; punch biopsy, sterile for culture and nonsterile for histopathology.	Giemsa (leishmaniae); H&E, routine histology (*Acanthamoeba* spp., *Entamoeba histolytica*).
Eye	Biopsy, corneal scrapings, contact lens and lens solution; sterile or nonsterile for histopathology; unopened commercial solutions not acceptable.	Calcofluor for cysts only (amebae [*Acanthamoeba*]); Giemsa for trophozoites and cysts (amebae); H&E for routine histology (cysticerci, *Loa loa*, *Toxoplasma gondii*); silver methamine stain, PAS, acid-fast, EM (for microsporidia).
Intestinal tract	Stool, fresh or preserved; sigmoidoscopy material, duodenal contents.	Trichrome or iron hematoxylin (intestinal protozoa); modified trichrome

(continued)

Collection and Transport

Table 3.5 Parasitology: specimen guidelines[a] *(continued)*

Body site	Specimen and procedures[b]	Recommended stain(s) and relevant parasites[b]
		(microsporidia); modified acid-fast (*Cryptosporidium* spp., *Cyclospora cayetanensis*, *Isospora belli*); immunoassays, e.g., EIA, FA, cartridge formats (*Entamoeba histolytica*, the *Entamoeba histolytica*/*E. dispar* group, *Giardia lamblia*, *Cryptosporidium parvum*, microsporidia [experimental]). Routine histology and/or wet squash preparations could reveal eggs of *Schistosoma* spp.
	Anal impression smear	No stain; cellulose tape, anal swab, or other collection device. Four to six consecutive negative tapes required to rule out infection with pinworm (*Enterobius vermicularis*).
	Adult worm or worm segments	Proglottids can usually be identified to the species level without using tissue stains.
	Biopsy	H&E, routine histology (*Entamoeba histolytica*, *Cryptosporidium* spp., *Cyclospora cayetanensis*, *Isospora belli*, *Giardia lamblia*, microsporidia); less common findings would include *Schistosoma* spp., hookworm, or *Trichuris trichiura*.
Liver and spleen	Aspirates, sterile collected in four aliquots (liver); biopsy, sterile for culture and nonsterile for squash preparation, FA, PCR, and histopathology.	Giemsa (leishmaniae); H&E (routine histology).
Lungs	Sputum, induced sputum, bronchoalveolar lavage fluid, transbronchial aspirate, tracheobronchial aspirate,	Modified acid-fast stains (*Cryptosporidium* spp.); H&E, routine histology (*Strongyloides stercoralis*,

(continued)

Table 3.5 Parasitology: specimen guidelines[a] *(continued)*

Body site	Specimen and procedures[b]	Recommended stain(s) and relevant parasites[b]
	brush biopsy, open-lung biopsy; sterile for bronchoalveolar lavage fluid and air-dried smears.	*Paragonimus* spp., *Dirofilaria* spp., amebae); silver methenamine stain, PAS, acid-fast, tissue Gram stains, modified trichrome, EM (microsporidia); Giemsa, silver methenamine, toluidine blue stains available for *Pneumocystis jiroveci*.
		Some helminth larvae (*Ascaris lumbricoides*, *Strongyloides stercoralis*), eggs (*Paragonimus* spp.), or hooklets (*Echinococcus* spp.) can be recovered in sputum.
Muscle	Biopsy	H&E, routine histology (*Trichinella* spp., cysticerci); silver methenamine stain, PAS, acid-fast, tissue Gram stains, EM (microsporidia).
Skin	Aspirates, skin snip, scrapings, biopsy; aseptic, no preservatives; biopsy, sterile or non-sterile to histopathology.	See Cutaneous ulcer (above). H&E, routine histology (*Onchocerca volvulus*, *Dipetalonema streptocerca*, *Dirofilaria repens*, leishmaniae, *Acanthamoeba* spp., *Entamoeba histolytica*, microsporidia).
Urogenital system	Vaginal discharge, saline swab, transport swab (no charcoal), culture medium, plastic envelope culture, air-dried smear for FA; urethral discharge, prostatic secretions; urine, single unpreserved specimen, 24-h unpreserved specimen, early-morning specimen.	Giemsa, immunoassay reagents (FA) (*Trichomonas vaginalis*); Delafield's hematoxylin (microfilariae); modified trichrome (microsporidia); H&E, routine histology (*Schistosoma haematobium*, microfilariae); PAS, acid-fast, tissue Gram stains, EM or PCR (microsporidia).

[a] Adapted from P. R. Murray, E. J. Baron, J. H. Jorgensen, M. A. Pfaller, and R. H. Yolken (ed.), *Manual of Clinical Microbiology*, 8th ed., ASM Press, Washington, D.C., 2003.

[b] Abbreviations: CSF, cerebrospinal fluid; EIA, enzyme immunoassay; EM, electron microscopy; FA, fluorescent antibody; GAE, granulomatous amebic encephalitis; GI, gastrointestinal; H&E, hematoxylin and eosin; PAM, primary amebic encephalitis; PAS, periodic acid-Schiff stain.

Collection and Transport

Table 3.6 Guidelines for processing stool specimens for parasites[a,b]

Option	Pros	Cons
Rejection of stools from inpatients who have been in hospital for >3 days.	Patients may become symptomatic with diarrhea after they have been inpatients for a few days; symptoms are usually attributed not to parasitic infections but generally to other causes.	There is always the chance that the problem is related to a nosocomial parasitic infection (rare), but *Cryptosporidium* and microsporidia are possible considerations.
Examination of a single stool (O&P examination). Data suggest that 40–50% of organisms present will be found by only a single stool exam; any patient remaining symptomatic would require additional testing.	Some think that most intestinal parasitic infections can be diagnosed from examination of a single stool specimen. If the patient becomes asymptomatic after collection of the first stool specimen, subsequent specimens may not be necessary.	Diagnosis from a single stool exam depends on the experience of the microscopist, proper collection, and the parasite load in the specimen. In a series of three stool specimens, it is often the case that not all three specimens are positive and/or may be positive for different organisms.
Examination of a second stool specimen only after the first is negative and the patient is still symptomatic.	With additional examinations, the yield of protozoa increases (*Entamoeba histolytica*, 22.7%; *Giardia lamblia*, 11.3%; and *Dientamoeba fragilis*, 31.1%).	Assumes the second (or third) stool specimen is collected within the recommended 10-day time frame for a series of stools; protozoa are shed periodically. May be inconvenient for the patient.
Examination of a single stool and an immunoassay (EIA, FA cartridge) (*Giardia*); this approach is a mix: one immunoassay is acceptable; one O&P exam is not the best approach.	If the exams are negative and the patient's symptoms subside, probably no further testing is required.	Patients may exhibit symptoms (off and on), so it may be difficult to rule out parasitic infections with only a single stool specimen and immunoassay. If the patient remains symptomatic, then even if the *Giardia* immunoassay is negative, other protozoa may be missed (*E. histolytica/E. dispar*, *D. fragilis*).

Pooling of three specimens for examination; one concentrate and one permanent stain are performed.	Three specimens are collected over 7–10 days and may save time and expense.	Organisms present in small numbers may be missed due to the dilution factor.
Pooling of three specimens for examination; a single concentrate and three permanent stained smears are performed.	Three specimens are collected over 7–10 days; this would maximize recovery of protozoa in areas of the country where these organisms are most common.	Light helminth infection (eggs, larvae) might be missed due to the pooling of the three specimens for the concentration; however, with a permanent stain performed on each of the three specimens, this approach would probably be the next best option after the standard approach (concentration and permanent stained smear performed on every stool).
Collection of three stools; samples of stool from all three collections are placed in a single vial (patient is given a single vial only).	Pooling of the specimens would require only a single vial.	This would complicate patient collection and very probably result in poorly preserved specimens, especially regarding the recommended ratio of stool to preservative and the lack of proper mixing of specimen and fixative.
Perform immunoassays on selected patients by methods for *Giardia lamblia*, *Cryptosporidium parvum*, and/or the *Entamoeba histolytica/E. dispar* group or *Entamoeba histolytica*.	Would be more cost-effective than performing immunoassay procedures on all specimens; however, information required to group patients is often not received with specimens. Client education required for appropriate test orders.	Labs rarely receive information that would allow them to place a patient in a particular risk group such as children <5 yr old, children from day care centers (who may or may not be symptomatic), patients with immunodeficiencies, and patients from outbreaks. Performance of immunoassay procedures on every stool specimen is not cost-effective, and the positive

(continued)

Collection and Transport

Collection and Transport

Table 3.6 Guidelines for processing stool specimens for parasites[a,b] *(continued)*

Option	Pros	Cons
		rate will be low unless an outbreak situationL is involved.
Perform immunoassays and O&P examinations on request for *Giardia lamblia*, *Cryptosporidium parvum*, and/or *Entamoeba histolytica/E. dispar* group or *Entamoeba histolytica*.	Limits the number of stools on which immunoassay procedures are performed for parasites using this approach. Immunoassay results do not have to be confirmed by any other testing (such as O&P examinations or modified acid-fast stains).	Requires education of the physician clients regarding appropriate times and patients for whom immunoassays should be ordered. If the patient remains symptomatic, further testing (O&P exams) is required. A single O&P exam may not reveal all organisms present.

[a]Adapted from P. R. Murray, E. J. Baron, J. H. Jorgensen, M. A. Pfaller, and R. H. Yolken (ed.), *Manual of Clinical Microbiology*, 8th ed., ASM Press, Washington, D.C., 2003.

[b]Abbreviations: EIA, enzyme immunoassay; FA, fluorescent antibody; O&P, ova and parasite.

Table 3.7 Agents of bioterrorism: specimen guidelines[a]

Disease agent	Type of disease	Specimen selection	Transport time and temp
Anthrax	Cutaneous	Vesicular stage: Collect fluid from intact vesicles on sterile swab(s). The organism is best demonstrated in this stage.	≤2 h, RT
		Eschar stage: Without removing eschar, insert swab beneath the edge of eschar, rotate and collect lesion material.	≤2 h, RT
	Gastrointestinal	Stool: Collect 5–10 g in a clean, sterile, leakproof container.	≤1 h, RT
		Blood: Collect per institution's procedure for routine blood cultures.	≤2 h, RT
	Inhalation	Sputum: Collect expectorated specimen into a sterile, leakproof container.	≤2 h, RT
		Blood: Collect per institution's procedure for routine blood culture.	≤2 h, RT
Brucellosis	Acute, subacute, or chronic	Serum: Collect 10–12 ml of acute-phase specimen as soon as possible after disease onset. Collect a convalescent-phase specimen 21 days later.	~2 h, RT
		Blood: Collect per institution's procedure for routine blood culture.	≤2 h, RT
		Bone marrow, spleen, or liver: Collect per institution's surgical or pathology procedure.	≤15 min, RT
Plague	Pneumonic	Sputum/throat: Collect routine throat culture with a swab or collect expectorated sputum into a sterile, leakproof container.	≤2 h, RT
		Bronchial/tracheal wash: Collect per institution's procedure in an area dedicated to collecting respiratory specimens under isolation or containment circumstances, i.e., isolation chamber "bubble."	≤2 h, RT
		Blood: Collect per institution's procedure for routine blood cultures.	≤2 h, RT

(continued)

Collection and Transport

Collection and Transport

Table 3.7 Agents of bioterrorism: specimen guidelines[a] *(continued)*

Disease agent	Type of disease	Specimen selection	Transport time and temp
Smallpox	Rash	Biopsy specimens: Aseptically place two to four portions of tissue into a sterile, leakproof, freezable container.	~ 6 h, 4°C
		Scabs: Aseptically place scrapings or material into a sterile, leakproof, freezable container.	~ 6 h, 4°C
		Vesicular fluid: Collect fluid from separate lesions onto separate sterile swabs. Be sure to include cellular material from the base of each respective vesicle.	~ 6 h, 4°C
Tularemia	Pneumonic	Sputum/throat: Collect routine throat culture with a swab or collect expectorated sputum into a sterile, leakproof container.	≤2 h, RT
		Bronchial/tracheal wash: Collect per institution's procedure in an area dedicated to collecting respiratory specimens under isolation or containment circumstances, i.e., isolation chamber or "bubble."	≤2 h, RT
		Blood: Collect per institution's procedure for routine blood cultures.	≤2 h, RT
VHF		Serum: Collect 10–12 ml of serum. Laboratory tests used to diagnose VHF include antigen capture ELISA, IgG ELISA, PCR, and virus isolation.	~2 h, RT

[a]Abbreviations: ELISA, enzyme-linked immunosorbent assay; IgG, immunoglobulin G; RT, room temperature; VHF, viral hemorrhagic fever.

Bacterial Diagnosis

This section provides guidelines for the selection and processing of specimens for the detection of specific bacteria. Testing can be subdivided into microscopy, culture, antigen tests (including immunoassays and molecular diagnostic tests), and antibody tests. Although it is impossible to provide guidelines for all possible infections, the most common bacteria associated with human disease are included. This section has been expanded to include summary tables of identification tests as well as a more detailed discussion of the immunological detection of organisms where appropriate.

Table 4.1 Detection methods for bacteria[a]

Organism	Microscopy	Culture	Antigen detection	Antibody detection	Molecular diagnostics
Aerobic gram-positive cocci					
Staphylococcus aureus	A	A	B	D	B
Streptococcus, group A	B	A	A	B	A
Streptococcus, group B	B	A	B	D	B
Streptococcus pneumoniae	A	A	B	C	C
Enterococcus spp.	A	A	D	D	A
Aerobic gram-positive rods					
Bacillus anthracis	A	A	C	D	B
Listeria spp.	B	A	C	D	C
Erysipelothrix spp.	A	A	D	D	D
Corynebacterium diphtheriae	B	A	D	D	C
Corynebacterium, other spp.	A	A	D	D	D
Gardnerella vaginalis	A	B	D	D	D
Tropheryma whipplei	B	D	D	D	A
Acid-fast and partially acid-fast gram-positive rods					
Mycobacterium tuberculosis	A	A	B	C	A
Mycobacterium avium complex	A	A	C	D	C

(continued)

Bacterial Diagnosis

Table 4.1 Detection methods for bacteria[a] (continued)

Organism	Microscopy	Culture	Antigen detection	Antibody detection	Molecular diagnostics
Nocardia spp.	A	A	D	D	D
Rhodococcus spp.	A	A	D	D	D
Aerobic gram–negative cocci					
Neisseria gonorrhoeae	A	A	D	D	A
Neisseria meningitidis	A	A	B	D	D
Moraxella catarrhalis	A	A	D	D	D
Aerobic gram–negative rods					
Actinobacillus spp.	A	A	D	D	D
Pasteurella spp.	A	A	D	D	D
Capnocytophaga spp.	A	A	D	D	D
Kingella spp.	A	A	D	D	D
Eikenella spp.	A	A	D	D	D
Cardiobacterium spp.	A	A	D	D	D
Streptobacillus spp.	A	A	D	D	D
Haemophilus influenzae	A	A	B	D	C
Haemophilus ducreyi	B	A	D	D	C
Escherichia coli	A	A	B	D	C
Salmonella enterica serovar Typhi	A	A	D	B	D
Salmonella, other serovars	A	A	D	D	D
Shigella spp.	A	A	D	D	D

Yersinia pestis	A	C	B	C
Yersinia enterocolitica	A	D	B	C
Other *Enterobacteriaceae*	A	D	D	D
Aeromonas spp.	A	D	D	D
Vibrio cholerae	A	D	D	D
Vibrio, other spp.	A	D	D	D
Pseudomonas aeruginosa	A	D	D	D
Burkholderia pseudomallei	A	B	C	C
Burkholderia cepacia complex	A	D	D	C
Stenotrophomonas spp.	A	D	D	D
Acinetobacter spp.	A	D	A	A
Bordetella pertussis	B	D	A	C
Francisella spp.	B	C	A	D
Brucella spp.	B	C	D	B
Legionella spp.	B	A	B	C
Bartonella spp.	C	D	A	C
Campylobacter spp.	B	A	D	C
Helicobacter pylori	B	A	A	C
Anaerobic bacteria				
Peptostreptococcus spp.	A	D	D	D
Clostridium perfringens	A	D	D	D
Clostridium botulinum	B	A	B	D
Clostridium tetani	A	D	D	D
Clostridium difficile	A	A	B	C

(continued)

Bacterial Diagnosis

Bacterial Diagnosis

Table 4.1 Detection methods for bacteria[a] (continued)

Organism	Microscopy	Culture	Antigen detection	Antibody detection	Molecular diagnostics
Actinomyces spp.	A	A	D	D	D
Mobiluncus spp.	A	B	D	D	D
Bacteroides fragilis group	A	A	D	D	D
Fusobacterium spp.	A	A	D	D	D
Curved and spiral-shaped bacteria					
Leptospira spp.	B	B	D	A	C
Borrelia burgdorferi	B	B	D	A	A
Borrelia, other spp.	A	B	D	D	D
Treponema pallidum	A	D	D	A	D
Mycoplasma spp. and obligate intracellular bacteria					
Mycoplasma pneumoniae	D	B	C	A	A
Chlamydia trachomatis	A	B	A	B	A
Chlamydophila psittaci	D	B	D	A	D
Chlamydophila pneumoniae	D	C	D	B	A
Rickettsia rickettsii	B	D	D	A	B
Ehrlichia spp.	B	D	D	A	B
Anaplasma spp.	B	D	D	A	B
Coxiella spp.	D	D	D	A	C

[a] A, test generally useful; B, test useful under certain circumstances or for the diagnosis of specific forms of infection; C, test seldom useful for general diagnostic purposes; D, test not generally useful.

Table 4.2 Recommendations for Gram stain and plating media[a,b]

Specimen or organism	Gram stain	Aerobic media	Anaerobic media	Comments[c]
Body cavity fluids				Blood culture bottles should be used to incubate large volumes of specimens for all body cavity fluids.
CSF (routine)	×	B C		
CSF (shunt)	×	B C Th		
Pericardial	×	B C	BBA	
Pleural	×	B C	BBA	
Peritoneal	×	B C Mac	BBA LKV BBE CNA	
CAPD	×	B C Th	BBA	
Synovial	×	B C		
Bone marrow	×	B	BBA	
Catheter tip		B C		
Ear external fluid/swab	×	B C Mac		
Ear internal fluid	×	B C	BBA	
Eye	×	B C		
Gastrointestinal tract				*C. jejuni/coli* in 5% O_2–10% CO_2–85% N_2 at 42°C for all gastrointestinal tract specimens
Feces		B Mac HE Ca EB		
Rectal swab		B Mac HE Ca EB		
Genital tract				
Vaginal/cervix		B TM		

(continued)

Bacterial Diagnosis

Bacterial Diagnosis

Table 4.2 Recommendations for Gram stain and plating media[a,b] *(continued)*

Specimen or organism	Gram stain	Aerobic media	Anaerobic media	Comments[c]
Urethra/penis	×	TM		
Other	×	B C Mac TM	BBA LKV BBE CNA	
Group B streptococcal screen		Selective broth, subculture to B		
Lower respiratory tract				
Sputum	×	B C Mac		
Tracheal aspirate	×	B C Mac		
Bronchoalveolar lavage fluid	×	B C Mac	BBA LKV CNA	
Bronchoscopy brushing, washing	×	B C Mac		Protected bronchoscope brushing required for anaerobic culture
Tissue	×	B C Mac Th	BBA LKV BBE CNA	
Upper respiratory tract				
Nasopharynx		B C		
Nose		B		
Throat		B or SSA		Add chocolate agar for epiglottitis
Urine		B Mac		
Wound or abscess				
Swab	×	B C Mac		Anaerobic culture only if separate swab transported in appropriate system
Aspirate	×	B C Mac	BBA LKV BBE CNA	

Selected organisms		
Bordetella pertussis and	Regan Lowe	
B. parapertussis		
Brucella spp.	B C	
Corynebacterium diphtheriae	Cysteine-tellurite	
	or Loeffler's serum	
Clostridium difficile	CCFA	
E. coli O157:H7 (EHEC)	Sorbitol-Mac	Shiga toxin EIA more sensitive
Francisella tularensis	C or BCYE	
Group B *Streptococcus*	LIM broth	
Haemophilus ducreyi	C + vancomycin	Gram stain resembling "school
	(3 µg/ml)	of fish"
Helicobacter pylori ×	B	*Campylobacter* gaseous atmo-
		sphere at 35–37°C
Legionella spp.	BCYE	
Leptospira spp.	Fletcher's medium	30°C for up to 13 wk
	or EMJH	
Neisseria gonorrhoeae	TM	
Nocardia	BCYE	
Vibrio spp.	TCBS	
Yersinia spp.	CIN	

[a] Adapted from P. R. Murray, E. J. Baron, J. H. Jorgensen, M. A. Pfaller, and R. H. Yolken (ed.), *Manual of Clinical Microbiology*, 8th ed., ASM Press, Washington, D.C., 2003.

[b] CAPD, fluid from chronic ambulatory peritoneal dialysis; B, blood agar; C, chocolate blood agar; Mac, MacConkey agar; Th, thioglycolate broth; Ca, campylobacter agar; HE, Hektoen enteric; EB, enrichment broth; SSA, group A *Streptococcus* selective agar; TM, Thayer-Martin; BCYE, buffered charcoal yeast extract; TCBS, thiosulfate citrate bile salt sucrose; CIN, cefsulodin-Irgasan-novobiocin; BBA, brucella blood agar; LKV, laked blood with kanamycin and vancomycin; BBE, bacteroides bile esculin; CNA, anaerobic colistin-nalidixic acid; CCFA, cycloserine-cefoxitin-fructose agar; EMJH, Ellinghausen-McCullough-Johnson-Harris medium.

[c] Set up anaerobic culture upon request, if specimen is collected and transported appropriately. Call physician if appropriate specimen does not have request for anaerobic culture.

Bacterial Diagnosis

Table 4.3 Screening specimens for routine bacterial culture[a]

Specimen	Screening method	Results of screen[b]	
		Acceptable	Unacceptable
Sputum	Microscopic examination of Gram-stained smear	<10 SEC/average 10× field	>10 SEC/average 10× field
Endotracheal aspirate	Microscopic examination of Gram-stained smear	<10 SEC/average 10× field and bacteria detected in at least 1 of 20 fields (100×)	>10 SEC/average 10× field and no bacteria detected in 20 fields (100×)
Bronchoalveolar lavage fluid	Microscopic examination of Gram-stained smear	<1% of cells present are SEC	>1% of cells present are SEC
Urine	Urinalysis, Gram stain of urine sediment	<3 + SEC by urinalysis; positive LE test result with >10 polymorphonuclear leukocytes/mm^3 from symptomatic patients (patients with asymptomatic bacteriuria may not have increased number of leukocytes)	≥3 + SEC on urinalysis or more than 3 potential pathogens by Gram stain implies gross contamination
Superficial wound	Microscopic examination of Gram-stained smear	<2 + SEC, polymorphonuclear leukocytes present	>2 + SEC and no polymorphonuclear neutrophils
Stool for bacterial pathogens	Location of patient? Duration of hospitalization?	Outpatient or inpatient for ≤3 days	In hospital >3 days, or diarrhea developed while in hospital

[a] Adapted from P. R. Murray, E. J. Baron, J. H. Jorgensen, M. A. Pfaller, and R. H. Yolken (ed.), *Manual of Clinical Microbiology*, 8th ed., ASM Press, Washington, D.C., 2003.
[b] LE, leukocyte esterase; SEC, squamous epithelial cells.

Table 4.4 Processing specimens for mycobacterial identification

Specimen type[a]	Smear[b]	Solid and liquid media at: 35°C	30°C
Abscess	R	×	
Blood/bone marrow	N	×	
Biopsy specimen			
Lung	R	×	
Not lung, lymph node, skin, or synovium	O	×	
Skin, synovium, and lymph node	O	×	×
Superficial skin, wound, or tissue[c]	R	×	×
Eye	O	×	×
Fluids			
Not joint or synovial fluid	O	×	
Joint and synovial fluid	O	×	×
Gastric washing	R	×	
Respiratory (not mouth)	R	×	
Stool	O	×	
Urine	O	×	

[a] Sources not generally recommended for mycobacterial culture include genital sites, ears, catheter, mouth, and rectal swabs. Consult laboratory prior to making a request.

[b] R, staining should be performed routinely; O, staining is optional and should be performed if requested; N, staining should not be performed unless the request is discussed with the physician.

[c] Suspect rapidly growing mycobacteria, *M. haemophilum*, or *M. marinum*.

Acridine Orange Stain

Acridine orange is a fluorescent dye that intercalates into nucleic acid (native and the denatured). At neutral pH, bacteria, fungi, and cellular material (e.g., leukocytes and squamous epithelial cells) stain red-orange. At acidic pH (pH 4.0), bacteria remain red-orange but the background material stains green-yellow. Optimal detection of fluorescence requires the use of a 420- to 490-nm excitation filter and a 520-nm barrier filter.

Auramine-Rhodamine Stain

Auramine and rhodamine are fluorochromes that bind to mycolic acids and are resistant to decolorization with acid-alcohol (acid-fast stain). Acid-fast organisms appear orange-yellow. Potassium permanganate is used as a counterstain. It is a strong oxidizing agent that inactivates the unbound fluorochrome dyes, producing a black background for the stained specimens. Fluorochrome-stained smears can be restained by the Kinyoun or Ziehl-Neelsen methods. Optimal detection of fluorescence requires use of a 420- to 490-nm excitation filter and a 520-nm barrier filter.

Direct Fluorescent-Antibody Stain

A variety of organisms (e.g., *Streptococcus pyogenes*, *Bordetella pertussis*, *Francisella tularensis*, *Legionella* spp., and *Chlamydia trachomatis*) are directly detected in clinical specimens by using specific fluorescein-labeled antibodies. The labeled antibodies bind to the organisms and fluoresce green under UV light. The sensitivity and specificity of the stain are determined by the quality of the antibodies used in the reagents. Optimal detection of fluorescence requires the use of either a 420- to 490-nm (wide-band) or 470- to 490-nm (narrow-band) excitation filter and a 510- to 530-nm barrier filter.

Gram Stain

Gram stain is the most commonly used stain in clinical microbiology laboratories. It is used to separate bacteria into gram-positive (blue) and gram-negative (red) groups. Variations in the performance of this stain are commonplace; however, the staining principle is constant. After the specimen is fixed to a glass slide (by either heating or treatment with 95% methanol), it is exposed to the basic dye crystal violet. Iodine is added and forms a complex with the primary dye. During the decolorization step, this complex is retained in gram-positive organisms but lost in gram-negative organisms. The gram-negative organisms are detected with a counterstain (e.g., safranin). The degree to which an organism retains the stain is a function of the species, culture conditions, and staining skills of the microbiologist. Older cultures tend to decolorize readily.

Kinyoun Stain and Modified Acid-Fast Stain

The presence of long-chain fatty acids (e.g., mycolic acid) in some organisms makes these organisms both difficult to stain with water-soluble dyes and resistant to decolorization with acid solutions (acid-fast). The Kinyoun method of staining uses phenol to facilitate the penetration of basic carbol fuchsin into the cells. This stain is also referred to as a cold acid-fast stain because the specimen does not have to be heated for the stain to penetrate, as it does with the Ziehl-Neelsen stain. Basic carbol fuchsin is used as the primary stain, 3% sulfuric acid in 95% ethanol (acid-alcohol) is the decolorizing agent, and methylene blue is the counterstain. Acid-fast organisms appear pink-red on a pale blue background. The contrast between organisms and background is sometimes poor, and the fluorochrome stain is generally preferred for specimen examination. Acid-fast stains are used for detecting bacteria including *Mycobacterium*, *Nocardia*, *Rhodococcus*, *Tsukamurella*, and *Gordonia* spp. Because some of these organisms lose the primary stain when exposed to 3% sulfuric acid, the decolorizing agent can be reduced to 0.5 to 1%. Organisms that retain this modified stain are referred to as being partially acid-fast.

Ziehl-Neelsen Stain

Ziehl-Neelsen stain is an acid-fast stain which requires that the specimen be heated during staining so that the basic carbol fuchsin can penetrate into the organisms. Once this penetration is accomplished, decolorization and counterstaining are the same as for the Kinyoun method. The sensitivity and specificity of this stain are essentially the same as those of the Kinyoun method.

Primary Plating Media: Bacteria

Bacteroides Bile-Esculin (BBE) Agar

Bacteroides bile-esculin agar is a selective, differential agar medium used for the recovery of the *Bacteroides fragilis* group and *Bilophila wadsworthia*. The medium contains oxgall (bile), esculin, ferric ammonium citrate, hemin, vitamin K_1, and gentamicin in a casein and soybean agar base. Growth of non-*B fragilis* group organisms is inhibited by the bile and the gentamicin. Supplementation of the agar with hemin and vitamin K_1 stimulates the growth of *Bacteroides* spp. Esculin hydrolysis is detected when esculin is converted to esculetin and reacts with ferric ammonium citrate to produce black colonies.

Bile-Esculin (Enterococcal Selective) Agar

Bile-esculin agar can be made selective for the recovery of vancomycin-resistant enterococci by adding 6 µg of vancomycin per ml to it. Enterococci are able to grow in the presence of bile and hydrolyze esculin. Vancomycin-resistant strains produce black colonies on this agar, but susceptible strains fail to grow.

Bismuth Sulfite Agar

Bismuth sulfite agar is a differential, selective medium used for the isolation and identification of *Salmonella enterica* serovar Typhi and other enteric rods. The medium contains digests of casein and animal tissue, beef extract, glucose, ferric sulfate, and bismuth sulfite. Most commensal organisms are inhibited by the bismuth sulfite. *S. enterica* serovar Typhi colonies appear black with a metallic sheen. This medium may be inhibitory for some species of *Shigella*.

Blood Agar

Many types of blood agar media are used in clinical laboratories. The two basic components are the basal medium (e.g., brain heart infusion, brucella, Columbia, Shaedler's, tryptic soy) and blood (e.g., sheep, horse, rabbit). Additional supplements are commonly used to enhance the growth of specific organisms or to suppress the growth of unwanted organisms.

Bordet-Gengou Agar

Recovery of *Bordetella pertussis* and *Bordetella parapertussis* is inhibited by factors such as fatty acids, metal ions, sulfides, and peroxides that are commonly present in media. Starch, charcoal, serum albumin, blood, or similar components are added to the medium to neutralize these inhibitors. Bordet-Gengou agar is a potato infusion-glycerol-based agar medium supplemented with 20 to 30% sheep, horse, or rabbit blood. Potato infusion is required for the growth of *Bordetella* spp., and glycerol is added to conserve moisture in the medium. Antibiotics such as methicillin or cephalexin are commonly added to suppress the growth of bacteria such as staphylococci, which inhibit the growth of *Bordetella* spp. Because this medium must be made fresh (it has a shelf life of less than 1 week), it has largely been replaced by Regan-Lowe agar.

Brain Heart Infusion Agar and Broth

Brain heart infusion agar is a general-purpose medium used for the isolation of a wide variety of pathogens. The basic formula includes infusion from brains and beef heart, as well as meat peptones, yeast extract, and dextrose. Vitamin K and hemin can be added for the enriched growth of anaerobes. The anaerobic formulation is inferior for the isolation of anaerobic gram-negative organisms. Broth formulations supplemented with 6.5% sodium chloride are used for the isolation of salt-tolerant streptococci and enterococci. Fildes enrichment can be added to the broth formulations for the isolation of fastidious organisms such as *Haemophilus* and *Neisseria* spp.

Brilliant Green Agar

Brilliant green agar is a selective, differential medium used for the isolation of *Salmonella* serovars except *S. enterica* serovar Typhi. The nutritive base contains meat and casein peptones. Brilliant green dye at a high concentration inhibits most gram-positive and gram-negative bacteria, including *Shigella* spp. and *S. enterica* serovar Typhi. Phenol red is the pH indicator. Yeast extract provides additional nutrients. Acid production from the fermentation of sucrose or lactose produces yellow-green colonies with a yellow-green zone around the colony. Nonfermenters may range in color from white to reddish pink with a red zone.

Bacterial Diagnosis

Brucella Agar and Broth

Brucella agar is a medium designed originally for the isolation of *Brucella* spp. Brucella agar supplemented with 5% horse blood can be used as a general-purpose medium for the isolation of both aerobic and anaerobic organisms. The nutritive base includes meat peptones, dextrose, and yeast extract. The agar formulation can be supplemented with hemin and vitamin K for recovery of fastidious anaerobes or with cefoxitin and cycloserine for the selective recovery of *Clostridium difficile*. The broth contains sodium bisulfite as a reducing agent and has been used for cultivation of *Campylobacter* spp.

Buffered Charcoal-Yeast Extract (BCYE) Agar

Buffered charcoal-yeast extract agar is selective for the recovery of *Legionella*, *Nocardia*, and *Francisella* spp. It contains agar, yeast extract, charcoal, and salts and is supplemented with L-cysteine, ferric pyrophosphate, ACES [*N*-(2-acetamido)-2-aminoethanesulfonic acid] buffer, and α-ketoglutarate. The charcoal detoxifies the medium, the yeast extracts are rich in nutrients, and the L-cysteine, ferric pyrophosphate, and α-ketoglutarate stimulate the growth of *Legionella* spp. The addition of ACES is required to buffer the medium because *Legionella* spp. have a narrow pH tolerance (growth is optimal at pH 6.9). Various antibiotics such as polymyxin B, anisomycin, cefamandole, vancomycin, and cycloheximide are added to inhibit the growth of other bacteria when nonsterile clinical and environmental specimens are cultured.

Burkholderia cepacia Selective Agar (BCSA)

Burkholderia cepacia selective agar is an enriched, selective medium used for the isolation of *B. cepacia*. Trypticase peptone, yeast extract, sodium chloride, sucrose, and lactose form the nutritive base, and polymyxin B, gentamicin, vancomycin, and crystal violet are added as selective agents. This agar is the most sensitive and selective medium for the recovery of *B. cepacia*.

Campylobacter Selective Medium

A large number of media have been developed for the selective isolation of *Campylobacter* spp. from stool specimens. Most contain a brucella basal medium, which preferentially supports the growth of *Campylobacter* spp. Blood is added, as are various combinations of antibiotics (e.g., cephalothin, vancomycin, trimethoprim, amphotericin, and polymyxin in the Blaser-Wang formulation; cycloheximide, cefazolin, novobiocin, bacitracin, and colistin in the Butzler formulation; cycloheximide, cefoperazone, and vancomycin in the Karmali formulation; and cycloheximide, rifampin, trimethoprim, and polymyxin in the Preston formulation).

Cefsulodin-Irgasan-Novobiocin (CIN) Agar

Cefsulodin-Irgasan-novobiocin agar is a selective, differential agar medium used for the isolation of *Yersinia* and *Aeromonas* spp. The medium consists of digests of animal tissue and gelatin, beef and yeast extracts, sodium pyruvate, sodium deoxycholate, neutral red, crystal violet, cefsulodin, Irgasan, and novobiocin. The antibiotics and sodium deoxycholate inhibit the growth of most organisms in stool specimens. However, *Yersinia* and *Aeromonas* spp. are resistant and can ferment mannitol in the medium. This fermentation produces colonies with a bull's-eye appearance, i.e., deep red centers with transparent edges.

Chocolate Agar

Chocolate agar is an enriched medium that derives its name from its color. Blood or hemoglobin is added immediately after the medium is heated, and the heat causes the added component to lyse and turn brown. This medium supports the growth of most bacteria and is required for the recovery of many *Haemophilus* spp. and some pathogenic *Neisseria* strains. A variety of formulations of this medium have been used, but the most common consists of a peptone base enriched with 2% hemoglobin or IsoVitaleX. Catalase-negative bacteria (e.g., *Streptococcus pneumoniae*) grow less well on this medium than on blood agar because catalase from ruptured erythrocytes in blood agar is not available to protect the bacteria from peroxides that accumulate in the medium.

Chopped-Meat Broth

Chopped-meat broth is an enriched broth used for the recovery of a variety of bacteria, particularly anaerobes, from clinical specimens. Extracts as well as solid particles of beef or horse meat are suspended in broth with peptones, yeast extract, sugars, starch, and L-cysteine. The L-cysteine helps maintain a low

E_h (oxidation-reduction potential), which supports the growth of anaerobes.

Colistin-Nalidixic Acid (CNA) Agar

Colistin-nalidixic acid agar is a selective medium used for the recovery of aerobic and anaerobic gram-positive bacteria. The medium consists of Columbia agar base supplemented with nalidixic acid, colistin, and blood. Nalidixic acid inhibits most aerobic gram-negative rods, as does colistin. The *B. fragilis* group is usually resistant to these antibiotics, but other anaerobic gram-negative rods can be inhibited by colistin.

Columbia Agar and Broth

Columbia agar with 5% sheep blood is a general-purpose medium used for the isolation of common bacteria. The medium contains meat and casein peptones, beef extract, yeast extract, and cornstarch as the nutritive base. Sheep blood allows the determination of hemolytic reactions and provides X factor. However, the substantial carbohydrate content may make beta-hemolytic streptococci appear to be alpha-hemolytic or take on a greenish hue. Use of horse or rabbit blood improves the hemolysis. NADase in sheep blood destroys the V factor (NAD); therefore, organisms that require this factor do not grow. Salt and Tris buffers are added to the broth formulation to enhance the growth of organisms and increase the buffering capacity, respectively.

Cycloserine-Cefoxitin-Egg Yolk-Fructose Agar (CCFA)

Cycloserine-cefoxitin-egg yolk-fructose agar is a selective, differential medium used for the recovery of *Clostridium difficile*. The medium consists of animal tissue digest, fructose, cycloserine, cefoxitin, and neutral red. Cycloserine and cefoxitin inhibit most intestinal bacteria. *C. difficile* can ferment fructose, producing a more acidic pH, which is detected by the indicator dye neutral red (shift from red to yellow medium surrounding the colonies). Various modifications of this medium are used, including supplementation with egg yolk to stimulate the growth of clostridia.

Cystine Lactose Electrolyte-Deficient (CLED) Agar

Cystine lactose electrolyte-deficient agar is a nonselective differential medium used for the recovery of urinary tract pathogens. The medium consists of casein and gelatin digests, beef extract, L-cystine, lactose, and bromthymol blue. Lactose-fermenting bacteria have yellow colonies, and the swarming of motile gram-negative bacilli is inhibited.

Cystine Tellurite Blood Agar

Cystine tellurite blood agar medium is a selective, differential medium used for the recovery of *Corynebacterium diphtheriae*. The medium consists of heart infusion agar, potassium tellurite, L-cystine, and rabbit blood. Potassium tellurite inhibits the growth of most commensal organisms and allows *C. diphtheriae* to grow. The organism produces hydrogen sulfide from cystine, and the reaction of tellurite with hydrogen sulfide results in brown halos surrounding the colonies of *C. diphtheriae*.

Egg Yolk Agar

Egg yolk agar (modified McClung-Toabe agar) is a selective, differential medium used for the isolation and differentiation of *Clostridium* spp. Degradation of lecithin results in an opaque precipitate around the bacterial colony, and lipase destroys fats in the egg yolk, resulting in an iridescent sheen on the colony surface. Proteolysis can also be determined on the basis of a translucent clearing of the medium around the colony. Addition of neomycin makes the egg yolk agar moderately selective by inhibiting some facultative anaerobic gram-negative rods.

Ellinghausen & McCullough Modified Bovine Albumin Tween 80 Medium

The modified bovine albumin Tween 80 medium is selective for the growth of *Leptospira* spp. The basal medium, consisting of glycerol, sodium pyruvate, and thiamine, is supplemented with bovine albumin, Tween 80, vitamin B_{12}, and salts of iron, calcium, magnesium, zinc, and copper.

Eosin-Methylene Blue (EMB) Agar

Eosin-methylene blue agar is a differential, selective medium used for the isolation and differentiation of lactose-fermenting and -nonfermenting gram-negative rods. The agar medium consists of casein digests, lactose, sucrose, eosin Y, and methylene blue. The Levine formulation does not include sucrose. Growth of gram-positive bacteria is suppressed by the methylene blue, which, together with eosin Y, also serves as an indicator for carbohydrate fermentation (dyes precipitate at an acidic pH). Bacteria that ferment lactose (e.g., *Escherichia*, *Klebsiella*, and *Enterobacter* spp.) form colonies that have a green metallic sheen or that are blue-black to brown. Non-fermentative bacteria (e.g., *Proteus*, *Salmonella*, and *Shigella* spp.) have colorless or light purple colonies.

Fletcher Medium

Fletcher medium is a semisolid medium used for the recovery of *Leptospira* spp. The medium consists of 0.15% agar, salt, peptones, beef extract, and rabbit serum. *Leptospira* spp. usually grow within 1 to 2 weeks in this medium.

Gram-Negative (GN; Hajna) Broth

Gram-negative broth is a selective enrichment broth used for the recovery of small numbers of salmonellae and shigellae from stool specimens. The medium consists of digests of casein and animal tissues, mannitol, glucose, sodium citrate, and sodium deoxycholate. The sodium citrate and sodium deoxycholate inhibit the growth of many gram-positive and gram-negative bacteria. The fact that the concentration of mannitol is higher than that of glucose limits the growth of *Proteus* spp. However, commensal organisms will overgrow the enteric pathogens if the broth is incubated for more than 4 to 6 h.

Haemophilus Test Medium (HTM) Agar and Broth

Haemophilus test medium is an enriched medium used for susceptibility testing of *Haemophilus* spp. The medium contains beef and casein extracts. Yeast extract, hematin, and NAD provide the necessary growth factors and enrichments. Antagonists to sulfonamides and trimethoprim are removed by thymidine phophorylase. The advantage of the agar medium is that it is a clear agar base so that sharp growth end-point interpretations can be made. The calcium and magnesium concentrations are adjusted to the concentrations recommended by the NCCLS.

Hektoen Enteric (HE) Agar

Hektoen enteric agar is a selective medium used for the isolation of *Salmonella* and *Shigella* spp. and differentiation of these organisms from other gram-negative rods that may be recovered on this medium. It consists of a peptone base agar supplemented with bile salts, lactose, sucrose, salicin, ferric ammonium citrate, and the pH indicators bromthymol blue and acid fuchsin. The bile inhibits all gram-positive bacteria and many gram-negative rods. Acids produced by fermentation of lactose, sucrose, or salicin react with bromthymol blue to produce a yellow color and with acid fuchsin to produce a red color. Hydrogen sulfide produced by the metabolism of sodium thiosulfate is detected when a black precipitate forms after the addition of ferric ammonium citrate. Lactose-fermenting bacteria (e.g., *E. coli*) are slightly inhibited on this agar and appear as orange or salmon pink colonies. *Salmonella* colonies typically appear blue-green with black centers. *Shigella* colonies appear green with no black center. *Proteus* spp. are inhibited; their colonies are colorless.

Kanamycin-Vancomycin Laked Blood (LKV) Agar

Kanamycin-vancomycin laked blood agar is a selective, differential medium used for the recovery of anaerobic gram-negative rods, especially *Bacteroides* and *Prevotella* spp. The medium consists of casein and soybean meal agar supplemented with kanamycin, vancomycin, vitamin K_1, and lysed (laked) sheep blood. Kanamycin inhibits most facultative, gram-negative rods, and vancomycin inhibits most gram-positive organisms and *Porphyromonas* spp. Vitamin K_1 stimulates the growth of some *Prevotella* strains, which also develop a black pigment in the presence of lysed blood.

Kelly Medium

Kelly medium is used for the isolation of *Borrelia* spp. from human specimens and arthropod vectors. The success of these cultures depends on the quality of the medium. In general, specimens should be submitted to reference laboratories for processing. A modified version (Barbour-Stoenner-Kelly II medium) of the original formulation is currently used. The medium consists of peptone and casein digests, albumin, gelatin, rabbit serum, hemin, yeast extracts, glucose, and a complex mixture of buffers, amino acids, vitamins, nucleotides, and other growth factors. Kanamycin and 5-fluorouracil have been added to the medium for the selective isolation of borreliae from contaminated specimens. Recovery of the organisms requires prolonged incubation in a microaerophilic atmosphere at 30 to 37°C. Organisms are detected by examining the broth at weekly intervals by dark-field microscopy.

Lactobacillus MRS Broth

Lactobacillus MRS broth is a nonselective liquid medium used for the isolation of lactobacilli. The nutritive base includes peptones, yeast extract with buffers, and glucose. Polysorbate 80 (Tween 80) supplies fatty acids and magnesium for additional growth requirements. Sodium acetate and ammonium citrate may inhibit member of the normal flora, including gram-negative bacteria, oral flora, and fungi, and improve the growth of the lactobacilli. The growth of lactobacilli is favored when the pH is adjusted to 6.1 to 6.6.

LIM Broth

LIM broth is a selective enrichment broth used for the recovery of group B streptococci. The medium consists of Todd-Hewitt broth supplemented with yeast extract, colistin, and nalidixic acid. Most aerobic and anaerobic gram-negative rods are inhibited by the antibiotics, while group B streptococci grow well in this broth.

Loeffler Medium

Loeffler medium is an enriched medium used for the recovery of *Corynebacterium diphtheriae*. The medium consists of animal digests, heart muscle infusion, beef serum, egg, and glucose. *C. diphtheriae* grows rapidly on this medium, and Gram stains of colonies demonstrate characteristic metachromatic granules.

MacConkey (MAC) Agar

MacConkey agar is a selective agar medium used for the isolation and differentiation of lactose-fermenting and -non-fermenting gram-negative rods. The medium consists of digests of peptones, bile salts, lactose, neutral red, and crystal violet. Bile salts and crystal violet inhibit the growth of gram-positive bacteria and some fastidious gram-negative bacteria. Colonies that ferment lactose (e.g., *Escherichia*, *Klebsiella*, and *Enterobacter* spp.) produce acid, which causes a red color shift in the neutral red pH indicator and precipitates the bile salts. Colonies appear red to pink, while nonfermenting colonies (e.g., *Proteus*,

Salmonella, and *Shigella* spp.) appear yellow, colorless, or translucent.

MacConkey Agar with Sorbitol — *see* Sorbitol-MacConkey Agar

Mannitol Salt Agar

Mannitol salt agar is a selective medium used for the isolation of staphylococci. The medium consists of digests of casein and animal tissue, beef extract, mannitol, salt, and phenol red indicator. If the organism can grow in the presence of 7.5% salt and ferment mannitol, the acid turns the indicator yellow. Most strains of *Staphylococcus aureus* produce yellow colonies, while coagulase-negative staphylococci do not ferment the mannitol and thus remain red. Most other organisms are inhibited by the high salt concentration.

Martin-Lewis Agar

Martin-Lewis agar, a formulation of the modified Thayer-Martin (MTM) agar, is an enriched selective medium for the isolation of *Neisseria gonorrhoeae*. The nutritive base is chocolate agar. The specific differences from MTM agar are a higher concentration of vancomycin (4 versus 3 µg/ml) and replacement of nystatin with anisomycin. Trimethoprim and colistin are also incorporated. Some pathogenic *Neisseria* strains have been reported to be inhibited by vancomycin and trimethoprim.

Mueller-Hinton Agar and Broth

Mueller-Hinton agar and broth are recommended by NCCLS for the routine susceptibility testing of nonfastidious organisms. Supplementation of this agar with 5% sheep blood is used for susceptibility testing of fastidious organisms such as *Streptococcus pneumoniae*. Beef and casein extracts and soluble starch form the nutritive base. Calcium and magnesium concentrations are controlled.

New York City Agar

New York City agar is a selective medium used for the isolation of pathogenic *Neisseria* spp. The medium consists of peptones, cornstarch, yeast dialysate, glucose, hemoglobin, horse plasma, and a mixture of antibiotics (vancomycin, colistin, amphotericin B, and trimethoprim). It can be used instead of Thayer-Martin agar.

Oxidative-Fermentative Polymyxin B-Bacitracin-Lactose (OFPBL) Agar

Oxidative-fermentative polymyxin B-bacitracin-lactose agar is a selective, differential medium used for the isolation of *Burkholderia cepacia*. The nutritive base is an oxidative-fermentative medium with peptones. When acid is produced from the utilization of lactose, as with *B. cepacia*, the bromthymol blue indicator changes the colony from green to yellow. Polymyxin B and bacitracin are selective agents that inhibit some gram-negative and gram-positive organisms, respectively. Other organisms may grow on this medium and are differentiated from *B. cepacia* by the inability to produce acid from lactose.

Phenylethyl Alcohol (PEA) Blood Agar

Phenylethyl alcohol blood agar is a selective medium that consists of casein and soybean agar supplemented with phenylethyl alcohol and blood. Facultative gram-negative rods are inhibited by the phenylethyl alcohol (e.g., the growth of swarming *Proteus* spp. is suppressed). Most gram-positive and gram-negative anaerobes, as well as aerobic gram-positive bacteria, will grow on this medium. *Pseudomonas* spp. are not inhibited.

Pseudomonas cepacia (PC) Agar

P. cepacia agar is a selective, differential medium used for the isolation of *Burkholderia* (*Pseudomonas*) *cepacia* from clinical specimens contaminated with other organisms. The medium consists of salt solutions, phosphate buffer, pyruvate, proteose peptones, bile, crystal violet, ticarcillin, polymyxin B, and phenol red. *Burkholderia* spp. are able to grow on this medium and metabolize pyruvate, producing alkaline by-products. Pink to red colonies are observed after 2 days of incubation. Other bacteria are inhibited by the crystal violet and antibiotics.

Regan-Lowe Agar Medium

Regan-Lowe agar medium, for the selective isolation of *Bordetella* spp., contains beef extract, gelatin digest, starch, charcoal, niacin, 10% horse blood, and cephalexin (40 µg/ml). The charcoal and horse blood are required to neutralize fatty acids and other inhibitory factors present in the medium. Sheep but not human blood can replace horse blood. Cephalexin can delay the detection of *Bordetella* spp. on this medium, but the use of an additional nonselective medium is not considered necessary. The shelf life of this medium is 6 to 8 weeks.

Salmonella-Shigella (SS) Agar

Salmonella-shigella agar is a highly selective medium for the recovery of *Salmonella* and *Shigella* spp. The medium consists of beef extract and peptone digests, lactose as a carbohydrate source, bile salts, sodium citrate, sodium thiosulfate, neutral red, brilliant green, and ferric citrate. Bile salts, sodium citrate, and brilliant green are inhibitory for all gram-positive and selected gram-negative bacteria. Bacteria that grow on the medium and produce hydrogen sulfide from the metabolism of sodium thiosulfate are detected by the black precipitate formed with ferric citrate. Acid produced from lactose fermentation is detected with the pH indicator neutral red. All lactose-fermenting bacteria form pink or red colonies, while nonfermenting bacteria form either colorless (e.g., *Shigella* spp.) or black (e.g., *Salmonella* spp.) colonies.

Schaedler's Agar

Schaedler's agar is a general-purpose medium used for the isolation of anaerobic bacteria. The nutritive base includes vegetable and meat peptones, dextrose, and yeast extract. Sheep blood, vitamin K_1, and hemin provide other additives that stimulate the growth of fastidious anaerobes. Because of the high carbohydrate content, colonies with beta-hemolytic reactions may have a greenish hue. Acid production may also lead to rapid cell death.

Selenite Broth

Selenite broth is a selective enrichment broth used for the isolation of *Salmonella* spp. from stools and other contaminated specimens. It consists of peptones, sodium phosphate, lactose, and sodium selenite. *E. coli* and other gram-negative rods are inhibited by sodium selenite. The broth should be subcultured within 8 to 12 h after inoculation with the specimen, or else the enteric pathogens will be overgrown with commensal organisms.

Skirrow Medium

Skirrow medium is an enriched selective blood agar medium used for the isolation of *Campylobacter* spp. The nutritive agar base is brucella agar. Hematin is provided by sheep blood. The selective agents are trimethoprim, vancomycin, and polymyxin B, which inhibit the normal flora found in fecal specimens.

Sorbitol-MacConkey Agar

Sorbitol-MacConkey agar is a selective differential agar used for the isolation of *E. coli* O157. Lactose is replaced with sorbitol. Most *E. coli* strains ferment sorbitol; however, *E. coli* O157 does not, and therefore its colonies are colorless on this agar.

Tetrathionate Broth

Tetrathionate broth is a selective enrichment broth used for the recovery of *Salmonella* spp. from stool specimens. It consists of a peptone base supplemented with yeast extract, mannitol, glucose, sodium deoxycholate, sodium thiosulfate, calcium carbonate, and brilliant green. The sodium deoxycholate, sodium thiosulfate, and brilliant green inhibit gram-positive and gram-negative bacteria. The broth should be subcultured for 12 to 24 h after inoculation to prevent overgrowth of *Salmonella* spp. with commensal organisms.

Thayer-Martin (Modified) Agar

Many modifications of Thayer-Martin medium have been developed for the isolation of pathogenic *Neisseria* spp. The blood agar base medium is enriched with hemoglobin and supplements. The growth of unwanted bacteria can be suppressed by the addition of antibiotics such as colistin (which inhibits most gram-negative bacteria except *Proteus* spp.), trimethoprim (which inhibits *Proteus* spp.), vancomycin (which inhibits most gram-positive bacteria), and nystatin (which inhibits yeasts). Some strains of *N. gonorrhoeae* are inhibited by vancomycin, and so nonselective media (e.g., chocolate agar) should be used for primary isolation.

Thioglycolate Broth

Thioglycolate broth is an enrichment broth used for the recovery of aerobic and anaerobic bacteria. Various formulations are used, but most include casein digest, glucose, yeast extract, cysteine, and sodium thioglycolate. Supplementation with hemin and vitamin K_1 will enhance the recovery of anaerobic bacteria.

Thiosulfate Citrate Bile Salts Sucrose (TCBS) Agar

Thiosulfate citrate bile salts sucrose agar is a selective, differential medium used for the recovery of *Vibrio* spp. The medium consists of digests of casein and animal tissue, yeast extract, sodium citrate, sodium cholate, oxgall (bile), sucrose, ferric citrate, thymol blue, and bromthymol blue. Sodium citrate, sodium cholate, and bile inhibit commensal organisms. *Vibrio cholerae* colonies are yellow on this medium due to fermentation of sucrose with the acid, resulting in a yellow color shift of the indicator, bromthymol blue. *Vibrio parahaemolyticus* fails to ferment sucrose, and the colonies are therefore blue-green. Some enteric rods and enterococci may grow, but the colonies are usually small and translucent. Sucrose-fermenting *Proteus* strains produce yellow colonies that are similar to *Vibrio* colonies.

Tinsdale Agar

Tinsdale agar is a selective differential medium used for the isolation of *Corynebacterium diphtheriae* from upper respiratory specimens. The medium consists of peptones, salt, yeast extract, L-cysteine, potassium tellurite, and serum. The potassium tellurite inhibits the growth of most commensal organisms in the upper respiratory tract and allows the growth of *C. diphtheriae* and related *Corynebacterium* species. *C. diphtheriae* colonies can be distinguished by the brown halo that develops around the black colonies. These halos result from the reaction of tellurite with hydrogen sulfide, which *C. diphtheriae* produces from the cysteine in the medium.

Tryptic or Trypticase Soy Agar (TSA) and Broth (TSB)

Tryptic(ase) soy agar with 5% sheep blood is a general-purpose medium used for the isolation of a wide variety of organisms.

The medium contains soybean and casein peptones as the nutritive base. The addition of sheep blood enriches the medium and allows the growth of more fastidious organisms by providing hemin (X factor). V factor (NAD) is inactivated by enzymes in the sheep blood. Sheep blood is used for the interpretation of hemolytic reactions. The broth formulation is recommended for preparation of inocula for susceptibility testing. Addition of 6.5% sodium chloride to the broth formulation can be used for isolation of salt-tolerant organisms, and Fildes enrichment can be added to the broth for recovery of fastidious organisms such as *Haemophilus* spp.

Xylose-Lysine-Deoxycholate (XLD) Agar

Xylose-lysine-deoxycholate agar is a moderately selective medium used for the isolation and differentiation of enteric pathogens. The medium consists of yeast extract with xylose, lysine, lactose, sucrose, sodium deoxycholate, sodium thiosulfate, ferric ammonium citrate, and phenol red. The majority of the nonpathogenic enteric rods ferment lactose, sucrose, or xylose, producing yellow colonies (the phenol red indicator is yellow at acidic pH). Because *Shigella* spp. do not ferment these carbohydrates, the colonies are red. *Salmonella* and *Edwardsiella* spp. ferment xylose, but they also decarboxylate lysine to an alkaline diamine, cadaverine. This diamine neutralizes the acid products of fermentation by decarboxylation of lysine and produces red colonies. If the organism produces hydrogen sulfide (e.g., *Salmonella* and *Edwardsiella* spp.), the center of the colonies will blacken. Sodium deoxycholate inhibits the growth of many nonpathogenic organisms (in the presence of acid, it precipitates, producing yellow, opaque colonies).

Primary Plating Media: Mycobacteria

American Thoracic Society Medium

American Thoracic Society medium contains coagulated egg yolks, potato flour, glycerol, and malachite green. The concentration of malachite green is lower than in Löwenstein-Jensen medium, allowing earlier detection of mycobacterial colonies, but the medium is also more easily overgrown by contaminants.

Bacterial Diagnosis

Dubos Broth

Dubos broth, a nonselective broth, contains casein digests, salt solutions, L-asparagine, ferric ammonium citrate, albumin or serum, and Tween 80. The growth of most species of mycobacteria is rapid in this medium, although the addition of antibiotics is required when specimens from contaminated sites are processed. Tween 80 is a surfactant that facilitates the dispersal of clumps of mycobacteria and results in more rapid, homogeneous growth.

Löwenstein-Jensen (LJ) Medium

Löwenstein-Jensen medium consists of glycerol, potato flour, defined salts, and coagulated whole eggs (to solidify the medium). Malachite green is added to inhibit contaminating bacteria, particularly gram-positive bacteria. LJ medium has a long shelf life (several months) and supports the growth of most mycobacteria, in part because lecithin in the eggs neutralizes many toxic factors present in clinical specimens. A problem with LJ medium is that the contaminants that grow on this medium can completely hydrolyze it.

Löwenstein-Jensen Medium, Gruft Modification

The Gruft modification of LJ medium contains RNA, penicillin, and nalidixic acid, which further suppress the growth of contaminating organisms. Because the growth of mycobacteria can be delayed with this selective medium, it should always be used with a tube of nonselective medium.

Löwenstein-Jensen Medium, Mycobactosel Modification

The Mycobactosel modification of LJ medium contains cycloheximide, lincomycin, and nalidixic acid to suppress the growth of contaminants.

Middlebrook 7H9 Broth

The 7H9 formulation of Middlebrook broth is the same as Middlebrook 7H10 agar, except that the agar and malachite green are absent. The growth of most mycobacteria is rapid in this medium, although antibiotics must be added to suppress the growth of contaminants.

Middlebrook 7H10 Agar

Middlebrook 7H10 agar is a nonselective medium that contains defined salts, vitamins, cofactors, oleic acid, albumin, catalase, glycerol, glucose, and malachite green. The addition of glycerol enhances the growth of *Mycobacterium avium-intracellulare*. Pyruvic acid can be added if *M. bovis* is suspected, and 0.25% L-asparagine or 0.1% potassium aspartate must be added for maximal production of niacin. The medium has a relatively short shelf life (approximately 1 month), and exposure to heat or light may result in its deterioration and in the release of formaldehyde. Growth of mycobacteria can be detected earlier on this medium than on egg-based media.

Middlebrook 7H10 Agar, Mycobactosel Modification

The Mycobactosel modification of Middlebrook 7H10 agar contains malachite green, cycloheximide, lincomycin, and nalidixic acid. As with the selective LJ media, the presence of antibiotics may delay the detection of mycobacteria, so a nonselective isolation medium should also be used.

Middlebrook 7H11 Agar

Middlebrook 7H11 agar is preferred over 7H10 agar because the addition of casein hydrolysates improves the recovery of isoniazid-resistant strains of *M. tuberculosis*, which have become prevalent in some communities.

Middlebrook 7H11 Agar, Mitchison's Modification

Mitchison's modification of 7H11 medium contains carbenicillin, polymyxin B, trimethoprim, and amphotericin B. The carbenicillin is particularly useful for suppressing the growth of *Pseudomonas* spp.

Middlebrook 7H13 Broth

Middlebrook 7H13 broth is based on the 7H9 broth formulation supplemented with casein hydrolysate, polysorbate 80, sodium polyanetholesulfonate, catalase, and [^{14}C]palmitic acid. This broth is used in the BACTEC system.

Petragnani Medium

Petragnani medium is a nonselective mycobacterial medium that contains coagulated whole eggs, egg yolks, whole milk, potato, potato flour, glycerol, and malachite green. This medium is more inhibitory than LJ medium because it contains a higher concentration of malachite green. It should be restricted to use with heavily contaminated specimens.

Mycobacterial Systems Media

ESP Culture System II.   ESP Culture System II has a modified 7H9 broth with cellulose sponge to increase the culture's surface area. Growth is detected by generation of pressure changes in the headspace above the broth medium in a sealed bottle as a result of gas production or oxygen consumption during the growth of microorganisms. Contaminating bacteria are suppressed by the addition of their mycobacterial antimicrobial supplement ESP MYCO AS (amphotericin B, azlocillin, nalidixic acid, polymycin B, and fosfomycin).

MB/BacT ALERT 3D.   MB/BacT ALERT 3D, a modified 7H9 broth, includes a colorimetric carbon dioxide sensor in each bottle to detect the growth of mycobacteria. Contaminating bacteria are suppressed by addition of their mycobacterial antimicrobial supplement MAS (amphotericin B, azlocillin, nalidixic acid, polymycin B, trimethoprim, and vancomycin).

BACTEC 12B Broth.   BACTEC 12B broth is used in the BACTEC AFB automated culture system. The formulation is Middlebrook 7H9 broth supplemented with albumin, casein hydrolysate, catalase, and ^{14}C-labeled palmitic acid. As the mycobacteria grow, palmitic acid is metabolized and $^{14}CO_2$ is released and is detected by the BACTEC instrument. Contaminating bacteria are suppressed by the addition of PANTA (polymyxin B, azlocillin, nalidixic acid, trimethoprim, and amphotericin B).

BACTEC 13A Broth.   BACTEC 13A broth medium is also used in the BACTEC system. The formulation is Middlebrook 7H12 medium supplemented with sodium polyanetholesulfonate. This broth can be used for blood and bone marrow aspirate specimens.

BACTEC Myco/F Media.   The BACTEC Myco/F media series has two types of supplemented 7H9 broth. Myco/F-Lytic can be inoculated directly at the bedside and is designed for rapid detection of mycobacteria in blood and of yeast and fungi in blood and sterile body fluids, while the Myco/F-sputa culture vials are for clinical specimens other than blood. Contaminating bacteria in the Myco/F-sputa vials can be suppressed by the addition of PANTA/F. The BACTEC 9000 MB series media use the same fluorescence quenching-based oxygen sensor as the MGIT system to detect growth.

Mycobacterial Growth Indicator Tube (MGIT). The Mycobacterial Growth Indicator Tube contains a modified Middlebrook 7H9 broth in conjunction with a fluorescence quenching-based oxygen sensor (silicon rubber impregnated with ruthenium pentahydrate) to detect the growth of mycobacteria. The large amount of oxygen initially present in the medium quenches the fluorescence of the sensor. Growth of mycobacteria or other bacteria depletes the oxygen, and the indicator fluoresces brightly when the tubes are illuminated with UV light at 365 nm. Contaminating bacteria are suppressed by the addition of PANTA/MGIT.

Specific Diagnostic Tests

Aerobic Gram-Positive Cocci

***Enterococcus* spp.**   Microscopy and culture are the most commonly used detection methods. Selective media (e.g., BE azide agar and Pfizer selective agar) can be used to recover the bacteria from specimens contaminated with gram-negative bacteria, and selective media supplemented with vancomycin can be used to recover vancomycin-resistant enterococcal strains. At least one company has developed a molecular probe for detection of vancomycin-resistant enterococci in clinical specimens.

Staphyloccus aureus.   Microscopy and culture are the most commonly used detection methods. Selective media (e.g., mannitol salt agar, colistin-nalidixic acid agar, and phenylethyl alcohol agar) can be used for recovery from heavily contaminated specimens. Molecular probes are available for detecting methicillin-resistant *S. aureus*. Detection of antibodies directed against species-specific teichoic acid was formerly done but is now considered insensitive.

***Streptococcus*, Group A.** Group A *Streptococcus* grows readily in culture. Microscopy is not useful for diagnosis of pharyngitis but is useful for cutaneous infections. Numerous direct antigen tests are available for streptococcal pharyngitis. Although the tests are highly specific (for *S. pyogenes* but not other species of group A *Streptococcus*), the sensitivity is <80% and negative reactions must be confirmed by culture. Antibody tests are used to confirm antecedent group A streptococcal pharyngitis or pyoderma in patients with suspected rheumatic fever or nephritis. The most popular tests are the anti-streptolysin O (ASO) and anti-DNase B tests. Both tests have a sensitivity of 85%, and they should be performed together. The ASO test is nonreactive in patients with nephritis following streptococcal pyoderma. False-positive ASO titers can occur in patients with liver disease and infections with streptococcal groups C or G. Anti-DNase B is specific for group A streptococci; there is no reactivity with other streptococcal groups. Peak ASO and anti-DNase B titers occur 2 to 3 weeks after the primary infection and persist for 6 months or more. Positive titers are two or more dilutions above the upper limit of normal. Other tests (e.g., Streptozyme) are less sensitive and reproducible.

***Streptococcus*, Group B.** Group B *Streptococcus* grows readily in culture, although 10% of strains are nonhemolytic and may not be detected in mixed cultures. Enrichment broth (i.e., LIM broth) can be used to recover small numbers of organisms. Microscopy is not helpful for detection of genital carriage. Numerous direct antigen tests have been developed for the detection of genital carriage, but the test sensitivity is too low to justify its use. At least one company has developed a direct nucleic acid amplification test that is specific and rapid and has a sensitivity approaching that of culture.

Streptococcus pneumoniae. Microscopy and culture are sensitive detection methods, although the bacteria can undergo spontaneous lysis and hence will not be recovered in specimens when processing is delayed. A variety of tests have been developed for detecting pneumococcal capsular antigens in cerebrospinal fluid (CSF) and urine. Urine tests are less sensitive than CSF tests, and all antigen tests are generally no more sensitive than a Gram stain. Type-specific anticapsular antibody titers can be measured to assess the response to vaccination but are not measured for diagnostic purposes.

Aerobic Gram-Positive Rods

Bacillus anthracis. Microscopy is useful if positive, but the test is insensitive and the capsule is generally not seen when the Gram stain is used. Fluorescein-labeled anticapsular antibodies have been developed. The organism grows rapidly in culture and has a characteristic colony morphology (large, irregular, sticky, nonhemolytic colonies). Antigen tests and molecular diagnostic tests have been developed and are available through State Public Health laboratories. These tests are generally specific but lack sensitivity, especially for asymptomatic patients exposed to *B. anthracis*. The serologic response to anthrax toxin (i.e., protective antigen) can be used to assess the response to vaccination but not as a diagnostic tool.

Corynebacterium diphtheriae. Diagnosis is based on clinical parameters. Microscopy is generally not useful. The organism grows readily on nonselective sheep blood agar; selective media (cysteine-tellurite blood agar or Tinsdale medium) should also be used for primary cultures. The Centers for Disease Control and Prevention (CDC) offer a direct PCR test for diphtheria toxin; this test is recommended for confirming the diagnosis of diphtheria but should not be used alone. Immunoassays have been developed to measure the level of antibodies against *C. diphtheriae* toxin in patients immunized with toxoid. These tests assess immunity and cannot be used for the diagnosis of diphtheria. Antitoxin levels of ≥ 0.01 IU/ml are considered protective. Lower levels indicate that immunization with toxoid may be required.

Corynebacterium, **Other spp.** Microscopy and culture are the most commonly used detection methods. Some species are slow growing unless the isolation media are supplemented with lipids.

Erysipelothrix **spp.** Microscopy is generally insensitive, but the presence of long, slender, gram-positive rods in the tissue of a patient suspected of having erysipeloid is helpful. Growth on blood agar plates is slow, and incubation should be extended for 7 days. Antigen and molecular diagnostic tests have not been developed, and serologic testing is not useful because patients do not develop antibodies after an episode of erysipeloid.

Gardnerella vaginalis. Gram stains of vaginal specimens are helpful if thin gram-variable coccobacilli or rods are seen. The organism grows poorly in culture and may not be detected.

Listeria **spp.** Microscopy is insensitive for patients with meningitis (generally, small numbers of organisms are present in CSF) and nonspecific (the organism can be confused with *Corynebacterium* or *Streptococcus*). The organism grows well on most nonselective media, but hemolysis may not be obvious on sheep blood agar. Special selective agars have been developed for the recovery of *Listeria* from stools and food products. Antigen detection kits have also been developed for food products but are not licensed for clinical specimens. Molecular assays for the detection of bacterial DNA in CSF have been developed but are not extensively used.

Tropheryma whipplei. Microscopy was the method of choice for diagnosing infections caused by this organism (Whipple's disease) but has now been replaced with molecular diagnostic techniques. The organism has not been cultured in vitro except in human macrophages and fibroblast cell cultures.

Acid-Fast and Partially Acid-Fast Gram-Positive Rods

Mycobacterium avium **Complex.** Microscopy and culture are sensitive detection methods. Disseminated infections are common in immunocompromised patients, with organisms recovered in high concentrations in blood and many body tissues.

Mycobacterium tuberculosis. Tuberculosis is most commonly diagnosed by microscopy (acid-fast stain) and culture. Mycobacteria can also be detected directly by using DNA probes and molecular amplification methods. The amplification methods are useful for use with smear-positive respiratory specimens but cannot be used with nonrespiratory specimens and have low sensitivity for smear-negative specimens, although some methods are now approved for smear-negative specimens. Antigen capture tests (i.e., enzyme-linked immunosorbent assay [ELISA], radioimmunoassay, and agglutination) with purified antigens (i.e., 38-kDa antigen, lipoarabinomannan, antigen 60, and antigen 85 complex) have been developed but are not widely used and cannot replace traditional methods. Serologic methods in addition to the skin test are being developed. The QuantiFERON-TB test (QFT) has received Food and Drug Administration approval. The QFT is a whole-blood test for diagnosing latent tuberculosis infection and measures the patient's immune reactivity to *M. tuberculosis*. Before the QFT is performed, arrangements should be made with a qualified laboratory to ensure proper processing of blood within the required 12 h. The role of the QFT has not yet been defined clearly. Refer to the CDC for current guidelines (http://www.cdc.gov).

***Nocardia* spp.**   Diagnosis of nocardiosis relies on microscopic detection of the organism in clinical specimens and isolation in culture. Filamentous forms stain poorly with the Gram stain and weakly with the acid-fast stain (even when a weak decolorizing solution is used). Although the organism grows on most nonselective enriched media, recovery is best on buffered charcoal yeast extract (BCYE) agar and Thayer-Martin agar. Serological testing methods have been handicapped by the antigenic heterogeneity of pathogenic *Nocardia* spp., poor serologic response of the patient, high levels of immunoreactivity to *Nocardia* spp., in healthy individuals, and cross-reactivity with other microbial antigens.

***Rhodococcus* spp.**   *Rhodococcus* spp. are weakly acid-fast, with relatively few cells staining acid-fast unless the organism is cultured on Löwenstein-Jensen medium or Middlebrook agar. Bacteria grown in broth cultures incubated for a few hours will appear as long rods, while those grown for longer periods will appear as cocci or coccobacilli. Prolonged incubation of culture may be required for the isolation of this organism.

Aerobic Gram-Negative Cocci

Moraxella catarrhalis.   Microscopy and culture are the most commonly used detection methods. Large numbers of organisms associated with polymorphonuclear leukocytes and mucus are typically observed in patients with respiratory tract infections.

Neisseria gonorrhoeae.   Historically, microscopy and culture were the diagnostic tests of choice. For patients with genital infections, the Gram stain has a sensitivity of 90 to 95% and a specificity of 95 to 100% in symptomatic males but a sensitivity of only 50 to 70% in symptomatic females and much lower in

Bacterial Diagnosis

asymptomatic females. The organism grows on chocolate agar, but selective media are used most commonly to suppress the urethral flora. Immunoassays have also been used to detect *N. gonorrhoeae* but are plagued with cross-reactions with saprophytic bacteria (e.g., other *Neisseria* spp., *Moraxella* spp., *Bacteroides* spp., *Peptostreptococcus* spp., and others). For the most part, culture and immunoassays have now been replaced by molecular tests, initially with molecular probes (Gen-Probe PACE2 and the Digene assay) and more recently with amplification methods (Abbott LCx, Roche AMPLICOR, and Becton Dickinson BDProbeTec). The amplification assays are the most sensitive, but care must be taken to eliminate inhibitors present in specimens (particularly in urine) and prevent cross-contamination of specimens. Antibody testing is not useful.

Neisseria meningitidis. Microscopy and culture are the most commonly used detection methods. Tests are available for detecting meningococcal capsular polysaccharide antigens in CSF, serum, and urine. The tests detect serogroups A, B, C, Y, and W135 (serogroup B antibodies cross-react with *E. coli* K1 antigen), and false-positive urine antigen tests have been reported. The test sensitivity approaches 90% for serogroups A, C, Y, and W135 but is much lower for serogroup B. A PCR assay for meningococcal DNA in CSF has been developed but is not commercially available.

Aerobic Gram-Negative Rods

Acinetobacter **spp.** The organisms are gram-negative coccobacilli, occasionally appearing gram positive, and are typically arranged in pairs. Growth on blood agar media is usually good. Most strains are able to grow on MacConkey agar, but there is no growth anaerobically (strict aerobic growth).

Actinobacillus **spp.** The microscopic morphology of the organisms is coccoid to coccobacillary, arranged singly, in pairs, or in short chains. Growth requires enriched media and is enhanced by a CO_2-rich atmosphere. Growth is variable on MacConkey agar; the organism is a facultative anaerobe.

Aeromonas **spp.** Most species grow readily in culture. Selective media (e.g., blood agar with ampicillin [20 µg/ml] and

CIN agar) improve recovery from contaminated specimens. Enrichment broth (e.g., alkaline peptone water) enhances recovery, but its use is generally not indicated. Serological assays have a low sensitivity and specificity and are not recommended.

***Bartonella* spp.** Bacilli may be observed in clinical specimens from diseased patients (e.g., those with cat scratch disease [CSD], bacillary angiomatosis, or peliosis) with the Warthin-Starry silver stain, although this is not commonly used in clinical microbiology laboratories. Some reference laboratories offer PCR assays for these bacteria. Culture is not recommended for patients with CSD but has been successful in other settings. Blood should be processed in the Isolator system, although some success has been achieved with broth-based blood culture systems. Prolonged incubation is required. Tissues should be cultured on heart infusion agar supplemented with rabbit or horse blood. These media are preferred to blood or chocolate agar. Cultures should be maintained in a humid atmosphere for 3 to 4 weeks. Serologic testing is the mainstay of diagnosis, particularly in patients with CSD, with tests performed at the CDC, State laboratories, and some reference laboratories. Commercial test kits are not available in the United States. Cross-reactions are observed in patients with infections caused by *Coxiella* and *Chlamydia* spp.

Bordetella pertussis. Microscopy and culture are relatively insensitive detection methods compared with PCR-based assays. The organisms appear as small gram-negative coccobacilli. They are best observed using a DFA test; commercial monoclonal and polyclonal (for *B. pertussis* and *B. parapertussis*) DFA tests (directed against cell wall lipooligosaccharides) are available. Both tests have a low sensitivity (30 to 70% compared with culture) and specificity. *B. pertussis* is a fastidious, strictly aerobic organism which does not grow on blood agar media or MacConkey agar (*B. parapertussis* grows on blood agar and has variable growth on MacConkey agar). Growth on Regan-Lowe medium is more reliable than on Bordet-Gengou medium. Detection generally requires a minimum of 3 to 4 days of incubation, which should be extended for a week or more. The PCR assay is clearly the most sensitive method for detecting *B. pertussis*. A variety of target genes have been used, including the pertussin toxin promoter region.

Positive tests are observed even after 7 days of effective therapy. Many serologic tests are available, with ELISA being the method of choice. Immunoglobulin G (IgG) and IgA responses to pertussis toxin (PT) or filamentous hemagglutinin (FHA) are reliable indicators of infection. Antibodies to PT are specific for *B. pertussis*; antibodies to FHA are specific to *B. pertussis* and *B. parapertussis* (with cross-reactions with other bacteria). Serologic testing (IgG versus PT) appears to be the most sensitive measure of *B. pertussis* infection in an unimmunized individual, but seroconversion must be demonstrated.

***Brucella* spp.** The organism is a small coccobacillus, with cells arranged typically singly or, less commonly, in pairs and small chains. DFA stains are not available. The organism is a strict aerobe, requiring complex media containing several amino acids, thiamine, nicotinamide, and magnesium ions. The presence of serum and a CO_2-enriched atmosphere enhance growth, and prolonged incubation is required. Various serologic assays have been developed, with the serum agglutination test being the most commonly used. A single titer of $\geq 1:160$ is suggestive of infection (with *B. abortus*, *B. suis*, or *B. melitensis*). Cross-reactions are observed with *F. tularensis, V. cholerae*, and *Y. enterocolitica*. A rapid dipstick assay for IgM antibodies has been developed.

***Burkholderia cepacia* Complex.** Selective media have been used to improve recovery from contaminated specimens. *B. cepacia* selective agar is the most sensitive and selective medium. PCR assays have been developed but are used for organism identification rather than detection. Serologic tests are not available.

Burkholderia pseudomallei. The organisms appear on direct Gram stain as small gram-negative rods with bipolar staining. The cells resemble "safety pins," and this characteristic can be used to make a presumptive identification. Direct detection methods include latex agglutination and enzyme immunoassays (EIA) for antigens excreted in urine (EIA is the more sensitive assay), DFA stains, and PCR. EIA has a sensitivity of 71%, but cross-reactions with *K. pneumoniae* and *E. coli* occur. The DFA test has a similar sensitivity and appears to be specific (the DFA reagents are not commercially available). The currently devel-

Bacterial Diagnosis

oped PCR tests are sensitive but not species specific. The organism grows on blood agar and MacConkey agar, but better recovery is found on Ashdown medium. An enrichment broth of Ashdown medium supplemented with colistin (incubated for 7 days before subculture) improves recovery. A noncommercial indirect hemagglutination assay has been developed; however, cross-reactions with *B. cepacia* complex occur, and high antibody titers are found in healthy individuals living in areas of endemic infection. A single titer cannot be interpreted, and so seroconversion must be demonstrated.

***Campylobacter* spp.**   The bacteria are curved rods typically arranged in pairs (resembling "gull wings" or S-shaped). The bacteria are thin and may not be observed in clinical specimens. Growth of most species requires a microaerophilic atmosphere, and selective medium is recommended for the recovery of *C. jejuni* and *C. coli* from fecal specimens. *C. upsaliensis* may be a common enteric pathogen, but its recovery is compromised because it is inhibited on most selective media for campylobacters. *C. fetus* is more commonly recovered in the blood. A commercial system is available for the detection of *Campylobacter* antigen in stool specimens with a reported sensitivity and specificity of 80 to 89% and 99%, respectively. PCR assays have limited utility because inhibitors in fecal specimens compromise the test sensitivity. Serologic testing is useful for epidemiologic investigations but not for diagnostic purposes.

***Capnocytophaga* spp. (includes former DF-1 and DF-2).** The organisms are fusiform; curved, coccoid, and spindle-shaped forms are also observed. Growth requires enriched media and CO_2; good growth occurs in 2 to 4 days; adherent colonies may be slightly yellow and have either a regular edge or a spreading edge. There is no growth on MacConkey agar; the organism is a facultative anaerobe.

***Cardiobacterium* spp.**   Rods are arranged singly or in pairs, short chains, or rosettes. The organism is facultatively anaerobic, with no growth on MacConkey agar. It is fastidious and slow growing, and requires CO_2.

***Eikenella* spp.**   The organisms are slender, straight rods that are facultatively anaerobic. There is no growth on MacConkey agar; growth requires hemin and is enhanced by CO_2.

Bacterial Diagnosis

Escherichia coli.   Selective media (e.g., MacConkey agar with sorbitol) can be used to detect enterohemorrhagic *E. coli* strains, and immunoassays can be used to detect the Shiga toxins. Commercial assays are also available to detect the heat-labile and heat-stable toxins of enterotoxigenic *E. coli* strains. Molecular tests have been developed to detect virulence factors in these and other *E. coli* strains.

Francisella **spp.**   Microscopy is relatively insensitive. The organism is a very small coccobacillus that retains the safranin counterstain poorly. A polyclonal DFA reagent is available, although the sensitivity and specificity are not well characterized. *Francisella* spp. are fastidious, strict aerobes that fail to grow on blood agar or MacConkey agar. Growth requires media supplemented with sulfhydryl compounds (e.g., cysteine, cystine, thiosulfate, and IsoVitaleX). Growth is slow but good on chocolate agar, Mueller-Hinton agar, and BCYE agar. Media should be incubated for up to 2 weeks. Antigen and PCR tests have been developed, but their sensitivities are low (antigen test, 10^6 bacteria/ml; PCR, 10^2 bacteria/ml). Serologic testing is the most commonly used diagnostic method. Antibodies are detected as early as 1 week after the onset of symptoms and may persist for years. Tube agglutination (TA) and microagglutination (MA) are the standard assays. A single TA titer of $\geq$1:160 or MA titer of $\geq$1:128 is considered a presumptive positive reaction. A fourfold titer change is considered diagnostic.

Haemophilus ducreyi.   The Gram stain morphology of this organism has been described as "long chains ('schools of fish')," but this description is more characteristic of in vitro cultures than of specimens collected from genital ulcers. The Gram stain sensitivity is <50%. Direct fluorescent-antibody (DFA) assay reagents have been prepared, but polyclonal antisera have poor specificity and monoclonal antisera are not commercially available. Culture requires the use of selective media (e.g., GC agar supplemented with vancomycin, hemoglobin, fetal bovine serum, and IsoVitaleX) and has variable sensitivity. PCR-based assays have been developed but are not widely available.

Haemophilus influenzae.   The organisms are pleomorphic rods (i.e., coccoid, coccobacillary, or short rods); they are facultatively anaerobic, with no growth on sheep blood agar or MacConkey agar. Detection of type-specific capsular antigen

Bacterial Diagnosis

has been used to diagnose disseminated disease (i.e., meningitis); however, this test is no more sensitive than a Gram stain, and vaccination has dramatically reduced the incidence of *H. influenzae* disease. PCR-based tests have also been developed but are rarely used. Serologic testing is generally restricted to demonstration of a response to vaccination.

Helicobacter pylori. Microscopy is useful for examination of tissue biopsy specimens but is performed primarily in cytology laboratories. Diagnosis is most commonly made using antigen tests, particularly the detection of urease activity in tissue biopsy specimens or by breath analysis. The tests vary widely in sensitivity and specificity but generally are >90% sensitive and specific. PCR assays are available but offer no more sensitivity than the antigen tests. Culture can also be performed (and is useful if drug resistance is suspected). The organism grows best on freshly prepared nonselective media (e.g., brucella or brain heart infusion agars supplemented with horse blood) incubated in a microaerophilic atmosphere for a minimum of 5 days. A variety of serologic tests are also available. Serum IgG assays are the tests of choice, although whole-blood assays are used with increasing frequency in physician offices (the tests have a sensitivity of 80 to 90% compared with serum assays). Serum IgA assays have a low sensitivity but may prove useful as a follow-up assay for patients with negative IgG assays.

***Kingella* spp.** The organisms are nutritionally fastidious, facultatively anaerobic short rods with square ends, arranged in pairs or chains. They decolorize unevenly on Gram staining. They do not require CO_2, but growth is enhanced; there is no growth on MacConkey agar.

***Legionella* spp.** *Legionella* spp. are small, poorly staining rods. If observed in clinical specimens, they typically appear as coccobacilli; long filamentous forms can be seen in culture. Monoclonal and polyclonal DFA stains are commercially available; their sensitivity compared with culture is poor (33 to 70%), and cross-reactions are observed with the monoclonal reagents (*Bacillus cereus*) and polyclonal reagents (*Bacteroides fragilis*, *Pseudomonas* spp., *Stenotrophomonas* spp., and *Bordetella pertussis*). Urinary antigen tests for *L. pneumophila* serogroup 1 are available (Wampole Laboratories, Bartels) and Binax and

Biotest market urinary antigen tests for non-serogroup 1 *L. pneumophila* and other *Legionella* spp. The sensitivity of these assays varies, but sensitivities are reported in the range of 70 to 80%. The specificity is good, although the Bartels test reacts with *S. pneumoniae* and false-positive reactions due to nonspecific protein binding have been reported for the Binax EIA. Reactivity persists in *Legionella*-infected patients for weeks to months after effective therapy. PCR assays are available but generally are not more sensitive than culture. The organism is fastidious, requiring media supplemented with L-cysteine and iron salts. BCYE, supplemented with antibiotics to suppress the growth of contaminating organisms, is the medium of choice. Incubation should be extended for a week or more. IFA tests and ELISA are available to measure an antibody response to infection. The test sensitivity and specificity are 75 and 96%, respectively. A titer of ≥1:256 is suggestive of current infection; however, titers at this level have been found in healthy individuals. A fourfold change in titer is presumptive evidence of recent disease.

Pasteurella spp.   The organisms are coccoid to coccobacillary, arranged singly, in pairs, or in short chains. Growth does not require hemin or CO_2, but some strains require V factor. The most commonly isolated species fail to grow on MacConkey agar; the organism is a facultative anaerobe.

Pseudomonas aeruginosa.   *P. aeruginosa* grows readily on a variety of laboratory media. PCR amplification methods have been developed for direct detection of the organism in respiratory specimens, particularly from cystic fibrosis patients. A fluorescent in situ hybridization (FISH) method has also been developed. The method is rapid but less sensitive than culture. Serologic testing is not useful.

Salmonella enterica Serovar Typhi.   Selective media must be used to optimize detection in fecal specimens. The Widal test measures agglutinating antibodies to the O and H antigens of *S. enterica* serovar Typhi and is used for serodiagnosis; however, it lacks sensitivity and specificity. Tests using other antigens (e.g., Vi antigen) have been developed but are restricted to epidemiological studies.

Salmonella, Other Serovars.   Selective media must be used to optimize detection in fecal specimens.

***Shigella* spp.** Selective media must be used to optimize detection in fecal specimens. Serodiagnostic assays have been developed for epidemiological surveys but have not been used for diagnostic testing.

***Stenotrophomonas* spp.** Microscopy and culture are sensitive detection methods. PCR assays have been developed but are not used for organism detection.

***Streptobacillus* spp.** The organisms are rod shaped, but on extended incubation they can form very long filaments (100 to 150 µm long) and bulbous forms. Colonies develop slowly. The organism is facultatively anaerobic; no growth occurs on MacConkey agar.

Vibrio cholerae. The viability of *V. cholerae* is maintained at an alkaline pH but decreases in formed stools or at an acidic pH. If culture is delayed, the specimen should be stored in Cary-Blair transport medium but not in buffered glycerol saline. The organism grows well on blood agar, slowly on MacConkey agar (lactose-negative), and well on selective media (e.g., TCBS). A reverse passive latex agglutination test is commercially available for the detection of cholera toxin (reacts also with *E. coli* heat-labile enterotoxin). Reference laboratories are also able to measure antibody response to infection.

***Vibrio*, Other spp.** Most pathogenic vibrios grow well on blood agar and MacConkey agar. As with *V. cholerae*, specimens should be processed immediately or transported in Cary-Blair medium. *V. parahaemolyticus* hemolysin (Kanagawa toxin) can be detected directly in specimens by a commercial reverse passive latex agglutination test.

Yersinia enterocolitica. The use of enrichment methods (e.g., storage of specimens inoculated into phosphate-buffered saline for up to 21 days at 4°C) for recovery of *Y. enterocolitica* is generally not necessary for diagnosis of patients with diarrhea but has proven useful for diagnosis of patients with terminal ileitis or postinfectious arthritis. CIN agar is the preferred selective medium, and growth is better at 25 to 30°C than at 35°C. MacConkey agar (lactose-negative colonies) can also be used. PCR tests directed against plasmid and chromosomal virulence factors have been developed but are not widely available. Antibodies against serogroups O:3, O:9, O:5, 27, and O:8 can be detected by tube or microtiter agglutination tests. Titers of $\geq 1:40$ or a fourfold rise in titer is considered significant. Cross-reactions occur with *Brucella* spp. These tests are available through specialty laboratories but are not commercially available.

Yersinia pestis. A variety of stains have been used (i.e., Giemsa, Wright, Wayson, methylene blue) in addition to the Gram stain. The characteristic "bipolar, safety pin" morphology is not observed with the Gram stain. A DFA stain directed against the capsular F1 antigen is performed by State Health Department laboratories but is not commercially available. The organism can be isolated on nonselective agar (sheep blood agar or brain heart infusion agar) or from contaminated specimens on MacConkey agar or CIN agar (with a reduced cefsulodin concentration [4 μg/ml]). Pinpoint growth is seen at 24 h. PCR directed against the genes for the plasminogen activator protein (*pla*) and capsular F1 antigen (*caf1*) have been developed but are less sensitive than culture and an ELISA for capsular F1 antigen. Passive hemagglutination tests and ELISAs, available through the CDC, have been developed to detect antibodies directed against the F1 antigen. A titer of $\geq 1:10$ is presumptive evidence of disease, and a fourfold rise or fall in the antibody titer is confirmatory.

Anaerobic Bacteria

***Actinomyces* spp.** The organisms may grow slowly in an aerobic atmosphere, and some strains are difficult to isolate in culture. Microscopic examination of "sulfur granules" (macroscopic colonies present in clinical specimens) is helpful for making the diagnosis of actinomycosis.

***Bacteroides fragilis* Group.** The organisms typically appear as pleomorphic rods in clinical specimens. Growth is rapid on most anaerobic media, although selective media (e.g., laked kanamycin-vancomycin sheep blood agar and bacteroides bile esculin agar) should be used with contaminated specimens.

Clostridium botulinum. Microscopy is generally of little value except when examining implicated food products. The

CDC provides tests measuring the level of antibodies against *C. botulinum* toxin (antitoxin levels) in patients immunized with toxoid. These tests assess immunity and cannot be used for the diagnosis of botulism. The appropriate diagnostic test for food-borne botulism is demonstration of botulinal toxin in serum, feces, gastric contents, or vomitus or recovery of the organism in the feces of the patient. Demonstration of the organism or toxin in suspected foods provides indirect evidence of botulism. The presence of the organism or detection of toxin in wound exudates confirms the diagnosis of wound botulism.

Clostridium difficile. Microscopic examination of fecal specimens is of little clinical utility. Culture on selective media such as cycloserine-cefoxitin-fructose agar is a sensitive method for detecting the organism but does not differentiate between colonization and clinically significant disease. Detection of antigen (i.e., cytotoxin or enterotoxins) is the diagnostic test of choice. A variety of immunoassays have been developed that detect one or both toxins. The tests vary widely in sensitivity and specificity, but the accuracy of the better tests is generally >90%. PCR methods have been used to detect *C. difficile* in specimens and to differentiate between toxigenic and nontoxigenic strains. These tests are not commonly used.

Clostridium perfringens. The microscopic morphology is characteristic (large, short, fat, rectangular cells with no spores observed). Growth on anaerobic sheep blood agar is rapid, with a double zone of hemolysis typically observed. Antigen tests for detection of toxins have not been developed, and PCR assays are restricted to research laboratories.

Clostridium tetani. Microscopy and culture are typically of little use because relatively small numbers of organisms can cause clinical disease. However, observation of the organisms in clinical specimens or recovery in culture can be diagnostic in the appropriate clinical setting. Serologic testing is also not useful for diagnostic purposes because antibodies are not formed in patients with clinical disease. It can be useful for assessing the immune status of an individual, with antitoxin levels of ≥0.5 IU/ml generally considered protective.

***Fusobacterium* spp.** Some species (e.g., *F. nucleatum*) have characteristic thin, fusiform morphology. Culture may require prolonged incubation (5 days or more).

***Mobiluncus* spp.** Routine culture of vaginal specimens for *Mobiluncus* spp. is generally not clinically useful. The preferred diagnostic test is microscopy, with curved rods observed in vaginal smears.

***Peptostreptococcus* spp.** Prolonged incubation may be required for more astidious species. The same comments apply to newer genera of anaerobic cocci that were formerly classified in this genus.

Curved and Spiral-Shaped Bacteria

Borrelia burgdorferi. Microscopic examination of blood, CSF, and other specimens is not useful for patients with Lyme disease because the level of spirochetes is below the detection level. Culture on media such as modified Kelly medium can be performed, although extended incubation must be used and the yield is low. ELISAs have been developed to detect antigen in tissues, but the method is not recommended. PCR assays have been developed for the detection of *B. burgdorferi*. The sensitivity of the assay depends on the testing method, target gene, and stage of illness. The following test sensitivities have been reported: skin, 50 to 70% for culture or PCR; synovial fluid, 50 to 70% for PCR, culture seldom positive; CSF, 10 to 30% for culture or PCR; and urine, 0%. Serologic testing has been the method most commonly used for the diagnosis of Lyme disease. The early antibody response is primarily an IgM response and is directed against outer membrane-associated protein OspC, p35, and flagellum subunits p37 and p41. The antibody titers peak within a week of clinical onset but may persist for months, even after effective treatment. IgG antibodies appear after the first weeks of disease, with reactivity against p37, p41, and OspC early in disease; against p39 and p58 in the early disseminated stage; and against a wide variety of antigen in the late disseminated stage. Reactivity against other antigens is also commonly observed. Assay methods include IFA, EIA, and immunoblotting. The specificity of IFA is improved by adsorption of sera with *Treponema phagedenis* sonicate. IFA titers of ≥1:64 are regarded as positive. This assay is difficult to standardize, and EIA is the preferred testing method. Immunoblotting is used to identify which antigens are reactive. The recommended approach to serodiagnosis is to screen serum or CSF for IgG and IgM antibodies with EIA. If the reaction is positive or borderline,

Bacterial Diagnosis

IgG and IgM immunoblotting is performed. The sensitivity of serologic testing is as follows: stage 1 (early, localized disease), 20 to 50% with IgM predominant; stage 2 (early, disseminated disease), 70 to 90% with IgG predominant; stage 3 (late, disseminated disease), nearly 100% with IgG predominant. Antibodies persist for months despite treatment.

***Borrelia*, Other spp.**   Patients with relapsing fever have large numbers of borreliae in their blood during febrile attacks. The diagnostic method of choice is microscopy, with the blood examined by dark-field microscopy or stained with Giemsa. Small numbers of bacteria can be concentrated in buffy coat preparations. Culture on media such as modified Kelly medium can be performed, although the cultures should be incubated at 30°C for at least 6 weeks.

***Leptospira* spp.**   The organisms may be detected by dark-field microscopy or DFA, although large numbers of organisms (10^4/ml) must be present in the specimen. Culture of blood and CSF during the first week of illness and culture of urine beginning in the second week can be performed using Ellinghausen-McCullough-Johnson-Harris medium. Cultures are incubated at 28 to 30°C and examined weekly by dark-field microscopy for up to 13 weeks. PCR assays have been developed but are not used extensively. Serologic testing is the most commonly used diagnostic method. Antibodies are detected by using the microscopic agglutination test with blood 5 to 7 days after onset of symptoms. Paired sera are required to confirm the diagnosis, with a presumptive diagnosis being made if a single serum has a titer of ≥1:200. The test is technically complex, and other assays have been developed. The indirect hemagglutination assay was shown to have a sensitivity and specificity of 92 and 95%, respectively. Latex agglutination assays and ELISAs have also been developed but have not been adequately evaluated.

Treponema pallidum.   When available, dark-field microscopy is very sensitive for diagnosis based on a freshly sampled genital chancre or secondary-stage exudates. The DFA test for *T. pallidum* (DFA-TP) does not require viable spirochetes and can differentiate between *T. pallidum* and nonpathogenic spirochetes. The test sensitivity for primary or secondary syphilis approaches 100%. The organism has not been grown in vitro, and antigen tests are not available. PCR methods have been developed but currently are restricted to research laboratories. Serologic testing by nontreponemal and treponemal assays is the most common diagnostic method. The nontreponemal assays include the Venereal Disease Research Laboratory (VDRL) test, rapid plasma regain (RPR) card test, unheated serum regain (USR) test, and toluidine red unheated serum test (TRUST). Treponemal tests include fluorescent treponemal antibody-absorption (FTA-ABS) test, treponemal pallidum particle agglutination (TP-PA) test, and EIA. The test sensitivities vary with the method and stage of disease. In general, nontreponemal tests have a sensitivity of 72 to >90% for the primary stage, 100% for the secondary stage, 95 to 100% for latent disease, and <75% for the late stage, while treponemal tests have a sensitivity of 80 to >90% for the primary stage, 100% for the secondary and latent stages, and >95% for the late stage. A number of conditions affect the test specificity, with more false-positive reactions being observed with nontreponemal tests.

Mycoplasma spp. and Obligate Intracellular Bacteria

***Anaplasma* spp.**   *Anaplasma* spp. were formerly members of the genus *Ehrlichia*. Giemsa or Wright stains of peripheral blood or buffy coat cells have a sensitivity approaching 60%. As with *Ehrlichia* spp., PCR assays have been developed and have a wide range of sensitivities (50 to 86%). Their specificity is reported to be 100%. IFA is the serologic method of choice. The typical response during the acute phase of infection is a rapid rise in antibody levels, reaching titers of $\geq 1{:}640$ within the first month of disease. Antibodies can persist for many months to years. The test sensitivity is >90%. False-positive reactions have been encountered for patients with infections caused by *Rickettsia* spp., *Coxiella* spp., and Epstein-Barr virus. Patients with high *Anaplasma* titers will also have elevated titers to *B. burgdorferi*.

***Chlamydia trachomatis*.**   Infections have historically been confirmed by culture, observation of elementary bodies in specimens by DFA, or detection of chlamydial antigens (i.e., lipopolysaccharide and major outer membrane proteins) by EIA. DFA has a sensitivity and specificity of 75 to 85 and 99%, respectively. The sensitivity of EIAs is reported to be 60 to 70% compared with that of nucleic acid amplification assays. More recently, these methods have been replaced by molecular methods, initially probe tests and now amplification tests. Amplification tests are the most sensitive, although care must be taken to eliminate inhibitors (particularly in urine) and to avoid cross-contamination of specimens. Two serologic assays are in common use: CF and microimmunofluorescence (micro-IF). The CF test detects antibodies to *C. trachomatis* as well as to *Chlamydophila psittaci* and *Chlamydophila pneumoniae*. The micro-IF test is type specific. The CF test is positive in virtually all patients with lymphogranuloma venereum but generally not positive in patients with oculogenital infections and trachoma. A positive CF titer is ≥1:16. CF titers for patients with lymphogranuloma venereum generally exceed 1:128, while patients with inclusion conjunctivitis, cervicitis, or urethritis have antibody titers of <1:16. The micro-IF test is more sensitive than the CF test. Most patients with chlamydial infections show positive reactivity (90 to 100% of patients have detectable IgG antibodies). However, antibodies to past infections persist for years and are commonly detected in the assay.

Chlamydophila pneumoniae. Most infections are diagnosed by either PCR-based assays or serological testing. Commercial PCRs (or other nucleic acid amplification methods) are not commercially available, although the test is widely performed in reference laboratories. Micro-IF testing is the method of choice for diagnosing acute infections. Cross-reactivity with other bacteria is uncommon. Serum specimens are generally screened for IgM and IgG antibodies at 1:8, and those giving positive reactions are tested at increasing twofold dilutions. The diagnostic criteria for acute infections include at least a fourfold rise in titer and a single serum IgM titer of ≥1:16 and/or IgG titer of ≥1:512.

Chlamydophila psittaci. Most infections are diagnosed by serological methods, with the CF test being the most common.

***Coxiella* spp.** *C. burnetii* can be recovered in culture, although this is rarely attempted. PCR appears to be sensitive but is currently restricted to research laboratories. A variety of serologic methods, including microagglutination, CF, IFA, and ELISA, have been used, with IFA currently being the method of choice. ELISA appears to be more sensitive than IFA, but interpretive standards have not been defined. Antigenic phase variation occurs with *C. burnetii* infections. In acute self-limited infections, antibodies to the phase II antigen appear first and dominate the immune response. In chronic infections, antibodies to the phase I antigen predominate. Phase II antibodies appear first and peak within 1 month at 1:1,024 or greater. Phase I antibodies appear later and peak at 4 months. The ratio between phase I and phase II responses may be useful for distinguishing between acute and chronic infections. A phase I titer of 1:800 or greater is diagnostic of chronic Q fever (e.g., endocarditis).

***Ehrlichia* spp.**   *Ehrlichia* spp. have been successfully cultured from blood, although this test is rarely used for diagnosis. Likewise, infected monocytes can be detected by use of Giemsa- or Wright-stained peripheral blood or buffy coat cells, but this test has a sensitivity of only <30%. PCR is a widely used diagnostic test, with the 16S rRNA gene being targeted; it has a sensitivity of 79 to 100% for *E. chaffeensis* or *E. canis* compared with serologic testing. Serological testing is also useful, with IFA being the test of choice. Although a specific antibody titer has not been defined for significant disease, a titer of ≥1:64 is considered presumptive evidence of past or current disease.

Mycoplasma pneumoniae.   Microscopy is not useful, and isolation of *M. pneumoniae* in culture is slow and insensitive. For this reason, a variety of antigen-directed tests including DFA, EIA, and immunoblotting have been developed. These tests, as well as DNA probes, have poor sensitivity and specificity. In contrast, PCR assays are reported to be highly sensitive and specific. Specific serologic tests include complement fixation (CF), ELISA, IFA, and latex agglutination. CF detects primarily IgM antibodies. Seroconversion is observed for about 60% of culture-positive patients, while 80 to 90% of patients have a single titer of >1:32. ELISA detects both IgM and IgG antibodies and appears to be more sensitive than CF. Specificity can be improved by using purified P1 adhesin protein as the capture antigen. Immunofluorescence IgG and IgM antibody titers of ≥1:10 are considered positive, with active disease being indicated by a fourfold change in titer. The latex agglutination assay detects IgG and IgM antibodies. A single agglutination antibody titer of ≥1:320 or a fourfold change in titer is indicative of active or recent infection. The specificity of each of these tests is a problem because cross-reactions with other *Mycoplasma* spp. have been observed.

Rickettsia rickettsii. Members of the spotted fever group of rickettsiae can be detected in tissue specimens by immunofluorescence or PCR. The 17-kDa lipoprotein gene is the principal target of PCR, although other targets have also been used. These tests are restricted primarily to reference laboratories. A variety of group-specific serologic tests have been developed (e.g., IFA, CF, ELISA, RIA, latex agglutination, and hemagglutination), with the IFA being considered the "gold standard." A diagnostic titer of ≥1:64 is usually detected in the second week of illness. The Proteus OX agglutination test was used historically but has been replaced by the more specific serologic tests.

General Comments about Molecular Methods for the Identification of Bacteria

Refer to NCCLS document MM3-A (*Molecular Diagnostic Methods for Infectious Diseases*, 1995, NCCLS, Wayne, Pa.) for more detailed comments.

DNA Sequencing

DNA sequencing for microbial identification involves extraction of the nucleic acids, amplification of the target sequence by PCR, sequence determination, and a computer software-aided search of an appropriate sequence database. The most widely used targets are the 16S rDNA gene and the *hsp65* gene. The DNA sequence of the 16S rRNA gene is a stable genotypic signature that can be used to identify an organism at the genus or the species level. Comparative studies of the available phenotypic and genetic methods, which include well-characterized clinical and reference isolates, are needed to determine the best technique for identification of each major pathogen. Some bacterial species are very closely related and not separated by initial sequencing. This test is performed with isolates from solid media or from broth cultures.

PCR and Restriction Endonuclease Analysis

PCR and restriction endonuclease analysis is based on PCR of a sequence of the gene encoding the 65k-Da heat shock protein (*hsp65*), followed by restriction enzyme digestion and analysis of the digestion products. This method has been extensively used for *Mycobacterium* and *Nocardia* identification. It is performed using isolates from solid media or from broth cultures.

Nonamplified Nucleic Acid Probes

AccuProbe (GenProbe Inc.) acridinium ester-labeled DNA probes are based on the detection of rRNA specific for numerous organisms including mycobacteria, group A streptocoocci, *Neisseria gonorrhoeae*, and *Streptococcus pneumoniae*. Target 16S rRNA is released from the organism by sonication. The labeled DNA probe combines with the organism's rRNA to form a DNA-rRNA hybrid. The labeled product is detected in a luminometer. This test is performed using isolates from solid media or from broth cultures.

Bacterial Diagnosis

Table 4.5 Differential characteristics of catalase-positive gram-positive cocci

Genus	Strict aerobe	Adherent to agar	Growth in 6.5% NaCl	Oxidase	Motility	Lysostaphin (200 µg/ml)	Erythromycin (0.4 µg/ml)	Bacitracin (0.04-U disk)	Furazolidone (100-µg disk)
Staphylococcus	−	±	+	−[d]	−	S	R	R	S
Micrococcus[b]	+	−	+	+	−	R	S	S	R
Planococcus	+	−	+	NT[a]	+	R	NT	NT	S
Alloiococcus[c]	+	−	+	−	−	NT	NT	NT	NT
Rothia	−	+	−	−	−	R	NT	S	NT

[a] NT, not tested.
[b] Includes the related genera *Kocuria, Kytococcus, Nesterenkonia, Dermacoccus,* and *Arthrobacter.*
[c] *Alloiococcus* is weakly catalase positive or catalase negative.
[d] *Staphylococcus lentus, S. sciuri,* and *S. vitulus* are oxidase positive.

Table 4.6 Differential characteristics of common *Staphylococcus* species

Staphylococcus species	Coagulase	Clumping factor	Heat-stable nuclease	Alkaline phosphatase	PYR[a] hydrolysis	Ornithine decarboxylase	Urease	β-Galactosidase	Voges-Proskauer	Novobiocin	Polymyxin B
S. aureus	+	+	+	+	−	−	V	−	+	S	R
S. epidermidis	−	−	−	+	−	V	+	−	+	S	R
S. haemolyticus	−	−	−	−	+	−	−	−	+	S	S
S. hyicus	V	−	+	+	−	−	V	−	−	S	R
S. intermedius	+	V	+	+	+	−	+	+	−	S	S
S. lugdunensis	−	(+)	−	−	+	+	V	−	+	S	V
S. saprophyticus	−	−	−	−	−	−	+	+	+	R	S
S. schleiferi	−	+	+	+	−	−	−	(+)	+	S	S

[a]PYR, pyrrolidonyl arylamidase.

Bacterial Diagnosis

Table 4.7 Differential characteristics of catalase-negative gram-positive cocci

Genus	Pyrrolidonyl arylamidase	Leucine aminopeptidase	Morphology[a]	Growth in 6.5% NaCl	Satellite growth	Motility	Vancomycin	Arginine hydrolysis	β-Glucuronidase	Esculin hydrolysis
Enterococcus	+	+	Chains	+	−	V[d]	S/R	+	−	+
Abiotrophia	+	+	Clusters	−	+	−	S			
Gemella	+	+	Chains[b]	−	−	−	S			
Granulicatella	+	+	Chains	−	−	−	S			
Facklamia	+	+	Chains[c]	+	−	−	S	V[e]	V[e]	−
Vagococcus	+	+	Chains	V	−	+	S			
Globicatella	+	−	Chains	+	−	−	S			

Aerococcus viridans	+	–	Clusters	+	–	–	S
Aerococcus urinae	–	+	Clusters	+	–	–	S
Pediococcus	–	+	Clusters	V	–	–	R
Lactococcus	V	+	Chains	V	–	–	S
Streptococcus	V	+	Chains	V	–	–	S
Leuconostoc	–	–	Chains	+	–	–	R

[a] Cellular morphology in broth culture.
[b] *Gemella haemolysans* is arranged in clusters.
[c] *Facklamia languida* is arranged in clusters.
[d] *Enterococcus casseliflavus* and *E. gallinarum* are motile.
[e] *Granulicatella adiacens* is ARG negative and BGUR positive; *G. elegans* is ARG positive and BGUR negative.

Bacterial Diagnosis

Bacterial Diagnosis

Table 4.8 Differential characteristics of beta-hemolytic streptococci[a]

Streptococcus species	Lancefield group	PYR	Bacitracin	Voges-Proskauer	CAMP	Hippurate	BGUR
S. pyogenes	A	+	+	–	–	–	NT
S. agalactiae	B	–	–	–	+	+	NT
S. dysgalactiae subsp. equisimilis	C, G	–	–	–	–	–	+
S. anginosus group	A, C, F, G, nongrp	–	–	+	–	–	–

[a]PYR, pyrrolidonyl arylamidase; BGUR, ß-glucuronidase; NT, not tested.

Table 4.9 Differential characteristics of viridans streptococci

Streptococcus group[a]	Acid from:		Voges-Proskauer	Hydrolysis of:	
	Mannitol	Sorbitol		Arginine	Esculin
S. mitis group	−	−	−	−	−
S. sanguis group	−	V	−	+	V
S. salivarius group	−	−	+	−	+
S. mutans group	+	+	+	−	V
S. anginosus group	−	−	+	+	V
S. bovis group	+	−	+	−	+

[a]S. mitis group: S. mitis, S. oralis, S. crista, S. peroris, S. infantis; S. sanguis group: S. sanguis, S. parasanguis, S. gordonii; S. salivarius group: S. salivarius, S. vestibularis; S. mutans group: S. mutans, S sobrinus; S. anginosus group: S. anginosus, S. intermedius, S. constellatus; S. bovis group: S. bovis.

Bacterial Diagnosis

Table 4.10 Differential characteristics of common *Enterococcus* species

Group	Species	Arabinose	Mannitol[a]	Sorbitol[a]	Raffinose	Sucrose	Pyruvate	Arginine hydrolysis[a]	Growth in 0.04% tellurite	Motility	Pigment production	Methyl-α-D-glucopyranoside
				Acid from:								
I	*E. avium*	+	+	+	−	+	+	−	−	−	−	+
	E. raffinosus	+	+	+	+	+	+	−	−	−	−	+
II	*E. faecalis*	−	+	+	−	+	+	+	+	−	−	−
	E. faecium	+	+	>	>	+	−	+	−	−	−	+
	E. casseliflavus	+	+	>	+	+	>	+	−	+	+	+
	E. gallinarum	+	+	−	+	+	−	+	−	+	−	+
III	*E. durans*	−	−	−	−	−	−	+	−	−	−	−
	E. hirae	−	−	−	>	+	−	+	−	−	−	−
	E. dispar	−	−	−	+	+	−	+	−	−	−	+
IV	*E. cecorum*	−	−	+	+	+	+	−	−	−	−	−

[a]Key tests for grouping enterococci.

Table 4.11 Differential characteristics of gram-positive rods

Catalase negative
    Beta-hemolytic — *Arcanobacterium*
    Alpha-hemolytic — *Erysipelothrix*, *Lactobacillus*
    Nonhemolytic — *Actinomyces*

Catalase positive
    Regular shape, spore former — *Bacillus*, *Paenibacillus*
    Regular shape, non-spore former — *Listeria*
    Irregular shape, pink pigment — *Rhodococcus equi*
    Irregular shape, orange pigment — *Rhodococcus*, *Microbacterium*, *Nocardia*
    Irregular shape, yellow pigment — *Oerskovia*, *Brevibacterium*, *Cellulomonas*, *Aureobacterium*
    Irregular shape, no pigment
        Bacillary — *Corynebacterium*
        Coccobacillary — *Arthrobacter*, *Brevibacterium*, *Corynebacterium*, *Dermabacter*, *Rhodococcus*
        Branching — *Nocardia*, *Actinomyces*, *Propionibacterium*, *Rothia*, *Streptomyces*, *Turicella*

Bacterial Diagnosis

Bacterial Diagnosis

Table 4.12 Differential characteristics of selected *Corynebacterium* species

Species	Fermentation/oxidation	Lipophilism	Nitrate reduction	Urease	Esculin hydrolysis	Acid from: Glucose	Maltose	Sucrose	Mannitol	Xylose	Comments
C. jeikeium	O	+	−	+	−	+	V	−	−	−	Strict aerobe
C. urealyticum	O	+	−	+	−	−	−	−	−	−	Strong urease production
C. pseudodiphtheriticum	O	−	+	+	−	−	−	−	−	−	
C. diphtheriae	F	−	+	−	−	+	+	−	−	−	
C. ulcerans	F	−	−	+	−	+	+	−	−	−	CAMP inhibited
C. amycolatum	F	+	V	V	−	+	V	V	V	−	
C. macginleyi	F	+	+	−	−	+	−	+	V	−	From eye; may have rose color
C. minutissimum	F	−	−	−	−	+	+	V	V	−	
C. striatum	F	−	+	−	−	+	+	V	V	−	
C. glucuronolyticum	F	−	V	V	V	+	V	+	−	V	CAMP and BGUR positive, floral odor
C. pseudotuberculosis	F	−	V	+	−	+	+	V	−	−	CAMP inhibited

Table 4.13 Differential characteristics of selected coryneform bacteria

Organism	Fermentation/ oxidation	Catalase	Nitrate reduction	Esculin hydrolysis	Motility	Acid from: Glucose	Maltose	Sucrose	Mannitol	Xylose	Comments
Turicella otitidis	O	+	−	−	−	−	−	−	−	−	Ear, CAMP positive
Arthrobacter spp.	O	+	V	V	V	V	V	V	−	−	
Brevibacterium spp.	O	+	V	−	−	V	V	V	−	−	Cheese-like odor
Microbacterium spp.	O/F	V	V	V	V	+	+	V	V	V	Yellow pigment
Arcanobacterium bernardiae	F	−	−	−	−	+	+	−	−	−	
Arcanobacterium haemolyticum	F	−	−	−	−	+	+	V	−	−	CAMP inhibited
Arcanobacterium pyogenes	F	−	−	V	−	+	V	V	V	+	Weak hemolysis
Gardnerella vaginalis	F	−	−	−	−	+	+	V	−	−	Gram variable to gram negative
Dermabacter hominis	F	+	−	+	−	+	+	+	−	V	Coccoid to coccobacillary
Rothia dentocariosa	F	V	+	+	−	+	+	+	−	−	
Oerskovia turbata	F	+	+	+	V	+	+	+	−	+	Pale yellow

Bacterial Diagnosis

Table 4.14 Differential characteristics of selected *Bacillus* species and related genera

Organism	Growth:			Lecithinase (egg yolk)	Casein hydrolysis	Gelatin hydrolysis	Arginine dihydrolase	Acid from:					
	Anaerobic	50°C	60°C					D-Arabinose	Glycerol	Glycogen	Inulin	Mannitol	Salicin
B. anthracis	+	–	–	+	+	+	–	–	–	+	–	–	–
B. cereus	+	–	–	+	+	+	v	–	v	+	–	–	+
B. thuringiensis	+	–	–	+	+	+	+	–	+	+	–	–	+
B. mycoides	+	–	–	+	+	+	v	–	+	+	–	–	+
B. subtilis	–	v	–	–	+	+	–	–	+	+	+	+	+
B. licheniformis	+	+	–	–	+	+	+	–	+	+	v	+	+
B. circulans	+	–	–	–	–	–	–	–	v	+	+	+	+
B. stearothermophilus	–	+	+	–	v	+	–	–	+	+	–	–	–
Paenibacillus	–	–	–	–	v	+	–	v	+	+	v	+	v
Virgibacillus	–	v	–	–	+	+	–	+	+	–	–	–	+

Table 4.15 Differential characteristics of selected actinomycetes[a,b]

Genus	Vegetative filaments Substrate	Vegetative filaments Aerial	Conidia	Acid-fast nature	Mycolic acids	Metabolism of glucose	Growth at 50°C	Arylsulfatase	Growth in lysozyme
Actinomadura	+	V	V	–	–	O	–	–	–
Amycolatopsis	+	+	V	–	–	O	–	–	–
Corynebacterium	+	–	–	–	+	O, F	–	–	NT
Dermatophilus	+	–	–	–	–	F	–	–	V
Gordonia	+	–	–	W	+	O	–	–	–
Micromonospora	+	–	+	–	–	O	–	–	–
Mycobacterium	+	–	–	+	+	O	–	+	–
Nocardia	+	+	V	W	+	O	–	–	+
Nocardiopsis	+	+	+	–	–	O	–	–	–
Rhodococcus	+	–	–	W	+	O	–	–	V
Saccharomonospora	+	+	+	–	–	O	+	–	–
Saccharopolyspora	+	+	+	–	–	O	+	–	V
Streptomyces	+	+	+	–	–	O	–	–	–
Thermoactinomyces	+	+	+	–	–	O	+	–	+
Tsukamurella	+	–	–	W	+	O	–	–	+

[a] Adapted from P. R. Murray, E. J. Baron, J. H. Jorgensen, M. A. Pfaller, and R. H. Yolken (ed.), *Manual of Clinical Microbiology*, 8th ed., ASM Press, Washington, D.C., 2003.

[b] W, weak or partially acid fast; O, oxidative; F, fermentative.

Bacterial Diagnosis

Bacterial Diagnosis

Table 4.16 Differential characteristics of selected *Nocardia* species[a]

| Species | Arylsulfatase (14 day) | Hydrolysis of: | | | | | Susceptibility to: | | | | | | | |
		Acetamide	Casein	Tyrosine	Xanthine	Opacification of Middlebrook agar	Amikacin	Cefotaxime	Ceftriaxone	Ciprofloxacin	Erythromycin	Gentamicin	Imipenem	Tobramycin
N. abscessus	NT	NT	–	–	–	NT	S	S	S	R	R	S	R	NT
N. cyriacigeorgica	–	V	–	–	–	–	S	S	S	R	R	I	S	NT
N. farcinica	–	+	–	–	–	+	S	R	R	NT	R	R	R	R
N. nova	V	–	–	–	–	–	S	I	I	R	S	NT	S	NT
N. brasiliensis	–	–	+	+	–	–	S	V	V	I/R	NT	NT	NT	NT
N. pseudobrasiliensis	–	–	+	+	–	–	S	V	V	S	NT	NT	NT	NT
N. otitidiscaviarum	–	–	–	–	+	–	NT	NT	NT	NT	NT	NT	NT	NT
N. asteroides IV/ *N. transvalensis*	NT	NT	NT	NT	NT	NT	R	NT	NT	NT	NT	R	NT	R

[a]The taxonomy of this genus has been extensively modified; molecular testing is required for identification of most species.

Table 4.17 Differential characteristics of selected weakly acid-fast *Rhodococcus*, *Gordonia*, and *Tsukamurella* species

Species	Hydrolysis of:					Utilization of:							
	Adenine (4 wk)	Tyrosine (4 wk)	Hypoxanthine (4 wk)	Xanthine (3 wk)	Acetamide	Cellobiose	Citrate	D-Galactose	i-*myo*-Inositol	Maltose	D-Mannitol	L-Rhamnose	D-Sorbitol
R. equi[a]	+	−			(+)		−	+	−	−	−	V	−
G. bronchialis					+		−	−	+		−	−	−
G. sputi					−		−	+	−		+	−	+
G. terrae					−		+	+	−		+	+	+
T. paurometabola		−	−	−	−	−	−		−	−	−	−	−
T. pulmonis		−	−	−	+	−	−		−	−	+	−	+
T. tyrosinosolvens		+	+	+	+	−	V		+	+	+	+	+

[a] Pink, mucoid colonies; early growth appears as rods but converts to cocci at 24 h.

Bacterial Diagnosis

Table 4.18 Differential characteristics of nonchromogenic, slow-growing *Mycobacterium* species[a,b]

Descriptive term	Species	Optimal temp (°C)	Usual colony morphology[c]	Pigmentation[d]	Niacin	Growth on T2H (10 μg/ml)[e]	Nitrate reduction	Semiquantitative catalase (mm of bubbles)	68°C catalase	Tween hydrolysis	Tolerance to 5% NaCl	Arylsulfatase, 3 days	16S rRNA ref. no.	Urease	Pyrazinamidase, 4 days	Nucleic acid probes available
TB complex	*M. tuberculosis*	37	R	N (100)	+(95)	+	+(97)	<45 (89)	−(1)	±(68)	−(0)	−(0)	X58890	±(64)	+	+
	M. africanum	37	R	N	V	V	V	<45	−	±	−	−	IDEM	+	−	+
	M. bovis	37	Rt	N (100)	−(4)	−	−(9)	<45 (69)	−(2)	−(21)	−(0)	−(0)	IDEM	±(50)	−	+
	M. bovis BCG	37	R	N	−	−	+	<45	−	±	−	−	IDEM	+	+	+
	M. canettii	37	Sm	N	+	+	+	ND	−	−	ND	−	IDEM	ND	+	+
Non-chromogens	*M. avium*	35–37	Smt/R	N	−	+	−	<45	±	−	−	−	X52198	−	+	+
	M. intracellulare	35–37	Smt/R	N	−	+	−	<45	±	−	−	−	X52927	−	+	+

M. haemophilum[g]	30	R	N	ND	+	−	−	<45	−	−	+(99)	−	X88923	−	+
M. malmoense	30	Sm	N (88)	−(0)	+	−(1)	<45 (99)	−/+	+(99)	−(0)	−(0)	X52930	−(9)	+
M. shimoidei	37	R	N	−	+	−	<45	−	+	ND	−	AJ005005	−	+
M. genavense	37	Smt	N	−	+	−	>45	+	+	ND	−	X60070	+	+(100)
M. celatum	35	Sm/Smt	N (100)	−	+	−(0)	<45 (100)	+(100)	−(0)	−(0)	+(100)	L08170, L08169	−(0)	−
M. ulcerans	30	R	N	−	+	±(67)	<45	+	−	−	−	X58954	V	V
M. terrae complex	35	Sm/R	N (93)	−(1)	+	+(67)	>45 (93)	+(92)	+(99)	−(2)	−(2)	X52925 (*M. terrae*)	−(13)	V
M. triviale	37	R	N (100)	−(0)	+	+(89)	>45 (100)	+(100)	+(100)	+(100)	±(56)	X88924	−/+(33)	V
M. gastri	35	Sm/SR/R	N (100)	−(0)	+	−(0)	<45 (100)	−(11)	+(100)	−(0)	−(0)	X52919	−/+(44)	−
M. triplex	35	Sm	N (100)	−(0)	+(100)	+(100)	>45(100)	+(100)	−(0)	−	−(0)+(50)[h]	U57632	+(100)	ND

[a] Adapted from P. R. Murray, E. J. Baron, J. H. Jorgensen, M. A. Pfaller, and R. H. Yolken (ed.), *Manual of Clinical Microbiology*, 8th ed., ASM Press, Washington, D.C., 2003.
[b] ±, usually present; −/+, usually absent; ND, not determined. The percentage of strains positive in each test is given in parentheses, and the test result is based on these percentages.
[c] R, rough; Sm, smooth; SR, intermediate in roughness; Smt, smooth and transparent; Rt, rough and thin, or transparent.
[d] N, nonchromogenic.
[e] T2H, thiophene-2-carboxylic acid hydrazide.
[f] Probe identifies *M. tuberculosis* complex.
[g] Requires hemin as growth factor.
[h] Arylsulfatase reaction at 14 days is positive; number in parentheses is the day.
[i] A MAC nucleic acid probe that recognizes *M. avium*, *M. intracellulare*, and the "X" strains is commercially available.

Bacterial Diagnosis

Bacterial Diagnosis

Table 4.19 Differential characteristics of chromogenic, slow-growing *Mycobacterium* species[a,b]

Descriptive term	Species	Optimal temp (°C)	Usual colony morphology[c]	Pigmentation[d]	Niacin	Nitrate reduction	Semiquantitative catalase (mm of bubbles)	68°C catalase	Tween hydrolysis	Arylsulfatase, 3 days	16S rDNA ref. no.	Urease	Pyrazinamidase, 4 days	Nucleic acid probes available
Chromogens	M. kansasii	35	Sm/SR/R	P (96)	−(4)	+(99)	>45 (93)	+(91)	+(99)	−(0)	X15916	−/+(49)	−	+
	M. marinum	30	Sm/SR/R	P (100)	−/+(21)	−(0)	<45	−(30)	+(97)	−/+(41)	X52920	+(83)	+	−
	M. avium	35–37	Sm/R	S	−	−	<45	±	−	−	X52198	−	+	+
	M. intracellulare	35–37	Sm/R	S	−	−	<45	±	−	−	X52927	−	+	+
	M. simiae	37	Sm	P (90)	±(63)	−(28)	>45 (93)	+(95)	−(9)	−(0)	X52931	±(69)	+	−
	M. asiaticum	37	Sm	P (86)	−(0)	−(5)	>45 (95)	+(95)	+(95)	−(0)	X55604	−(10)	−	−

M. xenopi	42	Sm	N/S^g	–	–	<45	+/–	+(97)	+	X52929	–	ND	–
M. gordonae	37	Sm	S (99)	–(0)	–(1)	>45 (90)	+(96)	+(100)	V	X52923	V (31)	–/+	+
M. scrofulaceum	37	Sm	S (97)	–(0)	–(5)	>45 (84)	+(94)	–(2)	V	X52924	V (31)	±	–
M. szulgai	37	Sm or R	S/P (93)	–(0)	+(100)	>45 (98)	+(93)	–/+(49)	V	X52926	+(72)	+	–
M. flavescens	37	Sm	S (100)^g	–(0)	+(92)	>45 (94)	+(100)	+(100)	–(0)	X52932	+/–(V)	+	+
M. intermedium	35	Sm	P	–	–	ND	+	+	+^e	X67847		–	–
M. lentiflavum	35	Sm	P	–	–	±(V)	±(V)	–	–^f	AF317658	ND	±(V)	–
M. interjectum	35	Sm	S	–	–	V	+	V	V	X70961	+	+	–

^a Adapted from P. R. Murray, E. J. Baron, J. H. Jorgensen, M. A. Pfaller, and R. H. Yolken (ed.), *Manual of Clinical Microbiology*, 8th ed., ASM Press, Washington, D.C., 2003.

^b ±, usually present; –/+, usually absent; ND, not determined. The percentage of strains positive in each test is given in parentheses, and the test result is based on these percentages.

^c R, rough; Sm, smooth; SR, intermediate in roughness.

^d P, photochromogenic; S, scotochromogenic; N, nonchromogenic (*M. szulgai* is scotochromogenic at 37°C and photochromogenic at 24°C).

^e Results for 3-day arylsulfatase not available; 10-day arylsulfatase positive.

^f Results for 3-day arylsulfatase not available; 10-day arylsulfatase negative.

^g Young cultures may be nonchromogenic or possess only pale pigment that may intensify with age.

Bacterial Diagnosis

Bacterial Diagnosis

Table 4.20 Differential characteristics of rapidly growing *Mycobacterium* species[a,b]

Descriptive term	Species	Optimal temp (°C)	Usual colony morphology[c]	Pigmentation[d]	Niacin	Growth on T2H (10 µg/ml)	Nitrate reduction	Semiquantitative catalase (mm of bubbles)	68°C catalase	Tween hydrolysis	Tolerance to 5% NaCl	Iron uptake	Arylsulfatase, 3 days	16S rDNA ref. no.	Urease	Nucleic acid probes available
Nonchromogens	*M. fortuitum* group[e]	28–30	R/Sm	N (100)	−	+	+(100)	>45 (93)	+(90)	−/+(43)	+(85)	+	+(97)	X52921	+(70)	−
	M. septicum	28–35	R	N (100)	−	ND	+	ND	ND	ND	+	+	V	AF111809	ND	−
	M. chelonae	28–30	Sm/R	N (100)	−/+	+	−(1)	>45 (92)	±(53)	−/+(39)	V	−	+(95)	X82236	+(89)	−
	M. senegalense	30	R	N	−	ND	+	ND	ND	ND	+	−	+	M29567	+	−

M. abscessus	28–30	Sm/R	N (100)	−	ND	−	>45	ND	V	±	−	+	X82235	+	−
M. immunogenum	30–35	R/Sm	N (100)	−	ND	−(100)	ND	ND	+	−	Tan	+(100)	AJ011771	ND	−
M. mucogenicum	28–30	Sm	N (100)	−	ND	V	>45	−(12)	+	−	+(67)	+(84)	X80771	+	−
M. smegmatis	28–35	Sm/R	LS (95)	−	+	+(95)	<45 (87)	−(0)	ND	+(100)	+	−(5)	X52922	ND	−
M. wolinskyi	28–35	Sm	N (100)	−	ND	+(100)	<45 (89)	−/+(100)	+(100)	+(100)	+	−(5)	Y12871	ND	−
M. goodii	28–35	Sm/R	LS (78)	−	ND	+(100)	<45 (50)	−(7)	ND	+(88)	+(40)	−(0)	Y12872	ND	−
M. mageritense	30–37	Sm	N (100)	ND	ND	+(70)	ND	−(0)	−(100)	+(80)	+	+(80)	X99838	+(60)	−
Chromogens — *M. phlei*	30	R	S	−	+	+	>45	+	+	+	+	−	M29566	ND	−
Chromogens — *M. vaccae*	30	Sm	S	−	+	+	>45	+	+	V	+	−	X55601	ND	−

a Adapted from P. R. Murray, E. J. Baron, J. H. Jorgensen, M. A. Pfaller, and R. H. Yolken (ed.), *Manual of Clinical Microbiology*, 8th ed., ASM Press, Washington, D.C., 2003.

b ±, usually present; −/+, usually absent; ND, not determined. The percentage of strains positive in each test is given in parentheses, and the test result is based on these percentages.

c R, rough; Sm, smooth.

d S, scotochromogenic; N, nonchromogenic; LS, late Scoto (7 to 10 days).

e Includes *M. fortuitum*, *M. peregrinum*, and *M. fortuitum* third-biovariant complex.

Bacterial Diagnosis

Table 4.21 Carbohydrate utilization tests of common rapidly growing *Mycobacterium* species[a,b]

Species or complex	Citrate	Mannitol	Inositol	Sorbitol
M. abscessus	−	−	−	−
M. chelonae	+	−	−	−
M. fortuitum	−	−	−	−
M. peregrinum	−	+	−	−
M. fortuitum third-biovariant complex				
Sorbitol (+)	−	+	+	+
Sorbitol (−)	−	+	+	−
M. mucogenicum	+	+	−	−
M. smegmatis sensu stricto	V	+	+	+
M. wolinskyi	V	+	+	+
M. goodii	V	+	+	+

[a] Adapted from P. R. Murray, E. J. Baron, J. H. Jorgensen, M. A. Pfaller, and R. H. Yolken (ed.), *Manual of Clinical Microbiology*, 8th ed., ASM Press, Washington, D.C., 2003.
[b] +, ≥80%; −, ≤20%; V, ≥21 to 79%.

Table 4.22 Differential characteristics of the gram-negative *Neisseria* and *Moraxella* species

Species	Growth on[a]:			Nitrate reductase	DNase	Acid from:					
	MTM, ML, NYC	CHOC, BA (22°C)	Nutrient agar (35°C)			Glucose	Maltose	Lactose	Sucrose	Fructose	
N. cinerea	V	−	+	−	−	−	−	−	−	−	
N. elongata	−	+	+	−	−	−	−	−	−	−	
N. flavescens	−	+	+	−	−	−	−	−	−	−	
N. gonorrhoeae	+	−	−	−	−	+	−	−	−	−	
N. lactamica	+	V	+	−	−	+	+	+	−	−	
N. meningitidis	+	−	V	−	−	+	+	−	−	−	
N. mucosa	−	+	+	−	−	+	+	−	+	+	
N. polysaccharea	−	+	+	−	−	+	+	−	V	−	
N. sicca	−	+	+	−	−	+	+	−	+	+	
N. subflava	V	+	+	−	−	+	+	−	V	V	
M. catarrhalis[b]	V	+	+	+	+	−	−	−	−	−	

[a]MTM, modified Thayer-Martin agar; ML, Martin-Lewis agar; NYC, New York City agar; CHOC, chocolate agar; BA, blood agar.
[b]*M. catarrhalis* is positive for butyrate esterase activity.

Bacterial Diagnosis

Table 4.23 Differential characteristics of selected members of the *Neisseriaceae*

Species	Oxidase	Catalase	Growth on MacConkey agar	Indole	Nitrate reductase	Arginine dihydrolase	Ornithine decarboxylase	Esculin hydrolysis	Alkaline phosphatase	Glucose	Lactose	Sucrose	Maltose	Mannitol	Xylose	Comments
										Acid from:						
Cardiobacterium hominis	+	−	−	+	−	−	−	−	−	+	−	+	+	+	−	Pleomorphic rods
Kingella kingae	+	−	−	−	−	−	−	−	+	+	−	−	+	−	−	Weak beta-hemolysis
Kingella denitrificans	+	−	−	−	+	−	−	−	−	+	−	−	−	−	−	
Kingella oralis	+	−	−	−	−	−	−	−	+	+	−	−	−	−	−	Slender rods; may pit agar
Eikenella corrodens	+	+	−	−	+	−	+	−	−	−	−	−	−	−	−	Coccobacillus; slight yellow color; may smell like popcorn
EF-4	+	+	>	−	+	>	−	−	−	+	−	−	−	−	−	
Simonsiella muelleri	+	−	−	−	>	−	−	−	−	+	−	−	−	−	−	Cells arrange in caterpillar-like filaments

Table 4.24 Differential characteristics of selected *Actinobacillus*, *Haemophilus*, and *Pasteurella* species

Species	Oxidase	Catalase	Growth on MacConkey agar	Urease	Esculin hydrolysis	Indole	ONPG	Gas from glucose	Acid from: Lactose	Maltose	Mannitol	Melibiose	Sucrose	Trehalose	Xylose	Comments
A. actinomycetemcomitans	–/W	+	–	–	–	NT	–	V	–	+	V	–	–	–	V	Coccobacillus; star shaped, adherent colonies
A. hominis	+	+	+	+	–	NT	+	–	+	+	+	+	+	+	+	Coccobacillus
A. ureae	+	+/–	–	+	–	NT	–	–	–	+	+	–	+	–	–	Pleomorphic, coccobacillus
H. aphrophilus	V	–	V	–	–	NT	+	+	(+)	+	–	NT	+	(+)	–	Adherent colonies
P. multocida	+	+	–	–	NT	+	NT	–	–	–	+	NT	+	NT	V	Coccobacillus
P. canis	+	+	–	–	NT	+	NT	–	–	–	–	NT	+	NT	–	Coccobacillus

Bacterial Diagnosis

Table 4.25 Differential characteristics of selected *Capnocytophaga, Dysgonomonas, Chromobacterium,* and *Streptobacillus* species

Species	Oxidase	Catalase	Indole	Nitrate reductase	Hydrolysis of: Arginine	Esculin	Starch	Gelatin	ONPG	Acid from: Glucose	Lactose	Sucrose	Xylose	Melibiose	Comments
C. ochracea	–	–	–	–	–	+	+	–	+	+	V	+	–	–	Fusiform; pleomorphic
C. sputigena	–	–	–	V	–	+	–	V	+	+	V	+	–	–	Fusiform; pleomorphic
C. gingivalis	–	–	–	–	–	–	NT	–	–	+	–	+	–	–	Fusiform; pleomorphic
C. canimorus	+	+	–	–	+	V	NT	–	+	+	+	–	–	–	Fusiform; pleomorphic
C. cynodegmi	+	+	–	V	+	+	NT	–	+	+	+	+	–	+	Fusiform; pleomorphic
D. capnocytophagoides	–	–	V	–	–	V	NT	–	+	+	–	+	+	+	Strawberry-like odor
C. violaceum	V	+	V	+	+	–	NT	V	–	+	–	V	–	NT	May be beta-hemolytic; most are purple
S. moniliformis	–	–	–	–	+	V	NT	–	–	+	–	–	–	NT	Typically form very long filaments

Table 4.26 Differential characteristics of *Haemophilus* species

Species	Growth requirement:			Hemolysis (horse blood)	Catalase	Acid from:			
	CO₂ enhances growth	Hemin (factor X)	NAD (factor V)			Glucose	Sucrose	Lactose	Mannose
H. influenzae	+	+	+	−	+	+	−	−	−
H. aphrophilus	+	−	−	−	−	+	+	+	+
H. haemolyticus	−	+	+	+	+	+	−	−	−
H. parahaemolyticus	−	−	+	+	+	+	+	−	+
H. parainfluenzae	V	−	+	−	V	+	+	−	+
H. paraphrophilus	+	−	+	−	−	+	+	+	+
H. segnis	−	−	+	−	V	+	+	−	−
H. ducreyi	−	+	−	−	−	−	−	−	−

Bacterial Diagnosis

Table 4.27 Differential characteristics of *H. aphrophilus*, *H. paraphrophilus*, and some related species[a]

Species	X factor required	V factor required	Indole	Urease	Ornithine decarboxylase	Lysine decarboxylase	Acid from: Glucose	Acid from: Sucrose	Acid from: Lactose	Acid from: Mannitol	Nitrate reduction	Catalase
H. aphrophilus	+[b]	−	−	−	−	−	+	+	+	−	+	−
H. paraphrophilus	−	+	−	−	−	−	+	+	+	−	+	−
A. actinomycetemcomitans	−	−	−	−	−	−	+	−	−	V	+	+
Eikenella corrodens	−	−	+	−	+	+	−	−	−	−	+	−
Cardiobacterium hominis	−	−	+	−	−	−	+	+	−	+	−	−
Suttonella indologenes	−	−	+	−	−	−	+	+	−	−	−	−
H. haemoglobinophilus	+	−	+	−	−	−	+	+	−	+	+	+

[a] Adapted from P. R. Murray, E. J. Baron, J. H. Jorgensen, M. A. Pfaller, and R. H. Yolken (ed.), *Manual of Clinical Microbiology*, 8th ed., ASM Press, Washington, D.C., 2003.

[b] The requirement for hemin is often lost on subcultivation, and the porphyrin test is weakly positive.

Table 4.28 Differential characteristics of selected members of the *Enterobacteriaceae*

Species	Indole production	Methyl red	Voges-Proskauer	Citrate utilization	Urease	Phenylalanine deaminase	Lysine decarboxylase	Arginine dihydrolase	Ornithine decarboxylase	Motility	Acid from: Glucose	Lactose	Sucrose	Mannitol	Dulcitol	Adonitol	Maltose	Xylose
Citrobacter freundii	V	V	−	V	V	−	−	V	−	+	+	V	+	+	−	−	+	+
Citrobacter koseri	+	+	−	+	V	−	−	V	+	+	+	V	V	+	V	+	+	+
Edwardsiella tarda	+	+	−	−	−	−	+	−	+	+	+	−	−	−	−	−	+	−
Enterobacter aerogenes	−	−	+	+	−	−	+	−	+	+	+	+	+	+	−	+	+	+
Enterobacter cloacae	−	−	+	+	V	−	−	+	+	+	+	+	+	+	V	V	+	+
Escherichia coli	+	+	−	−	−	−	+	V	V	+	+	+	V	+	V	−	+	+
Klebsiella oxytoca	+	V	+	+	+	−	+	−	−	−	+	+	+	+	V	+	+	+
Klebsiella pneumoniae	−	V	+	+	+	−	+	−	−	−	+	+	+	+	V	+	+	+
Morganella morganii	+	+	−	−	+	+	−	−	+	+	+	−	−	−	−	−	−	−

(continued)

Bacterial Diagnosis

Table 4.28 Differential characteristics of selected members of the *Enterobacteriaceae* (continued)

Species	Indole production	Methyl red	Voges-Proskauer	Citrate utilization	Urease	Phenylalanine deaminase	Lysine ecarboxylase	Arginine dihydrolase	Ornithine decarboxylase	Motility	Acid from: Glucose	Lactose	Sucrose	Mannitol	Dulcitol	Adonitol	Maltose	Xylose
Plesiomonas shigelloides	+	+	–	–	–	–	+	+	+	+	+	>	–	–	–	–	–	–
Proteus mirabilis	–	+	>	>	+	+	–	–	+	+	+	–	>	–	–	–	–	+
Proteus vulgaris	+	+	–	>	+	+	–	–	–	+	+	–	+	–	–	–	+	+
Providencia rettgeri	+	+	–	+	+	+	–	–	–	+	+	–	>	+	–	+	–	–
Providencia stuartii	+	+	–	+	>	+	–	–	–	>	+	–	+	–	–	–	–	–
Salmonella species	–	+	–	+	–	–	+	>	+	+	+	–	–	+	+	–	+	+
Serratia liquefaciens	–	+	+	+	–	–	+	–	+	+	+	–	+	+	–	–	+	+
Serratia marcescens	–	+	+	+	>	–	+	–	+	+	+	–	+	+	–	>	+	–
Shigella sonnei	–	+	–	–	–	–	–	–	+	–	+	–	–	+	–	–	+	–
Yersinia enterocolitica	>	+	–	–	>	–	–	–	+	–	+	–	+	+	–	–	>	>
Yersinia pestis	–	>	–	–	–	–	–	–	–	–	+	–	–	+	–	–	>	+

Table 4.29 Differential characteristics of *Citrobacter* species [a]

Species	Indole	ODC [b]	Malonate	Acid from: Sucrose	Dulcitol	Melibiose	Adonitol
C. amalonaticus	+	+	–	–	–	–	–
C. braakii	V	+	–	–	V	V	–
C. farmeri	+	+	–	+	–	+	–
C. freundii (sensu stricto)	V	–	–	V	–	+	–
C. koseri	+	+	+	V	V	–	+
C. rodentium	–	+	+	–	+	+	–
C. sedlakii	V	+	+	–	+	+	–
C. werkmanii	–	–	+	–	+	–	–
C. youngae	V	–	–	V	+	–	–
C. gillenii	–	–	+	V	–	V	–
C. murliniae	+	–	–	V	+	V	–

[a] Adapted from P. R. Murray, E. J. Baron, J. H. Jorgensen, M. A. Pfaller, and R. H. Yolken (ed.), *Manual of Clinical Microbiology*, 8th ed., ASM Press, Washington, D.C., 2003.
[b] ODC, ornithine decarboxylase.

Bacterial Diagnosis

Table 4.30 Differential characteristics of *Enterobacter* and *Pantoea* species[a]

Species	Lysine decarboxylase	Arginine dihydrolase	Ornithine decarboxylase	Voges-Proskauer	Acid from: Sucrose	Adonitol	Sorbitol	Rhamnose	α-Methyl glucoside	Esculin	Melibiose	Yellow pigment
E. aerogenes	+	−	+	+	+	+	+	+	+	+	+	−
P. agglomerans	−	−	−	V	V	−	V	V	−	V	V	V
E. amnigenus biogroup 1	−	−	V	+	+	−	−	+	+	+	+	−
E. asburiae	−	V	+	−	+	−	+	−	−	+	−	−
E. cancerogenus	−	+	+	+	−	−	−	+	−	+	−	−
E. cloacae	−	+	+	+	+	V	+	+	V	V	+	−
E. cowanii	+	−	−	+	+	−	+	+	−	+	+	−
E. gergoviae	+	−	+	+	+	−	−	+	−	+	+	V
E. hormaechei	−	V	V	+	V	−	+	+	V	−	+	−
E. intermedium	−	−	+	+	+	−	+	+	+	+	+	−
E. kobei	−	+	+	−	+	−	+	+	+	V	+	−
E. sakazakii	−	+	+	+	+	−	−	+	+	+	+	+

[a] Adapted from P. R. Murray, E. J. Baron, J. H. Jorgensen, M. A. Pfaller, and R. H. Yolken (ed.), *Manual of Clinical Microbiology*, 8th ed., ASM Press, Washington, D.C., 2003.

Table 4.31 Differential characteristics of *Klebsiella* and *Raoultella* species[a]

Species	Indole	Ornithine decarboxylase	Voges-Proskauer	Malonate	ONPG	Growth at: 10°C	Growth at: 44°C
K. oxytoca	+	−	+	+	+	−	+
K. ozaenae	−	−	−	−	V	NT	NT
K. pneumoniae	−	−	+	+	+	−	+
K. rhinoscleromatis	−	−	−	+	−	NT	NT
R. ornithinolytica	+	+	V	+	+	+	−
R. planticola	V	−	+	+	+	+	−
R. terrigena	−	V	+	+	+	+	−

[a] Adapted from P. R. Murray, E. J. Baron, J. H. Jorgensen, M. A. Pfaller, and R. H. Yolken (ed.), *Manual of Clinical Microbiology*, 8th ed., ASM Press, Washington, D.C., 2003.

Bacterial Diagnosis

Table 4.32 Differential characteristics of *Proteus*, *Providencia*, and *Morganella* species[a]

Organism	Indole	H$_2$S	Urea	Ornithine decarboxylase	Maltose	D-Adonitol	D-Arabitol	Trehalose	myo-Inositol
						Acid from:			
Proteus									
P. hauseri	+	V	+	−	+	−	−	+	−
P. mirabilis	−	+	+	+	−	−	−	+	−
P. penneri	−	V	+	−	+	−	−	V	−
P. vulgaris	+	+	+	−	+	−	−	V	−
Providencia									
P. alcalifaciens	+	−	−	−	−	+	−	−	−
P. heimbachae	−	−	+	−	V	+	+	−	V
P. rettgeri	+	−	+	−	−	+	+	−	+
P. rustigianii	+	−	V	−	−	−	−	−	+
P. stuartii	+	−	V	−	−	−	−	+	+
Morganella									
M. morganii subsp. morganii	+	−	+	+	−	−	−	−	−
M. morganii subsp. sibonii	V	−	+	+	−	−	−	+	−

[a]Adapted from P. R. Murray, E. J. Baron, J. H. Jorgensen, M. A., Pfaller, and R. H. Yolken (ed.), *Manual of Clinical Microbiology*, 8th ed., ASM Press, Washington, D.C., 2003.

Table 4.33 Differential characteristics of *Yersinia* species after incubation at 25°C for 48 h[a]

Species	Motility	Urease	Voges-Proskauer	Indole	Citrate	Ornithine	Acid from:				
							Sucrose	Rhamnose	Cellobiose	Melibiose	Sorbose
Y. pestis	−	−	−	−	−	−	−	−	−	V	−
Y. pseudotuberculosis	+	+	−	−	−	−	−	+	−	+	V
Y. enterocolitica	+	+	+	V	−	+	+	−	+	−	+
Y. intermedia	+	+	+	+	+	+	+	+	+	+	+
Y. frederiksenii	+	+	+	+	V	+	+	+	+	−	+
Y. kristensenii	+	+	−	V	−	+	−	−	+	−	−
Y. aldovae	+	+	+	−	V	+	−	+	−	−	+
Y. rohdei	+	(+)	−	−	+	+	+	−	+	V	−
Y. mollaretii	+	+	−	−	−	+	+	−	+	−	+
Y. bercovieri	+	+	−	−	−	+	+	−	+	−	−

[a] Adapted from P. R. Murray, E. J. Baron, J. H. Jorgensen, M. A. Pfaller, and R. H. Yolken (ed.), *Manual of Clinical Microbiology*, 8th ed., ASM Press, Washington, D.C., 2003.

Bacterial Diagnosis

Table 4.34 Differential characteristics of *Aeromonas* species[a]

Species	Voges-Proskauer	Lysine decarboxylase	Arginine dihydrolase	Ornithine decarboxylase	Gas (glucose)	Acid from: Arabinose	Acid from: Sucrose	Acid from: Mannitol	Esculin hydrolysis	Cephalothin resistance
A. caviae	–	–	+	–	–	+	+	+	+	R
A. hydrophila	+	+	+	–	+	V	+	+	+	R
A. jandaei	+	V	+	–	+	–	–	+	–	R
A. schubertii	V	+	+	–	–	–	V	–	–	S
A. veronii bv. sobria	+	+	+	–	+	–	+	+	–	S
A. veronii bv. veronii	+	+	–	+	+	–	+	+	+	S

[a] Adapted from P. R. Murray, E. J. Baron, J. H. Jorgensen, M. A. Pfaller, and R. H. Yolken (ed.), *Manual of Clinical Microbiology*, 8th ed., ASM Press, Washington, D.C., 2003.

Table 4.35 Differential characteristics of *Vibrio* species[a]

Species	Growth in: Nutrient broth	Growth in: Nutrient broth + 1% NaCl	Oxidase	Nitrate reduction	*myo*-Inositol fermentation	Arginine dihydrolase	Lysine decarboxylase	Ornithine decarboxylase
V. cholerae	+	+	+	+	–	–	+	+
V. mimicus	+	+	+	+	–	–	+	+
V. metschnikovii	–	+	–	–	V	V	V	–
V. cincinnatiensis	–	+	+	+	+	–	V	–
V. hollisae	–	+	+	+	–	–	–	–
V. damsela	–	+	+	+	–	+	V	–
V. fluvialis	–	+	+	+	–	+	–	–
V. furnissii	–	+	+	+	–	+	–	–
V. alginolyticus	–	+	+	+	–	–	+	V
V. parahaemolyticus	–	+	+	+	–	–	+	+
V. vulnificus	–	+	+	+	–	–	+	V
V. harveyi	–	+	+	+	–	–	+	–

[a] Adapted from P. R. Murray, E. J. Baron, J. H. Jorgensen, M. A. Pfaller, and R. H. Yolken (ed.), *Manual of Clinical Microbiology*, 8th ed., ASM Press, Washington, D.C., 2003.

Bacterial Diagnosis

Bacterial Diagnosis

Table 4.36 Differential characteristics of *Pseudomonas* species[a]

Species	Oxidase	Growth at 42°C	Nitrate reductase	Nitrate to gas	Arginine dihydrolase	Citrate	Acetamide	Hydrolysis of:			Acid from:			
								Esculin	Gelatin	Starch	Glucose	Maltose	Mannitol	Xylose
P. aeruginosa	+	+	+	+	+	+	+	–	V	–	+	–	V	+
P. fluorescens	+	–	V	–	+	+	–	–	+	–	+	–	V	+
P. putida	+	–	–	–	+	+	–	–	–	–	+	V	V	+
P. stutzeri	+	V	+	+	+	(+)	–	–	–	+	+	+	(+)	+
P. pseudoalcaligenes	+	+	+	–	V	V	NT	–	–	–	–	–	–	V
P. luteola	–	+	V	–	+	+	NT	+	V	–	+	+	(+)	+
P. oryzihabitans	–	–	–	–	–	+	NT	–	–	–	+	+	+	+

[a]Adapted from P. R. Murray, E. J. Baron, J. H. Jorgensen, M. A. Pfaller, and R. H. Yolken (ed.), *Manual of Clinical Microbiology*, 8th ed., ASM Press, Washington, D.C., 2003.

Table 4.37 Differential characteristics of *Ralstonia* species[a]

Species	Catalase	Oxidase	Growth at 42°C	Nitrate reduction	Motility	Hydrolysis of:		Acid from:									
						Tween 80	Urease	L-Arabinose	D-Arabitol	Glucose	Inositol	Lactose	Maltose	Mannitol	Sucrose	Xylose
R. pickettii	+	+	V	+	+	+	+	+	−	+	−	V	V	−	−	+
R. paucula	+	+	V	−	+	+	+	−	−	−	−	−	−	−	−	−
R. gilardii	+	−	+	−	+	NT	−	−	−	−	−	−	−	−	−	−
R. mannitolytica	+	+	+	−	+	+	+	+	+	+	−	+	+	+	−	+

[a]Adapted from P. R. Murray, E. J. Baron, J. H. Jorgensen, M. A. Pfaller, and R. H. Yolken (ed.), *Manual of Clinical Microbiology*, 8th ed., ASM Press, Washington, D.C., 2003.

Bacterial Diagnosis

Bacterial Diagnosis

Table 4.38 Differential characteristics of *Brevundimonas*, *Delftia*, *Comamonas*, and *Stenotrophomonas* species[a]

Species	Growth: Oxidase	MacConkey	42°C	Nitrate reduction	Nitrate to gas	Arginine dihydrolase	Lysine decarboxylase	Hydrolysis of: Citrate	Gelatin	Urea	Acid from: Glucose	Maltose	Mannitol	Xylose	Comments
B. diminuta	+	+	V	−	−	−	−	−	V	V	V	−	−	−	Brown-tan colonies
B. vesicularis	+	V	V	−	−	−	−	−	V	−	V	+	−	V	Colonies may be yellow-orange
D. acidovorans	+	+	V	+	−	−	−	+	V	−	−	−	+	−	Colonies may be yellow-tan
Comamonas spp.	+	+	V	+	−	−	−	V	−	−	−	−	−	−	
S. maltophilia	−	+	V	V	−	−	+	V	+	−	V	+	−	V	Lavendar-green colonies; ammonia odor

[a] Adapted from P. R. Murray, E. J. Baron, J. H. Jorgensen, M. A. Pfaller, and R. H. Yolken (ed.), *Manual of Clinical Microbiology*, 8th ed., ASM Press, Washington, D.C., 2003.

Table 4.39 Differential characteristics of selected nonfermentative gram-negative rods[a]

Organism	Oxidase	Catalase	Nitrate reductase	Arginine dihydrolase	Urease	Acid from: Glucose	Lactose	Maltose	Mannitol	Sucrose	Xylose
Acinetobacter											
Asaccharolytic	−	+	−	−	v	−	−	−	−	−	−
Saccharolytic	−	+	−	−	v	+	v	v	−	−	+
Bordetella holmesii	−	v	−	−	−	−	−	−	−	−	−
Bordetella parapertussis	−	+	−	−	+	+	−	+	+	−	−
Pseudomonas oryzihabitans	−	+	v	+	v	+	v	+	+	v	+
Pseudomonas luteola	−	+	v	−	v	+	v	+	(+)	−	+
CDC group EO-5	−	+	−	−	−	+	−	−	−	−	+
CDC group NO-1	−	+	+	−	−	−	−	−	−	−	−

[a]Adapted from P. R. Murray, E. J. Baron, J. H. Jorgensen, M. A. Pfaller, and R. H. Yolken (ed.), *Manual of Clinical Microbiology*, 8th ed., ASM Press, Washington, D.C., 2003.

Bacterial Diagnosis

Bacterial Diagnosis

Table 4.40 Differential characteristics of selected oxidase-negative, oxidative, gram-negative rods

Genus or species	Growth on MacConkey agar	Catalase	Motility	Arginine dihydrolase	Lysine decarboxylase	Urease	Indole production	Esculin hydrolysis	Nitrate reductase	D-Glucose	Acid from: OF-lactose	OF-sucrose	OF-mannitol	OF-maltose	OF-xylose
Acinetobacter	+	+	−	v	−	v	−	−	−	+	v	−	−	v	−
Chryseomonas	+	+	+	+	−	v	−	+	v	+	v	v	+	+	+
Flavimonas	+	+	+	v	−	v	−	−	−	+	v	v	+	+	+
Burkholderia cepacia	+	+	+	−	v	v	−	v	v	+	+	v	+	+	+
Roseomonas	+	+	v	−	−	+	−	−	−	v	−	−	v	−	v
Sphingomonas	v	+	v	−	−	−	−	+	−	+	+	+	−	+	+
Stenotrophomonas	+	+	+	−	+	v	−	v	v	+	v	v	−	+	v
Francisella	−	+	NT	−	NT	−	−	NT	−	+	NT	−	NT	−	−

Table 4.41 Differential characteristics of selected oxidase-positive, oxidative, gram-negative rods

Organism	Growth on MacConkey agar	Catalase	Arginine dihydrolase	Lysine decarboxylase	Urease	Indole production	Nitrate reductase	D-Glucose	OF-lactose	OF-sucrose	OF-mannitol	OF-maltose	OF-xylose
Agrobacterium	+	+	−	−	+	−	v	+	+	+	+	+	+
Alcaligenes xylosoxidans	+	+	v	−	−	−	+	v	−	−	−	−	+
Brucella	v	+	−	−	+	−	+	+	−	−	−	−	+
EF-4	v	+	−	−	−	−	+	+	−	−	−	−	−
Chryseobacterium meningosepticum	v	+	−	−	−	+	−	+	v	−	+	+	−
Methylobacterium	v	+	−	−	v	−	v	v	−	v	−	−	+
Ochrobactrum	+	+	v	−	+	−	+	+	−	v	v	v	+
Pseudomonas aeruginosa	+	+	+	−	v	−	+	+	−	−	v	−	+
Pseudomonas fluorescens	+	+	+	−	v	−	v	+	v	v	+	−	+
Burkholderia cepacia	+	+	−	−	v	−	v	+	+	v	+	+	+
Burkholderia pseudomallei	+	+	+	v	v	−	+	+	+	−	v	+	+
Roseomonas	v	+	−	−	+	−	−	v	−	−	−	−	v
Sphingomonas	−	+	−	−	−	−	−	+	+	+	−	+	+
Neisseria gonorrhoeae	−	+	−	NT	−	−	−	+	−	−	−	−	−
Neisseria meningitidis	−	+	−	NT	−	−	−	+	−	−	−	+	−
Neisseria lactamica	−	+	−	NT	−	−	−	+	+	−	−	+	−

Bacterial Diagnosis

Table 4.42 Differential characteristics of selected oxidase-positive, nonoxidative, gram-negative rods

Species	Growth on: MacConkey agar	Growth on: SS agar	Catalase	Motility	Flagella: 1–2 polar	Flagella: >2 polar	Flagella: Peritrichous	Urease	Indole production	Nitrate reductase	Nitrate to gas	H$_2$S on TSI^a	Acid from: Glucose	Acid from: OF-mannitol	Acid from: OF-xylose
Afipia felis	V	–	V	+	+	–	–	+	–	+	–	–	–	–	+
Alcaligenes faecalis	+	+	+	+	–	–	+	–	–	–	–	–	–	–	–
Alcaligenes xylosoxidans	+	+	+	+	–	–	+	–	–	+	+	NT	–	NT	–
Bordetella pertussis	–	–	+	–	–	–	–	–	–	–	–	–	–	–	–
Bordetella bronchiseptica	+	+	+	+	–	–	+	+	–	+	–	–	–	+	–
Brucella species	V	–	+	–	–	–	–	+	–	+	V	–	+	–	+
Campylobacter species	V	–	+	+	+	–	–	–	–	+	–	–	–	–	–
Methylobacterium species	V	–	+	+	+	–	–	V	–	V	–	–	V	–	+
Moraxella atlantae	+	–	+	–	–	–	–	–	–	–	–	–	–	–	–
Moraxella catarrhalis	–	–	+	–	–	–	–	–	–	V	–	–	–	–	–
Moraxella osloensis	V	–	+	–	–	–	–	–	–	V	–	–	–	–	–
Moraxella lacunata	–	–	+	–	–	–	–	–	–	–	–	–	–	–	–

Organism															
Moraxella phenylpyruvica	−	−	−	−	−	V	−	+	−	−	−	−	+	−	V
Neisseria flavescens	−	−	−	−	−	−	−	−	−	−	−	−	+	−	V
Neisseria mucosa	−	−	+	−	+	+	−	−	−	−	−	−	+	−	V
Neisseria sicca	−	V	+	V	−	−	−	−	+	−	−	+	V	+	V
Ochrobactrum anthropi	+	−	+	−	+	+	−	+	V	−	−	V	+	+	+
Oligella ureolytica	−	−	−	−	V	+	−	+	V	−	−	−	+	−	V
Oligella urethralis	−	−	−	−	−	−	−	−	−	−	+	+	+	−	+
Pseudomonas diminuta	−	−	V	−	−	V	−	V	−	−	+	+	+	−	+
Roseomonas species	V	V	V	−	−	−	−	+	−	−	+	−	+	−	+
Bartonella species	−	−	−	NT	−	+	−	−	−	−	−	−	−	−	−
Eikenella corrodens	−	−	−	−	−	+	−	−	−	−	−	−	−	−	−
Kingella denitrificans	−	−	+	−	V	−	−	−	−	−	−	−	−	−	−
Weeksella virosa	−	−	+	−	−	+	+	+	−	−	−	−	+	−	−
Weeksella zoohelcum	−	−	+	−	−	−	+	−	−	−	−	−	+	−	−

*a*TSI, triple sugar iron.

Bacterial Diagnosis

Table 4.43 Differential characteristics of selected *Campylobacter*, *Arcobacter*, and *Helicobacter* species

Species	Catalase	Nitrate reductase	Urease	Alkaline phosphatase	Hippurate hydrolysis	Indoxyl acetate hydrolysis	γ-Glutamyl transferase	Growth: 15°C	25°C	42°C	3.5% NaCl	1% Glycine
C. jejuni subsp. jejuni	+	+	–	NT	+	+	NT	–	–	+	–	+
C. coli	+	+	–	NT	–	+	NT	–	–	+	–	+
C. fetus subsp. fetus	+	+	–	NT	–	–	NT	–	+	–	–	+
C. upsaliensis	+	+	–	NT	–	+	NT	–	–	V	–	V
A. butzleri	+	+	–	NT	–	+	NT	+	+	+	V	+
A. cryaerophilus	+	V	–	NT	–	+	NT	+	+	–	–	–
H. pylori	+	–	+	+	–	–	+	–	–	–	–	+
H. cinaedi	+	+	–	–	–	–	–	–	–	–	–	–
H. fennelliae	+	–	–	+	–	+	–	–	–	–	–	+
H. pullorum	+	+	–	–	–	–	NT	–	–	+	–	+

Table 4.44 Differential characteristics of non-spore-forming, anaerobic, gram-positive rods

Genus	Strict anaerobe	Catalase	Motility	Nitrate reductase	Indole production	Metabolic products (GLC)[a]
Actinomyces	V	−	−	V	−	S, L, a
Bifidobacterium	+	−	−	−	−	A, L
Eubacterium	+	−	V	V	−	(A), (B)
Lactobacillus	V	−	−	−	−	L, (a), (s)
Mobiluncus	+	−	+	V	−	S, A, (L)
Propionibacterium	V	V	−	V	−	A, P, iv, s, l

[a]A, acetic acid; P, propionic acid; IB, isobutyric acid; B, butyric acid; IV, isovaleric acid; V, valeric acid; IC, isocaproic acid; C, caproic acid; L, lactic acid; S, succinic acid. Capital letters indicate a major acid peak, lowercase letters indicate a minor peak, and letters in parentheses indicate that the acids are irregularly observed.

Bacterial Diagnosis

Table 4.45 Differential characteristics of selected *Actinomyces* and *Propionibacterium* species

| Species | Catalase | Nitrate reductase | Indole | Urease | Hydrolysis of: | | Acid from: | | | | | | | | | Metabolic products (GLC) |
					Esculin	Gelatin	Glucose	Arabinose	Mannose	Raffinose	Trehalose	Inositol	Glycerol	Xylose	Mannitol	
A. israelii	–	v	–	–	+	–	+	+	+	+	v	+	–	+	+	A, L, S
A. meyeri	–	–	–	+	v	–	+	v	–	–	–	–	v	+	–	A, S
A. naeslundii	–	+	–	+	+	–	+	–	+	–	v	+	v	v	–	A, L, S
A. odontolyticus	–	v	–	+	v	–	+	v	–	–	–	v	v	v	–	A, S
A. pyogenes	–	–	–	–	–	+	+	v	v	–	v	v	v	v	–	A, S
P. acnes	+	+	+	–	–	+	+	–	+	–	–	–	+	–	+	A, P, (iv), (l), (s)
P. propionicus	–	+	–	–	–	–	+	–	v	+	v	v	v	–	v	A, P, (l), (s)

Table 4.46 Differential characteristics of selected *Clostridium* species

Species	Egg yolk agar		Gelatinase	Milk digestion	Indole	Acid from:				Metabolic products (GLC)
	Lecithinase	Lipase				Glucose	Maltose	Lactose	Sucrose	
C. perfringens	+	–	+	–	–	+	+	+	+	A, B, (P), (L)
C. baratii	+	–	–	–	–	+	+	+	+	A, B, (L)
C. novyi A	+	+	+	–	–	+	+	–	–	A, P, B, (V)
C. novyi B	+	–	+	–	–	+	+	–	–	A, P, B
C. novyi C	–	–	V	–	–	+	–	–	–	A, P, B
C. haemolyticum	+	–	+	–	+	+	+	–	–	A, P, B
C. bifermentans	+	–	+	+	+	+	+	–	–	A, IC, (P), (IB), (IV), PP
C. sordellii	+	–	+	+	+	+	+	–	–	A, IC, (P), (IB), (IV)

(continued)

Bacterial Diagnosis

Table 4.46 Differential characteristics of selected *Clostridium* species *(continued)*

Species	Egg yolk agar		Gelatinase	Milk digestion	Indole	Acid from:				Metabolic products (GLC)
	Lecithinase	Lipase				Glucose	Maltose	Lactose	Sucrose	
C. botulinum I	–	+	+	+	–	+	+	–	–	A, IB, B, IV, (P), (V), (IC), PP
C. botulinum II	–	+	+	+	–	+	+	–	+	A, B
C. botulinum III	–	+	+	V	–	+	V	–	–	A, P, B
C. sporogenes	–	+	+	+	–	+	+	–	–	A, IB, B, IV, (P), (V), (IC), PP
C. septicum	–	–	+	–	–	+	+	+	–	A, B
C. chauvoei	–	–	+	–	–	+	+	+	+	A, B, F
C. difficile	–	–	+	–	–	+	–	–	–	A, IB, B, IV, V, IC, (P), PP
C. tetani	–	–	+	+	+	–	–	–	–	A, P, B, (PP)
C. histolyticum	–	–	–	–	+	–	–	–	–	A, (PP)
C. sphenoides	–	–	–	–	–	+	+	+	+	A, F
C. tertium	–	–	–	–	–	+	+	+	+	A, B, (L), (PP)
C. butyricum	–	–	–	–	–	+	+	+	+	A, B
C. fallax	–	–	–	–	–	+	+	+	+	A, B, (L)
C. ramosum	–	–	–	–	–	+	+	+	+	A, L, (PY)

Table 4.47 Differential characteristics of anaerobic gram-negative bacteria

Species	Susceptibility to:											
	Kanamycin (1,000 μg)	Vancomycin (5 μg)	Colistin (10 μg)	Growth in 20% bile	Formate or fumate required	Nitrate reductase	Indole	Catalase	Lipase	Urease
Bacteroides fragilis group	R	R	R	+	–	–	v	v	–	–
Other *Bacteroides* spp.	R	R	v	v	–	–	v	v	–	–
Porphyromonas spp.[a]	R	S	R	–	–	–	+	–	–	–
Prevotella spp.[a]	R	R	v	–	–	–	v	–	v	–
Bilophila wadsworthia	S	R	S	+	–	+	–	+	–	+
Fusobacterium nucleatum	S	R	S	–	–	–	+	–	–	–
Other *Fusobacterium* spp.	S	R	S	v	–	–	v	–	v	–
Acidaminococcus fermentans	S	R	S	–	–	–	–	–	–	–
Megasphaera elsdenii	S	R	S	–	–	–	–	–	–	–
Veilonella spp.	S	R	S	–	–	+	–	v	–	–

[a] *Porphyromonas* and some *Prevotella* spp. initially fluoresce red and then develop pigmented colonies.

Bacterial Diagnosis

Table 4.48 Differential characteristics of the *Bacteroides fragilis* group

Species	Indole	Catalase	Esculin hydrolysis	α-Fucosidase	Acid from: Arabinose	Cellobiose	Rhamnose	Salicin	Sucrose	Trehalose	Xylan	Metabolic products (GLC)
B. fragilis	−	+	+	+	−	V	−	−	+	−	−	A, p, S, pa (ib, iv, l)
B. caccae	−	V	+	+	+	V	V	V	+	+	−	A, p, S (iv)
B. distasonis	−	V	+	−	V	+	V	+	+	+	−	A, p, S (pa, ib, iv, l)
B. merdae	−	V	+	−	V	V	+	+	+	+	V	A, p, S (ib, iv)
B. vulgatus	−	V	V	+	+	−	+	−	+	−	−	A, p, S
B. thetaiotaomicron	+	+	+	+	+	V	+	V	+	+	−	A, p, S, pa (ib, iv, l)
B. eggerthii	+	−	+	−	+	V	V	−	−	−	+	A, p, S (ib, iv, l)
B. ovatus	+	V	+	+	+	+	+	+	+	+	+	A, p, S, pa (ib, iv, l)
B. stercoris	+	−	V	V	V	V	+	V	+	−	V	A, p, S, f (ib, iv)
B. uniformis	+	V	+	+	+	+	V	V	+	−	V	a, p, l, S (ib, iv)

Viral Diagnosis

Viral infections have historically been diagnosed by culture in primary or continuous cell lines and by detection of antibody responses to infection. This has changed in recent years. Traditional cell cultures in glass test tubes or plastic petri dishes have been replaced in many laboratories by the shell vial culture method. That is, glass coverslips covered with monolayer cells are inoculated with the clinical specimen and, after 1 to 5 days of incubation, are stained with labeled virus-specific antibodies. This method has a sensitivity approaching that of traditional cell cultures and is significantly faster. Antigen capture immunoassays, which allow for the direct detection of viruses in clinical specimens, have also been developed. Additionally, nucleic acid amplification tests have been developed for a wide variety of important viral pathogens. Although these tests are restricted primarily to large clinical laboratories and reference centers, it is anticipated that they will become more widely available as the technology develops. Despite these changes, serology remains important for many viral infections. What we have witnessed in the last decade is a transition from the more labor-intensive complement fixation and neutralization tests to commercially prepared enzyme immunoassays. This technical change allows many smaller laboratories to perform tests that were previously available only in reference laboratories.

This section summarizes the tests currently available for the laboratory diagnosis of the most common viral infections. For additional information, the reader is referred to the ASM *Manual of Clinical Microbiology* and *Clinical Virology* by Richman et al. (see the Bibliography).

Viral Diagnosis

Table 5.1 Detection methods for viruses[a]

Virus[b]	Cell culture	Microscopy	Usefulness of detection by: Antigen detection methods	Antibody detection methods	Molecular diagnostics
RNA viruses					
Alphavirus	C	D	C	A	B
Arenavirus	C	C	C	B	C
Astrovirus, calicivirus, rotavirus	C	A	A	C	B
Bunyaviruses	D	D	D	A	C
Coronavirus	C	D	D	A	B
Coxsackievirus types A and B	A	D	D	D	A
Enterovirus	A	D	D	D	A
Filoviruses	D	D	C	C	C
Hantavirus	D	D	D	A	B
Hepatitis A virus	C	D	D	A	A
Hepatitis C virus	D	D	D	A	A
Hepatitis E virus	D	B	A	A	C
HTLV-I and -II	C	D	D	A	B
HIV-I and -II	C	D	B	A	A
Influenzavirus types A to C	A	B	A	B	C
Measles virus	B	B	C	A	B
Mumps virus	A	B	C	A	B
Parainfluenzavirus types 1 to 3	A	A	C	C	B

(continued)

Viral Diagnosis

Table 5.1 Detection methods for viruses[a] *(continued)*

Virus[b]	Cell culture	Microscopy	Usefulness of detection by:		
			Antigen detection methods	Antibody detection methods	Molecular diagnostics
Poliovirus	A	D	D	D	A
Rabies virus	C	A	D	B	B
Respiratory syncytial virus	A	A	A	C	C
Rhinovirus	A	C	C	C	C
Rubella virus	A	D	D	A	B
DNA viruses					
Adenovirus	A	C	A	C	C
Cytomegalovirus	A	B	A	A	B
Erythrovirus (B19 virus)	C	D	D	A	B
Epstein-Barr virus	C	B	D	A	B

Hepatitis B virus	D	A	C	A	B
Herpes simplex virus types I and II	A	A	B	B	B
Human herpesvirus 6	B	C	C	B	B
Orthopoxvirus	B	B	D	A	C
Papillomavirus	D	C	D	A	A
Polyomavirus (BK virus, JC virus)	D	C	D	D	A
Varicella-zoster virus	A	A	D	B	A
Transmissible spongiform encephalopathy agents					
Bovine encephalopathy agent	D	C	D	D	D
Creutzfeldt-Jakob agent	D	C	D	D	D
Kuru agent	D	C	D	D	D

[a] A, test is generally useful; B, test is useful under certain circumstances; C, test is seldom used for general diagnosis but may be available in reference laboratories; D, test is generally not used for laboratory diagnosis.

[b] HTLV, human T-cell leukemia virus; HIV, human immunodeficiency virus.

Viral Diagnosis

Table 5.2 Cells used for viral isolation[a]

Type of cell	Tissue of origin	Viruses isolated[b]
Primary cell lines		
African green monkey	Kidney	HSV, VZV, mumps virus, rubella virus
CBMC, PBMC[c]	Human	HIV-1, HIV-2, HTLV-1, HTLV-2, HHV-6
Neonatal, human	Kidney	HSV, VZV, adenoviruses, mumps virus
Rabbit	Kidney	HSV
Rhesus or cynomolgus monkey	Kidney	Enteroviruses, influenza viruses, parainfluenza viruses, RSV, mumps virus, measles virus
Low-passage/finite cell lines		
Foreskin fibroblasts	Human	HSV, CMV
Lung fibroblasts	Human embryo	HSV, CMV, VZV, rhinoviruses, coronavirus
Kidney fibroblasts	Human fetus	Coronavirus, HSV, rhinovirus
WI-38, MRC-5	Human fetal lung	HSV, VZV, CMV, adenoviruses, enteroviruses, RSV, rhinoviruses
Continuous cell lines		
293	Human kidney	Adenoviruses (types 5, 40, and 41)
A549	Human lung	Adenoviruses (except types 40 and 41), HSV
HeLa	Human cervix	Poxviruses, RSV, rhinoviruses, enteroviruses
HEp-2	Human larynx	Adenoviruses, RSV, measles virus
MDCK	Canine kidney	Influenza viruses, parainfluenza viruses
Mink lung	Mink lung	HSV
RD	Human rhabdomyosarcoma	Enteroviruses (coxsackievirus type A), coronavirus, poliovirus
RK_{13}	Rabbit kidney	Rubella virus, poxviruses
BGMK, Vero, CV-1	African green monkey kidney	HSV, VZV, enteroviruses, measles virus, poxviruses, rubella virus, RSV, parainfluenza viruses

[a]Adapted from P. R. Murray, E. J. Baron, J. H. Jorgensen, M. A. Pfaller, and R. H. Yolken (ed.), *Manual of Clinical Microbiology*, 8th ed., ASM Press, Washington D.C., 2003.

[b]CMV, cytomegalovirus; HHV, human herpesvirus; HIV, human immunodeficiency virus; HSV, herpes simplex virus; HTLV, human T-cell leukemia virus; RSV, respiratory syncytial virus; VZV, varicella-zoster virus.

[c]CBMC, cord blood mononuclear cells; PBMC, peripheral blood mononuclear cells

Specific Diagnostic Tests

RNA Viruses

Alphavirus (Eastern Equine Encephalitis Virus, Western Equine Encephalitis Virus, Venezuelan Equine Encephalitis Virus). Viruses grow in a variety of cell lines including Vero, A549, and MRC-5 cells. Virus can be found in blood at the time of clinical onset but is typically cleared when neurological symptoms develop. Additionally, antigen detection assays and reverse transcriptase PCR (RT-PCR) tests have been developed for some members of this group (e.g., Venezuelan equine encephalitis virus). The most sensitive serological assays detect virus-specific immunoglobulin M (IgM) antibodies by capture enzyme-linked immunosorbent assay (ELISA). IgM antibodies are detected in serum and cerebrospinal fluid (CSF) within the first 7 to 10 days of clinical illness. Because IgM antibodies may persist for months, seroconversion should be demonstrated. Virus-specific assays are available for Western and Venezuelan equine encephalitis virus. These do not cross-react with other alphaviruses.

Arenavirus (Lymphocytic Choriomeningitis Virus, Lassa Virus, Junin Virus, Machupo Virus). Arenaviruses are a family of 21 named viruses divided into two groups: Old World complex (e.g., lymphocytic choriomeningitis [LCM] virus, Lassa virus) and New World or Tacaribe complex (e.g., Junin virus, Machupo virus). Direct fluorescent-antibody (DFA) tests have been used with peripheral blood and urine sediment for detection of Junin virus. Antigen capture ELISAs have also been developed for detection of Lassa virus antigens in blood as well as for the identification of virus grown in cell cultures. The RT-PCR assay is a useful test for the rapid, definitive diagnosis of LCM and Lassa virus infections. The test sensivity is approximately 80% for Lassa virus; this reflects the genetic variation among Lassa virus strains. Cell culture is the most sensitive diagnostic method for Lassa and related viruses. The viruses grow in Vero cells (and other cell lines), with viral antigens detected by immunofluorescent-antibody (IFA) staining of inoculated cell cultures or ELISA. LCM virus also grows in cell culture, but intracranial inoculation of weanling mice is a more sensitive diagnostic procedure. The most sensitive and rapid method to diagnose infection with Lassa virus is to perform the antigen capture ELISA combined with serologic testing (ELISA) for IgM and IgG. The diagnosis of infection can be confirmed for most patients at the time of clinical onset. ELISAs have also been developed for detecting antibody responses to other arenaviruses and have replaced neutralization and IFA serologic tests. RT-PCR assays continue to be developed and will probably replace viral culture.

Astrovirus, Calicivirus, and Rotavirus.   Eight serotypes of astroviruses have been identified, with serotype 1 being the most common human pathogens. Caliciviruses are subdivided into Norwalk-like viruses and Sapporo-like viruses, with a large number of viruses in each group. Rotaviruses have been subdivided into groups A to G, with most human infections caused by group A. All of these viruses can be detected in stool specimens by electron microscopy. Only rotaviruses can be isolated in cell culture; however, growth is slow and culture is not generally performed. RT-PCR is a sensitive method for detection of these viruses, although inhibitors in fecal specimens can cause false-negative reactions. A wide range of ELISAs and latex agglutination tests have been developed for the detection of rotaviruses in fecal specimens, and an ELISA is commercially available for astroviruses.

Bunyavirus (Bunyamwera Virus, California Encephalitis Virus, La Crosse Virus).   Virus can grow in Vero and BHK-21 cell lines; however, attempts to isolate virus from clinical specimens are generally unsuccessful. Serologic testing (e.g., neutralization, hemagglutination inhibition [HI], complement fixation [CF] and ELISA) is primarily used to establish infection. Most patients are seropositive by IgM ELISA at the time of onset of illness. Neutralizing antibodies are detected at the end of the first week of illness and persist for life. In contrast, HI antibodies are detected at the end of the first week and CF antibodies develop a few weeks later; both antibodies disappear within 1 year.

Coronavirus.   Although coronaviruses are recognized as a common source of upper respiratory disease, interest in this group of viruses has been stimulated by the onset of severe acute respiratory syndrome (SARS). The viruses are difficult to grow in culture, so diagnosis has primarily depended on RT-PCR and serologic testing. RT-PCR is available through Public Health Laboratories, tertiary-care centers, and commercial laboratories. Commercial vendors have developed ELISAs, and it is likely that these tests will be available soon.

Enterovirus (Coxsackie A and B Viruses, Enterovirus, Poliovirus). Isolation in culture is the method of choice. Some serotypes of coxsackie A virus fail to grow in culture. These serotypes can be recovered by inoculation of suckling mice, but the procedure is not usually performed in clinical laboratories. For viruses able to grow in culture, human rhabdomyosarcoma cells, WI-38, and human embryonic lung cells are best for coxsackie A virus and monkey (e.g., Buffalo green, rhesus, and cynomolgus) kidney or HeLa cells are best for coxsackie B virus. Isolation in culture is the method of choice for enterovirus and poliovirus, with growth being observed in a wide range of cell lines. RT-PCR is also a useful assay, particularly for CSF samples, for which this assay is as sensitive as culture. Serological testing is restricted primarily to research laboratories.

Filovirus (Ebola Virus, Marburg Virus). Filoviruses are biosafety level 4 (BSL-4) pathogens, and so all work with the viruses is restricted to BSL-4 facilities. Virus can be cultured from serum at the time of clinical onset. Vero cells are permissive. Antigen capture ELISA has been used to detect viral antigens in serum. Filovirus-specific IgM capture and IgG ELISA are used to assess the serological response to infection. IgM and IgG appear 8 to 10 days after onset of disease. IgM antibody levels decrease over the first few months of infection, but IgG antibodies will persist for 2 years or more. RT-PCR can detect viral RNA in serum and tissues and appears to be at least as sensitive as antigen capture assays.

Flavivirus (Yellow Fever Virus, Dengue Virus, St. Louis Encephalitis Virus, West Nile Virus). Yellow fever virus antigen can be detected by antigen capture assays or RT-PCR; however, these assays are not commercially available. Most infections are diagnosed by IgM capture ELISA, with a presumptive diagnosis being based on the presence of IgM antibodies and the diagnosis being confirmed by the demonstration of a significant rise in antibody levels. Dengue virus infections are diagnosed on the basis of clinical presentation and detection of viral RNA by RT-PCR. Serological testing is generally of little value because most severe infections are in previously infected patients. Although antigen capture assays and RT-PCR tests have been developed for St. Louis encephalitis virus, serologic testing is the most sensitive diagnostic test. Cross-reactivity with West

Nile virus and Japanese encephalitis virus occurs, and so neutralization assays must be performed to demonstrate which virus is responsible for the infection. Likewise, West Nile virus infections are diagnosed primarily by serologic testing, except in immunocompromised patients, for whom RT-PCR assay may remain positive. Positive serologic tests must be confirmed by neutralization assays, and a fourfold change in antibody levels must be demonstrated because IgM and IgG antibodies can persist for months to years.

Flavivirus (Hepacivirus [Hepatitis C Virus]).   Diagnosis of infections caused by hepatitis C virus (HCV) is by either serologic testing or nucleic acid amplification (NAA) assays. The current enzyme immunoassays (EIAs) used for screening blood donors and patients are directed against core, NS3, and NS5 antigens. Seroconversion is detected by 10 weeks after exposure. False-positive reactions occur at a low rate. To improve the test specificity, a strip immunoassay (recombinant immunoblot assay [RIBA]) was developed. The strip incorporates HCV-specific antigens and superoxide dismutase. Reactions with two or more HCV-specific antigens are considered to indicate a positive result. Reaction with only one antigen or one antigen and superoxide dismutase is considered indeterminate. In the setting of acute hepatitis, qualitative and quantitative NAA tests have been developed for detecting viral nucleic acids in serum or plasma. In the setting of chronic hepatitis, EIAs are highly sensitive and specific, and confirmation by RIBA or NAA tests is not necessary. For patients presenting with acute hepatitis, qualitative NAA tests are used to confirm active infection. Quantitative NAA tests can be used to monitor the response to therapy or the progression of disease.

Hantavirus (Hantaan Virus).   Hantaviruses are difficult to grow in culture. Diagnosis is most commonly made by serologic testing. IgM and IgG antibodies are typically detected at the time of clinical presentation. ELISA, Western blot (WB) assay, and RIBA are the most commonly used techniques; RT-PCR assays have also been developed.

Hepatitis A Virus.   Hepatitis A virus (HAV) is difficult to culture, and so this is done only in research laboratories. Commercially available assays for anti-HAV IgM are the methods of choice for diagnosis of acute type A hepatitis, with solid-phase antibody capture immunoassay being the most commonly used method. Antibodies are detected at the time of onset of symptoms and have disappeared by 6 months following infection. EIAs are used to measure total anti-HAV antibody levels (IgM, IgG, and IgA), which increase during acute infections and then persist indefinitely. Detectable anti-HAV antibodies in the absence of IgM antibodies are indicative of past infection and immunity.

Hepatitis E Virus. Although hepatitis E virus (HEV) has been grown in culture, this is inefficient and is performed only in research laboratories. The method of choice for diagnosis of acute HEV infections is detection of IgM antibodies, which are detectable at the time of onset of symptoms and disappear within several weeks after symptoms resolve. IgG antibodies are also short-lived, typically becoming undetectable within several months of resolution of symptoms. Acute HEV infections may also be diagnosed by detecting HEV RNA in serum or plasma. This NAA assay remains positive for 2 to 7 weeks after onset, although viral RNA may be detected in some individuals for a more prolonged period.

Human Immunodeficiency Virus Types 1 and 2. Human immunodeficiency virus (HIV) infections can be diagnosed by culture, antigen or antibody detection, and NAA methods. Most infections are made initially by screening for HIV-specific antibodies that are produced within a few weeks after infection (50% of patients are detected as positive at 3 weeks by current EIAs and 95% are positive at 2 months). Assays for p24 antigen, PCR for proviral DNA, and PCR for viral RNA in plasma are slightly less sensitive. Rapid immunoassays and tests designed for home diagnosis are also available. Quantitative NAA methods are available for monitoring the viral load, which has prognostic implications. The complexity of the available diagnostic tests precludes a detailed discussion here; the user of this *Pocket Guide* is referred to the ASM *Manual of Clinical Microbiology*.

Human T-Cell Lymphotropic Virus Types 1 and 2. EIA measuring the serologic response to human T-cell lymphotropic virus type 1 (HTLV-1) and HTLV-2 infection is the primary diagnostic test, and a WB assay is used to confirm the diagnosis. It is recommended that a test giving an initial positive EIA result be repeated. If both tests are positive, the band profile observed in the WB assay is used to distinguish between HTLV-1 and HTLV-2.

Influenza Virus (Types A to C). The Madin-Darby canine kidney (MDCK) cell line is most commonly used for isolation of influenza viruses, although growth is observed in a variety of cell lines (e.g., Vero, MRC-5, and baby hamster kidney cells). Cytopathic effect (CPE) is typically observed within 2 to 3 days, but negative cultures should be tested by hemadsorption. Immunologic staining of infected cells at 1 and 2 days (shell vial assay) is more commonly used nowadays. DFA can be performed with nasopharyngeal washes, although this test has a sensitivity of only 80 to 90% compared with culture. Specific EIAs for either influenza A virus or influenza A plus B viruses are available. The sensitivities of the assays vary widely and are dependent on the quality of specimen, commercial assay system, and viral strain type that is circulating in the community. None of these assays can be reliably used alone. NAA assays are available in research laboratories and have been demonstrated to be the most sensitive detection system available. Serologic tests are used primarily for epidemiological surveys.

Measles Virus. Measles virus can be isolated from the conjunctiva, nasopharynx, and blood during the late prodromal period and early stage of rash development. Viremia clears within 2 to 3 days of the rash, but virus can be detected in urine for up to 7 days. B95-8 (B-lymphoblastoid) cells are used for isolation of virus. However, few clinical laboratories attempt to culture the virus. Virus-infected cells can be detected by cytologic examination (detection of intracytoplasmic and intranuclear inclusions and giant cells), and RT-PCR has been used by research laboratories. The recommended laboratory method for confirmation of infection is a serum-based IgM EIA. Commercial assays are available. Serum can be collected at the time of rash onset or up to 4 weeks later. IgG assays are also available and, in combination with IgM assays, can be used to assess immunity as well as primary disease.

Mumps Virus. Mumps is diagnosed by viral isolation, NAA, or serologic testing. Mumps virus is cultured most commonly in primary rhesus monkey kidney cells and human neonatal kidney cells. Cells are examined for CPE for 14 days, and negative cell cultures are tested by hemadsorption with guinea pig erythrocytes. Rapid antigen tests are infrequently used because mumps infections are uncommon in vaccinated populations. Mumps virus can be detected by RT-PCR, although this technique is not widely used. Serologic testing can be used to define an acute infection or immunity. A single positive IgG test is sufficient to identify an immune patient; seroconversion is necessary to identify a primary infection. EIAs are available for measuring IgM and IgG antibodies with whole virus, sonicated virus, or purified viral antigens (e.g., HN or nucleocapsid [NP]) used in the assays.

Parainfluenza Virus. Primary human embryonic kidney and primary monkey kidney cells are the most sensitive cell line for culture of parainfluenza virus (PIV). Other cell lines can support the growth of PIV but are not recommended for primary isolation. Cultures are examined for CPE for 10 to 14 days, with 50% of positive cultures being detected at 5 days. Positive cultures can also be detected as early as 48 h after inoculation if cultures have been stained with virus-specific fluorescent antibodies. In most clinical laboratories, culture has been replaced with the shell vial assay, which has comparable sensitivity and is more rapid. Direct and indirect immunofluorescent-antibody tests are commonly used to examine respiratory specimens for virus-infected cells. Specimens are typically examined with pooled reagents (for influenza A and B viruses, PIV-1 to PIV-3, respiratory syncytial virus [RSV], and adenoviruses), and those giving positive reactions are tested with virus-specific reagents. RT-PCR assays have been developed but are used primarily for epidemiological studies. A variety of serologic assays (CF, HI, IFA, neutralization, and EIA) have been developed. Cross-reactions with mumps virus limit the utility of these tests.

Rabies Virus. The preferred method for the diagnosis of rabies in animals is the DFA test for rabies virus antigen in brain tissue. Fluorescein isothiocyanate-labeled antirabies antibodies can be prepared against whole rabies viruses or purified RNA-nucleoprotein complex or nucleoproteins (N proteins). For the diagnosis of rabies in humans, the following specimens are collected: saliva (collected with an eye dropper and placed in a sterile container with no preservatives), neck biopsy specimen (collected from the hair line and of sufficient depth to include cutaneous nerves and placed in a sterile container with no preservatives), 0.5 ml of serum (not whole blood) or CSF, and brain biopsy specimen (only if the specimen was collected for other diagnostic procedures). The following tests are recommended: saliva, RT-PCR and culture; neck biopsy

Viral Diagnosis

specimen, RT-PCR, and IFA; serum and CSF, serologic testing; brain biopsy specimen, RT-PCR and IFA. Serologic testing can be used to assess the response to vaccination. The neutralization test is most commonly used, although a rabies surface glycoprotein (G)-specific ELISA is available in Europe.

Respiratory Syncytial Virus.　Nasal aspirates or washes give a better yield of RSV than do swab specimens. Viral infectivity is rapidly lost at room temperature, and so specimens for culture should be processed promptly. The most sensitive cell lines for culture are HEp-2 and HeLa; less sensitive cells include primary monkey kidney and human fibroblast cell lines. CPE is observed on average at 4 to 5 days. The shell vial assay is slightly more sensitive, and positive cultures are detected at 1 to 2 days. Direct antigen detection tests (IFA and EIA) have a sensitivity equivalent to that of culture, are more rapid, and are not adversely affected by specimen transportation problems. NAA assays are not widely available. Serologic testing is useful for epidemiological surveys but is not as sensitive as culture or antigen tests.

Rhinovirus.　The cell lines used most commonly for growth of rhinoviruses are WI-38 and MRC-5. Cultures should be incubated at 33°C, with CPE seen as early as 1 to 2 days after inoculation. Negative cultures should be held for 7 days or more. EIAs are insensitive because there are a large number of serotypes of rhinoviruses and no common antigen exists. RT-PCR assays are more sensitive than culture but are restricted primarily to research laboratories. The large number of serotypes also makes serologic testing impractical.

Rubella Virus.　Throat swabs and nasopharyngeal specimens are reliable sources of rubella virus, with positive cultures detected a few days before the rash develops to up to 4 days after onset. The virus grows in a variety of cell lines (e.g., Vero, BHK21, AGMK, and RK-13). Cultures are maintained for 1 week and then passaged. Viral growth is detected by IFA or RT-PCR. RT-PCR assays have also been used for primary detection of virus but are restricted primarily to research laboratories and are not used routinely for clinical diagnosis. Detection of rubella virus-specific IgM is the fastest and most efficient method to diagnose recent postnatal infection. However, only 50% of infected newborns are IgM positive on the day of symptom onset. By 8 days after the onset of rash, the infant should be positive for both IgM detectable by IgM capture ELISA and IgG detectable by indirect ELISA. False-positive tests can occur; care must be exercised in interpreting the test results.

DNA Viruses

Adenovirus. All adenoviruses except types 40 and 41 replicate and produce CPE in cell cultures (e.g., HeLa, KB, A549, HEp-2, and HEK cells). CPE usually appears in 2 to 7 days, but passage of cell cultures for up to 1 month is recommended for negative cultures. Shell vial assays are as sensitive as traditional culture and more rapid (taking 2 to 5 days). Clinical specimens can also be examined by IFA, but this is significantly less sensitive than culture. Commercial EIAs are also available and are particularly useful for detecting types 40 and 41 in patients with gastroenteritis. NAA assays have also been developed but are not widely available. Serologic tests are used primarily for epidemiological purposes. A seroconversion must be demonstrated to confirm a current infection, because seroreactivity to adenovirus is common.

Cytomegalovirus. Culture is a sensitive method for detecting cytomegalovirus (CMV) in respiratory specimens, urine, and anticoagulated whole blood (leukocytes). Intermittent shedding in urine is possible, and so multiple specimens should be processed. Recovery of CMV from leukocytes is a better indicator of symptomatic infection. Human fibroblast cell lines (e.g., WI-38, MRC-5, and IMR-90) are best, but growth is typically slow and may require serial passage of the cells and prolonged incubation (for up to 6 weeks). Assays to detect the CMV 65-kDa phosphoprotein (pp65) are commercially available and are useful for the determination of CMV viremia in recipients of solid-organ and bone marrow transplants and HIV-positive individuals. Results of this test compare favorably with the quantitative detection of CMV DNA in leukocytes or plasma by NAA methods (PCR). A variety of serologic tests are available (e.g., EIA, IFA, and passive latex agglutination), including IgM- and IgG-specific tests. IgM results must be interpreted with caution because IgM antibody is found in both primary and reactivated infections and can persist for months. Demonstration of IgG seroconversion is diagnostic of primary infection. Serologic testing is important in assessing organ donors and recipients but is not useful in diagnosing infections in immunocompromised patients.

Epstein-Barr Virus. Epstein-Barr virus (EBV) can be cultured in human cord blood lymphocytes, but this is rarely done for diagnostic purposes. Indirect, direct, and anticomplement immunofluorescence are the main methods used for the detection of EBV antigens in tissues and cell cultures. However, the test of choice for detection of virus is NAA. Detection of EBV genomes in serum or plasma is a more reliable sign of significant infection, and quantitative tests are more valuable than qualitative ones. EBV-positive CSF is significantly associated with primary lymphoma in HIV-positive individuals and with encephalitis in immunocompetent individuals. Serologic testing is the method of choice for the diagnosis of primary infection. For interpretation of serologic test results, refer to Table 5.3.

Erythrovirus (B19 Virus). B19 virus, a member of the *Parvoviridae*, is difficult to grow in vitro. Viral particles or DNA can be detected in blood about 6 days after infection, with peak viremia occurring 2 to 3 days later. Viral titers decrease, but B19 DNA can be detected by PCR for up to 2 months. Serologic tests to detect antibodies are commercially available and are the most commonly used methods for diagnosis of acute infections and immune status. In immunocompetent individuals, IgM antibodies develop 2 weeks after infection and persist for up to 30 weeks. In patients with aplastic crisis, antibodies appear several days after onset of clinical symptoms. In patients with fetal hydrops, detection of IgM antibodies at the time of clinical onset is more variable. In immunocompetent patients, IgG antibodies appear several days after IgM antibodies and persist for years. The presence of IgG antibodies is consistent with immunity. In immunocompromised patients, IgG and IgM antibody responses are unpredictable, and so serologic testing is not used for these patients. NAA and PCR are the most common methods used to detect B19 DNA. Serologic diagnosis of recent infection is generally performed by IgM capture EIAs. If IgM assays are negative for immunocompromised patients, DNA detection methods should be used. B19 IgG antibodies detected by EIA in the absence of seroconversion are indicative of past infection.

Hepatitis B Virus. Diagnosis of hepatitis B virus (HBV) infections is based primarily on the detection of virus-specific antigens and antibodies. A variety of assays have been developed to detect early and late antigens and the antibody response to each. Refer to Table 5.4 for interpretation of these assays in specific clinical presentations.

Viral Diagnosis

Table 5.3 EBV serologic profiles under different conditions[a,b]

Condition	Presence of antibodies to antigen and Ig isotype[c]:						
	VCA, IgG	VCA, IgM	VCA, IgA	EA/D, IgG	EA/R, IgG	EBNA, Ig	EBNA1, IgG
Seronegative	−	−	−	−	−	−	−
Ongoing primary infection	++	+++	++	++	±	−	−
Recent primary infection	++	++	++	++	++	−	−
Past primary infection	++	−	−	−	−	++	++
Chronic active EBV infection	+++	++	++	++	++	±	±

[a]Adapted from P. R. Murray, E. J. Baron, J. H. Jorgensen, M. A. Pfaller, and R. H. Yolken (ed.), *Manual of Clinical Microbiology*, 8th ed., ASM Press, Washington, D.C., 2003.

[b]The most frequently employed antigens and Ig isotypes are included. The characteristic reactivity is given. For all conditions apart from seronegativity, there are exceptions to the rule. Clinical data including other laboratory parameters supporting the likelihood of a diagnosis must always be kept in mind.

[c]−, antibodies completely absent; ±, antibodies absent or present in low titers; +, antibodies present in low titers; ++, antibodies present in medium titers; +++, antibodies present in elevated titers; ++++, antibodies present in strongly elevated titers. VCA, viral capsid antigen; EA/D, early antigen; EA/R, early antigen—restricted component; EBNA, Epstein-Barr nuclear antigen; EBNA1, Epstein-Barr nuclear antigen 1.

Viral Diagnosis

Viral Diagnosis

Table 5.4 Hepatitis B virus markers in different stages of infection and convalescence[a,b,c]

Stage of infection	HBV DNA	HBsAg	HBeAg	Anti-HBc			Anti-HBe	Anti-HBs
				Total	IgM			
Early incubation	+	–	–	–	–		–	–
Late incubation	+	+	+ or –	–	–		–	–
Acute infection	+	+	+	+	+		–	–
HBsAg-negative acute infection	+ or –	–	–	+	+		–	–
Chronic infection	+	+	–	+++	+ or –		–	–
Healthy HBsAg carrier	–	+	–	+++	+ or –		+	–
Recent infection	+ or –	–	–	++	+		+	+ or ++
Remote infection	–	–	–	+	–		–	+ or –
Vaccination response	–	–	–	–	–		–	+

[a] Adapted from P. R. Murray, E. J. Baron, J. H. Jorgensen, M. A. Pfaller, and R. H. Yolken (ed.), *Manual of Clinical Microbiology*, 8th ed., ASM Press, Washington, D.C., 2003.

[b] HBV, hepatitis B virus; HBsAg, hepatitis B surface antigen; HBeAg, hepatitis B e antigen; HBc, hepatitis B core antigen.

[c] –, antibodies absent; +, antibodies present; ++, antibodies present in moderately high titers; +++, antibodies present in very high titers.

Herpes Simplex Virus Types 1 and 2.   Culture is a sensitive method for detecting virus in mucocutaneous, genital, and ocular lesions. Viral growth, as indicated by a CPE, is rapid in most cell lines (95% of specimens are positive by 5 days). Some cell lines (e.g., mink lung cells) are better than others (e.g., MRC-5 and Vero cells). Culture is insensitive for CSF infections, for which PCR is the recommended test. DFA and IFA tests are available and provide a rapid result if positive, but they are relatively insensitive compared with culture and PCR. DFA and IFA can be used to distinguish between herpes simplex virus type 1 (HSV-1) and type 2 (HSV-2) when the viruses are isolated in culture. An EIA has also been developed but is less sensitive than culture, particularly for specimens from asymptomatic patients. PCR assays can detect all strains of HSV and can distinguish between HSV-1 and HSV-2. Type-specific IgG assays are also available commercially.

Human Herpesvirus 6.   Human herpesvirus 6 (HHV-6) causes roseola infantum (exanthem subitum) in children and opportunistic infections in immunocompromised patients. HHV-6 can be isolated from peripheral blood mononuclear cells by cocultivation with human cord blood lymphocytes; however, this test is not commonly performed. Quantitative PCR assays have been developed and have proved useful for monitoring viral concentrations in peripheral blood mononuclear cells. A variety of serologic assays (e.g., neutralization, immunoblot, IFA, and ELISA) are available for measuring IgG antibodies to HHV-6. Some cross-reactivity with HHV-7 and CMV occurs. Seroconversion can be used to define a primary infection.

Orthopoxvirus (Vaccinia Virus, Smallpox Virus, Monkeypox Virus).   Orthopoxviruses can grow in a variety of established cell lines (BSC-1, CV-1, and LLCMK-2 cells, monkey kidney cells, human embryonic lung fibroblasts, HeLa cells, chicken embryo fibroblasts, and MRC-5 cells). Growth is rapid, with most cultures being positive within 48 h. PCR-based NAA tests are also available for detecting virus in serum and vesicular lesions. Virus- and family-specific assays have been developed. Neutralizing antibodies can be detected as early as 6 days after infection or vaccination. The absence of antibodies does not define susceptibility to infection, because the level of antibodies required for protective immunity is not known.

Papillomavirus.   Human papillomavirus (HPV) cannot be grown in culture. Late-structure antigens have been detected in tissue biopsy specimens by using virus-specific polyclonal antibodies. This assay is specific but insensitive and is rarely used for diagnostic purposes. HPV DNA can be detected by using type-specific DNA or RNA probes in a variety of hybridization techniques. The use of target amplification to increase the sensitivity of this method has made this the diagnostic test of choice. Serologic tests are used for epidemiological studies because type-specific antibodies can be detectable for many years after exposure.

Polyomavirus (JC Virus, BK Virus). Viral culture is not routinely used for clinical diagnosis because JC virus and BK virus have long growth cycles and a limited range of host cells. Serologic testing has been used primarily for epidemiological studies. Most individuals are infected at a young age. IgM antibodies develop initially, as measured by EIAs. The role of this antibody response in recurrent infections is not well characterized. NAA tests are the primary tests used to document infection with JC virus and BK virus. JC virus DNA is detected in patients with progressive multifocal leukoencephalopathy, and BK virus DNA is detected in the blood and urine of renal transplant recipients.

Varicella-Zoster Virus. Diploid human cell lines (e.g., human fetal diploid kidney [HFDK] and human fetal diploid lung [HFDL] cells) are the most sensitive cells for isolation of varicella-zoster virus (VZV). Other cell lines can support the growth of VZV but are much less sensitive. CPE is generally observed in the first week of incubation, but prolonged incubation may be required. DFA tests are available and are much more sensitive than culture (98 and 50%, respectively) because the virus is highly labile. Cellular material from the base of a vesicular lesion must be collected; vesicle fluid alone is unsatisfactory. PCR is also more sensitive than culture. The value of serologic testing (many tests are commercially available) is limited because increases in the titer of heterotypic antibody to VZV may occur in HSV-infected patients who have had a prior infection with VZV. Serologic testing is used primarily to assess immunity in unvaccinated health care workers exposed to patients with documented VZV infections.

Transmissible Spongiform Encephalopathies

Bovine Encephalopathy. Diagnosis is based on clinical history and histopathologic examination of brain tissues. Early

Viral Diagnosis

diagnosis has also been made on the basis of examination of tonsillar and appendix biopsy specimens.

Creutzfeldt-Jakob Disease.   Diagnosis is based on clinical history and histopathologic examination of brain tissues.

Kuru.   Diagnosis is based on clinical history and histopathologic examination of brain tissues.

Fungal Diagnosis

Mycology: Specimen Collection and Transport Guidelines

General Guidelines

1. Although the recovery of some fungi in clinical specimens is always considered significant (e.g., dermatophytes, dimorphic fungi, *Cryptococcus neoformans*), most fungi are part of the patient's normal flora (e.g., *Candida* spp.) or found in the environment (e.g., most dematiaceous and moniliaceous fungi). Specimens must be carefully collected to avoid contamination with indigenous or exogenous fungi.

2. Bacteria can rapidly overgrow fungi, so care must be used in cleaning the site where the specimen will be collected (e.g., skin surface, nail beds). Transport conditions must be selected to minimize the risk of bacterial overgrowth.

3. Microscopic examination of specimens is important for the rapid detection of a fungal infection and for assessing the significance of an isolate.

Dematiaceous Fungi

Specimens submitted for microscopy and culture include aspirates, scrapings, and tissues. Swabs should not be used because an inadequate quantity of material is recovered and desiccation occurs. Transport medium is unnecessary if the specimen is processed immediately. Serologic testing is not available except for *Sporothrix* spp. (discussed below with dimorphic fungi).

Dermatophytes (*Epidermophyton, Microsporum, and Trichophyton* spp.)

Collect infected hairs with sterile forceps (guided by the use of a Wood's lamp if the suspected dermatophyte is fluorescent). Endothrix fungi may require the use of a sterile scalpel to collect the hair root. Sample skin lesions at the active border of the lesion with a sterile scalpel to collect the sample. Disinfect nails with alcohol before collecting the sample by clipping or scraping. Do not place hair, skin, or nail samples in closed tubes. The high humidity fosters overgrowth of contaminating bacteria. If possible, directly inoculate the sample to appropriate media.

Dimorphic Fungi (*Blastomyces, Coccidioides, Histoplasma, Paracoccidioides,* and *Sporothrix* spp.)

Process specimens (e.g., respiratory specimens and wound aspirates) promptly to avoid overgrowth of contaminating bacteria. Do not use swabs, because these organisms are susceptible to desiccation. *Histoplasma capsulatum* can be recovered in blood cultures, particularly from patients with AIDS and other immunosuppressive diseases. The lysis-centrifugation system (Isolator [Wampole]) and the MycoF/Lytic blood culture bottle (Becton Dickinson) are useful for the isolation of dimorphic moulds from blood.

Eumycotic Mycetoma Agents

Examine pus, exudate, or biopsy material for the presence of granules (sclerotia) consisting of the eumycotic agents and matrix material. Wash the granules with saline containing antibiotics (e.g., penicillin and streptomycin), and then culture them. Organisms can be visualized by examining crushed granules microscopically.

Moniliaceous Fungi

Process specimens (e.g., biopsy specimens, lower respiratory secretions, nails, eye specimens) promptly to avoid overgrowth of contaminating bacteria. Do not transport specimens on swabs, because organisms are susceptible to desiccation. Specimens should be examined microscopically and cultured. *Pseudallescheria boydii* and *Fusarium* spp. are among the few filamentous fungi that can be recovered in blood cultures. Collect blood specimens in the lysis-centrifugation system (Isolator) and/or the MycoF/Lytic blood culture bottle. Serologic tests are available for some of these fungi.

Pneumocystis (carinii) jiroveci

Respiratory specimens should be limited to induced sputa or bronchoscopy specimens. Patients can only rarely expectorate sputum, and throat washings are insensitive. Collect first morning specimens when possible. A 24-h collection is unacceptable. The presence of oral contamination, signified by squamous epithelial cells, does not invalidate the specimen.

Yeast

Yeasts are relatively easy to isolate from clinical specimens, although overgrowth of contaminating bacteria should be avoided. Yeasts are isolated commonly from blood specimens. Lysis centrifugation, biphasic systems, and the MycoF/Lytic blood culture bottle are reliable methods for isolating yeasts from blood. Automated continuous-monitoring systems are reliable for common yeasts but less reliable for *Cryptococcus neoformans.* Direct detection includes microscopy (Gram stain, KOH, India ink, Calcofluor white) and antigen tests. Serologic testing is available for antibodies to *Candida* spp. but is not commonly used.

Table 6.1 Methods for the identification of fungi

Organism	Applicability of [a]:				
	Direct microscopy	Culture	Antigen detection	Antibody detection	Nucleic acid detection [b]
Candida spp.	A	A	C	D	D
Cryptococcus spp.	A	A	A	B	D
Malassezia spp.	A	B	D	D	D
Trichosporon spp.	A	A	D	D	D
Blastomyces dermatitidis [c]	A	A	A	B	D
Coccidioides spp. [c]	A	A	A	A	D
Histoplasma capsulatum [c]	A	A	B	B	D
Paracoccidioides brasiliensis	A	A	A	A	D
Penicillium marneffei [c]	A	A	C	C	D
Sporothrix schenckii	A	A	C	C	D
Aspergillus spp.	A	A	B	B	D
Moniliaceous fungi (not *Aspergillus* spp.)	A	A	D	D	D
Dematiaceous fungi	A	A	D	D	D
Dermatophytes	A	A	D	D	D
Zygomycetes	A	A	D	D	D
Eumycotic mycetoma agents	A	A	D	D	D
Pneumocystis spp.	A	D	D	D	C

[a] A, test is generally useful for diagnosis; B, test is useful under certain circumstances; C, test is seldom useful for general diagnostic purposes but may be available in reference laboratories; D, test is generally not used for laboratory diagnosis of infection.

[b] Nucleic acid techniques will probably be used in the future as primary tools for the diagnosis of fungal infections. At present, further technical developments and clinical studies are needed.

[c] For laboratory safety purposes, please notify the laboratory if this agent is suspected. The conidia of the mycelial form of these dimorphic fungi are highly infectious and easily transmissible by aerosolization.

Fungal Diagnosis

Acridine Orange Stain

Acridine orange stains fungi red-orange, but the background material stains green-yellow. For stain details, see section 4.

Calcofluor White Stain

Calcofluor white is a nonspecific fluorochrome that binds to cellulose and chitin in the cell walls of fungi. The dye can be mixed with 10% potassium hydroxide so that mammalian cells can be dissolved, thus facilitating visualization of fungal elements. Fungi (including *Pneumocystis jiroveci*) appear green or blue against a dark background when the stained slide is examined under UV illumination. Care must be used to distinguish specific staining from stained debris. Optimal detection of fluorescence requires the use of a 400- to 500-nm excitation filter and 500- to 520-nm barrier filter.

Fluorescent-Antibody Stain

Direct and indirect fluorescein-conjugated monoclonal anti-*Pneumocystis* antibodies are used for immunofluorescence assays and target a family of surface glycoproteins that contain both common and distinct epitopes within and among *Pneumocystis* species. Depending on the monoclonal antibody supplied with the kit, staining may target only the cyst form or may target all forms of the organism. The typical fluorophore that is conjugated to the antibody or used in an indirect assay is fluorescein isothiocynate, which produces a brilliant apple green color. The staining reaction shows a diffuse pattern distributed over the surface of the entire cluster of organisms and often over the matrix in which the organisms are embedded. Single cysts usually appear with a distinctive rim of fluorescence and a duller interior fluorescence.

Giemsa Stain

The Giemsa stain combines methylene blue and eosin. It is useful for the detection of *Histoplasma capsulatum* in bone marrow, peripheral smears, and touch preparations, as well as intracystic bodies and trophozoites of *Pneumocystis jiroveci* in induced sputum, bronchoscopy specimens, and lung tissue. *H. capsulatum* appears as tiny blue-purple budding yeast cells. The cyst wall of *P. jiroveci* appears as a clear ring around spores or intracystic bodies. The nuclei stain red-purple, and the cytoplasm generally stains light to dark blue.

Fungal Diagnosis

Gram Stain

The Gram stain detects most fungi if present. Most yeast appear gram positive; however, *Cryptococcus* and *Malassezia* spp. stain weakly and in some instances exhibit only stippling. The hyphae of moulds generally appear gram negative. *Pneumocystis* produces a negative (pink) reaction with poorly defined organism morphology.

India Ink Stain (Nigrosin)

The use of India ink is not technically a staining method. Detection of encapsulated fungi (i.e., *Cryptococcus neoformans*) is made possible by exclusion of the ink particles by the polysaccharide capsule of the organism. Care in interpretation is required because artifacts (e.g., leukocytes, erythrocytes, powder, and bubbles) may be confused with yeast cells. The morphologic characteristics of the yeast cells must be recognized before the preparation can be interpreted. Although a rapid detection method for encapsulated yeasts, the India ink procedure is an insensitive method for the detection of *Cryptococcus neoformans*; cryptococcal antigen testing (latex or enzyme immunoassay) is recommended.

Kinyoun Stain

Some ascomycetous fungi produce ascospores when grown on a medium that promotes their formation. Ascospores are acid-fast and stain red, while the ascomycete cell wall and cytoplasm appear blue. (For stain details, see section 4.)

Potassium Hydroxide (KOH)

A 10 to 15% solution of potassium hydroxide can be used to dissolve cellular and organic debris and facilitate the detection of fungal elements, which are not affected by strong alkali solutions (although fungal elements dissolve after exposure for a few days). The hyphae of dematiaceous fungi can be distinguished from those of hyaline moulds by their brown melanin pigment on these direct preparations. Ink (e.g., permanent blue-black Parker Super Quick Ink) can be added as a contrasting agent to aid the detection of fungi. Lactophenol cotton blue (i.e., Poirrier's blue) can also be added to the KOH. The aniline blue stains the outer cell wall of fungi, and the lactic acid is a clearing agent.

Toluidine Blue-O Stain

Toluidine blue-O stain is used primarily for the detection of *Pneumocystis jiroveci* in respiratory specimens. *P. jiroveci* cysts

Fungal Diagnosis

stain reddish blue to dark purple against a light blue background. Trophozoites do not stain by this method. This staining method is rapid and inexpensive, but some skill is required to recognize *P. jiroveci* cysts (usually present in clumps). Many laboratories prefer the direct fluorescent-antibody test for the detection of *P. jiroveci* even though the stain is more expensive.

Table 6.2 Characteristic fungal elements seen by direct examination of clinical specimens

Morphologic fungal structure found	Organism(s)	Diam range (µm)	Characteristic features	Illustration[a]
Yeast forms	*Histoplasma capsulatum*	2–5	Oval to round budding cells; often found clustered within histiocytes	
	Sporothrix schenckii	2–6	Oval to round to cigar-shaped, single or multiple buds present; yeast uncommonly seen in clinical specimens	
	Cryptococcus neoformans	2–15	Cells vary in size; usually round to oval; buds usually single and "pinched off"; capsule may or may not be evident; pseudohyphal forms rare	

[a]Illustrations from D. H. Larone, *Medically Important Fungi, a Guide to Identification*, 4th ed., ASM Press, Washington, D.C., 2002.

(continued)

Fungal Diagnosis

Table 6.2 Characteristic fungal elements seen by direct examination of clinical specimens *(continued)*

Morphologic fungal structure found	Organism(s)	Diam range (μm)	Characteristic features	Illustration[a]
	Penicillium marneffei	3	Fission yeast; do not bud; round to oval with a central septum	
	Blastomyces dermatitidis	8–15	Cells usually large and spherical, doubly refractile; buds usually single but may remain connected to parent cells by broad base	
	Paracoccidioides brasiliensis	5–60	Cells usually large and surrounded by smaller buds around periphery (mariner's wheel appearance); small cells (2–5 μm) that resemble *H. capsulatum* may be present	

Yeast forms and pseudohyphae or true hyphae	*Candida* spp.	3–4 (yeast forms), 5–10 (pseudohyphae)	Cells usually exhibit single budding; pseudohyphae, when present, are constricted at ends and remain attached; true hyphae, when present, have parallel walls
	Malassezia spp.	3–4 (yeast forms), 2.5–4 (pseudohyphae)	Short, curved hyphal elements may be present along with round-oval yeast cells that are round at one end and have a flat collarette at the opposite end
Spherules	*Coccidioides* spp.	10–200	Spherules vary in size; some contain endospores; hyphae may be found in cavitary lesions

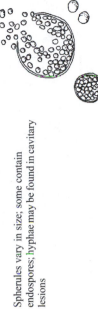

(continued)

[a]Illustrations from D. H. Larone, *Medically Important Fungi, a Guide to Identification*, 4th ed., ASM Press, Washington, D.C., 2002.

Fungal Diagnosis

Fungal Diagnosis

Table 6.2 Characteristic fungal elements seen by direct examination of clinical specimens *(continued)*

Morphologic fungal structure found	Organism(s)	Diam range (μm)	Characteristic features	Illustration[a]
Sporangium	*Rhinosporidium seeberi*	6–300	Large, thick-walled sporangia containing sporangiospores; mature sporangia are larger than *Coccidioides* spherules	
Adiaconidia	*Emmonsia crescens*	20–140	Large, round, thick walled, no budding; interior of adiacondium usually appears empty	
Wide nonseptate or rarely septate hyphae	Zygomycetes, *Pythium* spp.	10–30	Large, ribbonlike hyphae, often fractured or twisted, branching usually at right angles	

Hyaline septate hyphae	Dermatophytes	3–15	Branched, septate hyphae; chains of arthroconidia may be seen	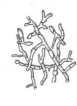
	Other hyaline moulds; *Aspergillus*, *Fusarium*	3–12	Hyphae are septate and may exhibit 45° (dichotomous) and 90° angle branching	
Dematiaceous septate hyphae	Organisms causing phaeohyphomycosis	2–6	Brown-pigmented septate hyphae, dark budding yeastlike forms may also occur	

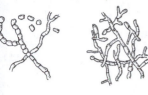

*Illustrations from D. H. Larone, *Medically Important Fungi, a Guide to Identification*, 4th ed., ASM Press, Washington, D.C., 2002.*

(continued)

Fungal Diagnosis

Fungal Diagnosis

Table 6.2 Characteristic fungal elements seen by direct examination of clinical specimens *(continued)*

Morphologic fungal structure found	Organism(s)	Diam range (μm)	Characteristic features	Illustration[a]
Dematiaceous sclerotic bodies	Organisms causing chromoblastomycosis	5–12	Sclerotic bodies are brown pigmented and thick walled and have horizontal and vertical septations	
Cysts and trophozoites	*Pneumocystis (carinii) jiroveci*	3–5	Nonbudding, round, ovoid, or collapsed crescent forms appear in small clusters against a foamy background	

[a]Illustrations from D. H. Larone, *Medically Important Fungi, a Guide to Identification*, 4th ed., ASM Press, Washington, D.C., 2002.

Primary Plating Media

Birdseed Agar

Birdseed (also called niger seed) agar is used for the selective isolation and identification of *Cryptococcus neoformans*. The agar medium contains an extract of *Guizotia abyssinica* seed, caffeic acid. *C. neoformans* produces phenol oxidase, and dark brown colonies develop in the presence of caffeic acid. The medium contains chloramphenicol to suppress the growth of bacteria.

Brain Heart Infusion Agar (BHI)

Brain heart infusion agar is a nutritionally enriched medium that can be used for the isolation of a variety of fastidious bacteria, yeast, and moulds. It is prepared with infusions of calf brains and beef hearts, peptones, glucose, sodium chloride, and disodium phosphate. Supplementation with 5 to 10% sheep blood can enrich the medium, and the addition of antibiotics (e.g., gentamicin, chloramphenicol, and penicillin) can make this medium selective for fungi.

CHROMagar *Candida*

CHROMagar *Candida* is a selective, differential agar medium for the isolation and presumptive identification of *Candida albicans*, *C. krusei*, and *C. tropicalis*. The medium consists of peptones, glucose, chloramphenicol, and "chromogenic mix." The antibiotic inhibits the growth of most bacteria. *C. albicans* forms green colonies, *C. krusei* forms pink colonies, and *C. tropicalis* forms purple colonies.

Dermatophyte Test Medium (DTM)

Dermatophyte test medium is a selective agar medium used for the isolation and identification of dermatophytes. It consists of digests of soybean meal supplemented with glucose, cycloheximide, chlortetracycline, gentamicin, and phenol red. The antibiotics suppress the growth of bacteria, saprophytic yeasts, and moulds. Dermatophytes growing on this medium produce alkaline by-products that change the phenol red indicator from yellow to red. This color change may be obscured when grossly contaminated specimens (e.g., nails) are processed on this medium. The pigment produced by dermatophytes, which is used for their identification, is obscured by the intense red color produced on this medium.

Inhibitory Mould Agar (IMA)

Inhibitory mould agar is an enriched, selective medium that is used for the isolation of pathogenic fungi other than dermatophytes. It consists of digests of animal tissue and casein, yeast extract, dextrin, starch, glucose, salts, and chloramphenicol. Contaminating bacteria are inhibited by chloramphenicol.

Mycosel (Mycobiotic) Agar

Mycosel (Mycobiotic) agar is a selective medium used for the isolation of pathogenic fungi from contaminated specimens. Mycosel and Mycobiotic (BD Diagnostic) agars consist of digests of soybean meal supplemented with glucose, cyclohex-imide, and chloramphenicol. Cycloheximide-susceptible fungi, including *Cryptococcus neoformans, Pseudallescheria boydii,* the zygomycetes, many species of *Candida* and *Aspergillus, Trichosporon* spp., and most saprophytic or opportunistic fungi, do not grow on this medium.

Sabouraud Agar-Brain Heart Infusion (SABHI)

Sabouraud agar-brain heart infusion (SABHI), an enriched agar medium, is a variation of Sabouraud dextrose agar (described below). The medium consists of infusions of beef heart and calf brains, peptones, salts, glucose, blood, and chloromycetin (chloramphenicol). It is used for the cultivation of dermatophytes and other pathogenic and nonpathogenic fungi.

Sabouraud Dextrose Agar (SDA)

Sabouraud dextrose agar is an enriched agar medium used for the isolation of saprophytic and pathogenic fungi. The original formulation of SDA consists of digests of casein and animal tissue supplemented with 4% glucose and adjusted to pH 5.6. The Emmons modification is preferred by many mycologists. It contains a reduced concentration of glucose (2%) and is buffered to neutrality (pH 6.9). Yeast, dermatophytes, and other filamentous fungi grow on these media. The original formulation of SDA was acidic to suppress the growth of bacteria. This problem can be circumvented by the addition of antibiotics (e.g., cycloheximide and chloramphenicol) to the media. However, cycloheximide-susceptible fungi (refer to Mycosel agar above) do not grow on this medium.

Fungal Diagnosis

Yeast Extract-Phosphate Agar

Yeast extract-phosphate agar is a selective medium used for the isolation of pathogenic fungi such as *Histoplasma* and *Blastomyces* spp. It consists of yeast extract and phosphate buffer supplemented with chloramphenicol to suppress the growth of bacteria. The pH is adjusted to 6.0.

Fungal Diagnosis

Fungal Diagnosis

Table 6.3 Mycology plating guide

Source	Direct exam[a] (wet mount, Calcofluor white, KOH)	MAF for Nocardia[b]	Enriched SABHI, SDA, BHI	Selective	Comments
Blood	N		× (or automated systems media)		Lysis and centrifugation; automated systems include BacT/Alert (bioMerieux), BACTEC (Becton Dickinson), and ESP (Trek); if *Malassezia* suspected, add olive oil to plates
Body fluids	O		×	IMA, Mycosel, yeast extract, phosphate	>2 ml, filtration or centrifugation at 2,000 × *g* for 10 min to concentrate fungal organisms; for quantification of urines, uncentrifuged urine can be streaked with a calibrated loop onto a plate of noninhibitory media
Bone marrow	N		×		
Eye					
Corneal scrapings	O		×		Inoculate media directly using C or X marks
Eyelid, conjunctiva	O		×	IMA, Mycosel	
Vitreous fluid	O		×		>2 ml, filtration or centrifugation at 2,000 × *g* for 10 min to concentrate fungal organisms
Exudates, pus, drainage	O	×	×	IMA, Mycosel, yeast extract	If granules present, wash, centrifuge, examine, and crush granules

Mouth	R or Gram stain			CHROMagar *Candida*, IMA	Candidiasis is usually diagnosed on the basis of clinical symptoms and direct microscopic examination
Nails, hair, skin scrapings	R			IMA, Mycosel, DTM	Cut into small pieces and embed directly into agar; if *Malassezia* suspected, add olive oil to plates
Respiratory secretions	R, O (PCP stain)	×	×	CHROMagar *Candida*, IMA, Mycosel, yeast extract, phosphate, birdseed	Liquefication with a mucolytic agent; necessary with centrifugation for induced sputum specimens for the detection of *Pneumocystis* spp.
Sinus	R		×	CHROMagar *Candida*, IMA	
Tissue	R, O (PCP stain, lung)	×	×	IMA, Mycosel, yeast extract, phosphate, bird-seed	Mincing (zygomycetes), grinding (*Histoplasma*), or use of stomacher
Vagina	R, Gram stain			CHROMagar *Candida*, IMA	Vaginal candidiasis is usually diagnosed on the basis of clinical symptoms and direct microscopic examination

[a] R, staining should be routinely performed; O, staining is optional and should be performed if requested; N, staining should not be performed unless the request is discussed with the physician.

[b] Although *Nocardia* is a bacterium, stains and cultures are commonly pursued through the Mycology Laboratory. For appropriate bacterial culture media, please see Primary Plating Media in section 4 of this handbook.

Fungal Diagnosis

Abbreviation Guide. CF, complement fixation; CIE, counter-immunoelectrophoresis; EIA, enzyme immunoassay; ID, immunodiffusion; IFA, indirect fluorescent-antibody test; LA, latex agglutination; RIA, radioimmunoassay; TA, tube agglutination; TP, tube precipitin.

Aspergillus **Species.** Microscopy and culture are sensitive detection methods for *Aspergillus* species. Molecular methods are being developed for both direct specimen and *Aspergillus* spp. identification. EIA and RIA for *Aspergillus* antigens and CF, CIE, and ID tests for antibodies have been developed. Antigen tests are used primarily to diagnose invasive aspergillosis. Commercial EIAs detect galactomannan (GM) in serum and urine. The tests have a sensitivity between 71 and 95% (higher when monoclonal antibodies are used) and good specificity. Clinical experience of interpreting antigen results is limited. A latex test measuring GM in serum only has also been developed but is less sensitive than EIA. The RIA is not commercially available. Antibody tests are most sensitive for immunocompetent patients with allergic bronchopulmonary aspergillosis (ABPA), pulmonary aspergilloma, and invasive aspergillosis (IA). The sensitivities of the ID and CIE tests are comparable, while ID is more specific. The CF test is more specific but less sensitive than ID. The sensitivity of ID is improved by the use of multiple antigens from *A. fumigatus*, *A. flavus*, *A. niger*, and *A. terreus*. Precipitins are present in more than 90% of patients with aspergillomas, 70% of patients with ABPA, and fewer patients with IA. A fourfold concentration of serum and retesting is recommended for patients with suspected IA and a negative ID result. The ID is highly specific, with false-positive precipitins developing only against C-reactive protein. A complement fixation antibody titer of $\geq 1:8$ is considered positive. Skin test reactivity to *Aspergillus* antigen extracts is useful for patients with suspected allergic bronchopulmonary aspergillosis, atopic dermatitis, or allergic asthma sensitized to aspergilli.

Blastomyces dermatitidis **(Blastomycosis).** Demonstration of broad-based budding yeast cells and culture are the most reliable detection methods for *B. dermatitidis*. This organism can be identified by using microscopic and macroscopic morphology as well as Accuprobe (Genprobe; see section 4) and exoantigen methods. Due to the lack of sensitivity and specificity of available serologic tests (ID, EIA, CF, and RIA), these tests are generally not helpful for diagnosing blastomycosis. The use of the A antigen, obtained from yeast culture filtrates, has improved the specificity of these tests. The commercially available EIA is more sensitive but less specific than ID. An EIA titer of 1:32 or greater is considered diagnostic for blastomycosis. Titers of 1:8 to 1:16 should be confirmed with ID or culture because cross-reactivity with *Histoplasma* antibodies can occur at this level. ID has a sensitivity of approximately 80% and a specificity approaching 100%. Antibodies are detected within 1 month of onset, and the level declines with successful treatment. RIA has a sensitivity and specificity similar to ID but is rarely used. A CF antibody titer of $\geq 1:8$ is considered positive. This test is relatively insensitive and nonspecific for blastomycosis and has generally been replaced by EIA and ID.

***Candida* Species (Candidiasis).** *Candida* species can be detected by direct examination with Gram stain, KOH, or Calcofluor white preparations. *Candida* species grow well on most culture media. The identification of *Candida* species can be pursued through use of color production on differential agars, germ tube production, sugar assimilation and/or fermentation, temperature tolerance, cycloheximide tolerance, and urea and nitrate testing. Currently yeast identification using nucleic acids is not widely practiced. LA, ID, and CIE tests for antibodies and EIAs for antigens have been developed for the diagnosis of candidiasis. In general, the sensitivity and specificity of available tests are low.

***Coccidioides* Species (Coccidioidomycosis).** Microscopy and culture are reliable detection methods for *Coccidioides* species. There are two species of *Coccidioides: C. immitis* and *C. posadasii. C. immitis* can be identified using microscopic and macroscopic morphology as well as Accuprobe and exoantigen methods, while molecular methods are required to definitively identify *C. posadasii.* CF, TP, ID, and EIA have been developed for detection of antibodies against *C. immitis.* The test antigens, called coccidioidin, are prepared from filtrates of mycelial cultures. Two primary antigens are used: a heat-stable 120-kDa glycoprotein (factor 2 antigen) located in the walls of arthroconidia and spherules, and a heat-labile 110-kDa chitinase enzyme (F antigen). The former protein is detected in the TP test, and the latter is detected in the CF test. Both antigens can be detected in the ID test and EIAs. Another antigen, spherulin, is prepared from spherules of *C. immitis* and has been used in CF tests. Factor 2 antigen is not specific for *C. immitis* and is also found in morphologically similar saprophytic fungi. The TP test is used to detect early disease (80% positive at 2 to 3 weeks, disappearing by 6 months), and the CF test detects persistent antibodies. TP remains positive in patients with disseminated disease. The combination of CF and TP tests is positive in more than 90% of infected patients. ID is comparable to CF and TP. The commercially prepared EIA measures both immunoglobulin M (IgM) and IgG antibodies. Both tests must be performed for maximum sensitivity. A positive EIA result must be confirmed by ID. CF antibody titers of 1:2 to 1:4 usually indicate early, residual, or meningeal disease. Antibody titers of $\geq$ 1:16 indicate disseminated disease. Negative titers do not exclude the disease. Coccidioidin skin tests are of limited usefulness, although failure to develop a positive skin test has been associated with poor response to therapy.

***Cryptococcus neoformans* (Cryptococcosis).** Microscopy and culture are useful detection methods for *C. neoformans*. *Cryptococcus* grows readily in culture but is inhibited by cycloheximide. Cryptococcal antigens can be measured by LA and EIA. EIA is more sensitive for capsular glucuronoxylomannan polysaccharide, and the method is suitable for testing of multiple specimens. Titers are generally determined using the LA method. A titer of 1:8 or greater in serum or cerebrospinal fluid (CSF) is considered diagnostic. Titers of 1:4 or less may be indicative of early disease or nonspecific reactions (prozone, patients with rheumatoid arthritis, syneresis fluid, platinum wire loops, *Capnocytophaga* [DF-1], *Trichosporon beigelii*, disinfectants, and soaps). These nonspecific reactions have been documented by LA only. Titers in CSF can be helpful in monitoring therapy when the titers are tested over appropriate intervals (at least 2 weeks). Interpretation of follow-up titers is sometimes difficult because the antigen is harbored within the body; therefore, the definitive decision often depends on the results of culture. More than 99% of patients with culture-confirmed cryptococcosis have positive antigen tests. IFA, EIA, and LA have been developed for measuring cryptococcal antibodies. These tests are not useful for diagnosis because capsular polysaccharide may inhibit antibody synthesis or mask the presence of antibody. Antibody testing may have prognostic value during the recovery of non-AIDS patients.

Fungal Diagnosis

Histoplasma capsulatum (**Histoplasmosis**).   Definitive diagnosis of histoplasmosis requires growth of the fungus. Mycelial forms mature within 20 days and display diagnostic tuberculate macroconidia. Identification is performed by mould-yeast conversion, Accuprobe, and exoantigen methods. CF, EIA, LA, and ID have been developed to measure antibodies to *H. capsulatum*. RIA and EIA have been developed to detect *Histoplasma* antigens in urine and serum. The CF test is sensitive (more than 90% of culture-confirmed patients have antibodies), but cross-reactions can occur in patients with blastomycosis, coccidiodomycosis, other mycoses, and leishmaniasis. Two antigens are used in the CF test: yeast phase antigen and mycelial phase antigen (histoplasmin). CF antibodies develop within 4 weeks after exposure in patients with pulmonary infections, with antibodies against the yeast phase being detected first and those against histoplasmin developing later. Patients with chronic histoplasmosis generally have higher titers to histoplasmin. Antibody titers between 1:8 and 1:32 are considered presumptive evidence of histoplasmosis; however, high titers can be observed in patients with other diseases so serology should be confirmed by culture. Antigen EIA and RIA provide rapid diagnosis, but cross-reactivity occurs with other mycoses. Cross-reactivity does not detract from the value of these tests since, depending of the severity of the clinical picture, antifungal therapy is essentially the same. If these tests are used, the results must be confirmed by ID tests. The ID test can detect as many as six precipitin bands when histoplasmin is used as the test antigen. Two bands, H and M, have diagnostic value. The M band generally appears first and is an indicator of early disease. The presence of both the M and H bands is indicative of active disease, past disease, or recent skin testing. The presence of both M and H bands is consistent with active disease. The LA test is used to detect acute histoplasmosis, with reactivity occurring 2 to 3 weeks after exposure. Positive reactivity should be confirmed with the ID test. A heat-stable polysaccharide antigen can also be detected in serum, urine, and CSF specimens in patients with disseminated histoplasmosis (90% sensitivity), as well as localized pulmonary disease (<50% sensitivity). The urine test is the most sensitive for disseminated disease, but false-positive reactions have been reported with other diseases (e.g., coccidioidomycosis paracoccidioidomycosis, penicilliosis, and blastomycosis). Positive reactions should be confirmed with culture.

Fungal Diagnosis

***Malassezia* Species.** Direct examination and culture are the methods of choice for the detection of *Malassezia* species. The genus *Malassezia* has been revised through use of morphology, ultrastructure, physiology, and molecular techniques. All species are lipophilic (except *M. pachydermatitis*) and require the addition of long-chain fatty acids (e.g., sterile olive oil) to culture media for growth. *Malassezia* exists both as a skin commensal and as an etiological agent of cutaneous and systemic disease. Differentiation of lipophilic species is not generally performed.

Paracoccidioides brasiliensis. Diagnosis is established when direct examination demonstrates the organism's characteristic "ship's wheel." Mycelial forms mature within 21 days, but their presence is not diagnostic. Mould-yeast conversion or exoantigen testing is necessary for definitive identification. CF, ID, EIA, and CIE have been developed to measure antibodies to *P. brasiliensis*. The CF test detects antibodies (titer of 1:32 or greater) in at least 80 to 95% of patients with paracoccidioidomycosis, while positive serologic test results are reported for 98% of patients when both the CF and ID tests are used. Cross-reactivity with *H. capsulatum* can occur in the CF test. Declining CF titers are consistent with a response to therapy, and the presence of persistently high titers indicates a bad prognosis. One to three unique precipitin bands are observed in the ID test. Antigen 1 has been characterized as a 43-kDa glycoprotein. This antigen has also been used in EIA. Both the CF and ID tests are available through the CDC.

***Penicillium marneffei* (Penicilliosis).** The diagnostic test of choice is demonstration of fission yeast cells in direct examinations and the recovery of *P. marneffei* in clinical specimens. These infections are usually disseminated, with multiple-organ involvement including lymphadenitis, subcutaneous abscesses, bone lesions, arthritis, splenomegaly, and lesions in the lungs, liver, or bowel. Serodiagnostic tests (antigen and antibody) are under development. The presence of a precipitin band(s) indicates a positive ID assay. Data regarding the sensitivity and specificity of this test are not currently available. The test should be used to confirm the clinical diagnosis of penicilliosis.

Pneumocystis jiroveci. Demonstration of the organism in clinical specimen by microscopy is diagnostic. *P. jiroveci* grows poorly in cell culture, and reliable antigen and antibody tests have not been developed. The presence of the PCR product has not been strictly correlated with disease. Toluidine blue O, Calco-fluor white, and methenamine silver stain the cyst wall; Gram Weigert and Papanicoalou stain the intracystic bodies and faintly stain trophozoite forms; Giemsa and fluorescein-labeled antibodies (IFA, DFA) stain both cysts and trophozoites.

Sporothrix schenckii **(Sporotrichosis).**   Isolation and mould-yeast conversion are required for the diagnosis of sporotrichosis. Although antigen and antibody tests are available, they are not widely used. EIA, LA, and TA can be used reliably to detect antibodies to *S. schenckii*, while the CF and ID tests are less reliable and are not recommended. Antibodies to at least two cell wall antigens (40- and 70-kDa antigens) are detected. EIA titers of at least 1:16 in serum and 1:8 in CSF are considered diagnostic. Elevated titers can be observed, which decline with successful therapy. LA titers of 1:4 or greater are consistent with disease, although nonspecific reactions can occur at titers of 1:8. Antibody titers in the LA test do not change predictably with therapy, so they cannot be used for prognostic purposes. Investigation into molecular identification is ongoing but is currently limited to taxonomic research.

Zygomycetes **(Zygomycosis, Mucormycosis).**   EIA and ID have been developed to detect antibodies in patients with active zygomycosis. The tests have a sensitivity of approximately 70% and a specificity of greater than 90%. They are rarely used because the etiologic agents of zygomycosis grow rapidly.

The following tables summarize organisms described in the eighth edition of the *Manual of Clinical Microbiology*. They are organized in parallel with the discussions of the organisms within the *Manual*. Due to the dependence on phenotypic growth characteristics for the identification of moulds, the information summarized includes colony morphology, line drawings, and key differential characteristics. All line drawings are used with the author's permission and come from the book *Medically Important Fungi, a Guide to Identification*, fourth edition (2002), by D. H. Larone. For further organism information, please refer to the eighth edition of the *Manual of Clinical Microbiology* and the fourth edition of *Medically Important Fungi, a Guide to Identification*.

Fungal Diagnosis

Table 6.4 Cultural and biochemical characteristics of yeasts frequently isolated from clinical specimens[a,b]

Species	Growth at 37°C	Pseudo- or true hyphae	Germ tubes	Assimilation of: Glucose	Maltose	Sucrose	Lactose	Galactose	Melibiose	Cellobiose	Inositol	Xylose	Raffinose	Trehalose	Dulcitol	Fermentation of: Glucose	Maltose	Sucrose	Lactose	Galactose	Trehalose	Urease	KNO$_3$ utilization	Phenol oxidase
Candida albicans	+	+	+	+	+	+*	–	+	–	–	–	+	–	+	–	F	F	–	–	F	F	–	–	–
C. catenulata	+*	+	–	+	+	–	–	+	–	–	–	+	–	–	–	F*	F	–	–	–	–	–	–	–
C. dubliniensis	+	+	+	+	+	+	–	+	–	–	–	+*	–	+	–	F	–	–	–	F	–	–	–	–
C. famata	+	–	–	+	+	+	+*	+	+	+	–	+	+	+	+*	W	F	W	–	–	W	–	–	–
C. glabrata	+	–	–	+	+	–	–	–	–	–	–	–	–	+	–	F	–	–	–	–	F	–	–	–
C. guilliermondii	+	+	–	+	+	+	+	+	+	+	–	+	+	+	+	F	–	F	–	F*	F	–	–	–
C. kefyr	+	+	–	+	–	+	–	+	+	+*	–	+*	+	–*	–	F	–	F	F*	F	–	–	–	–
C. krusei[c]	+	+	–	+	–	–	+	–	–	–	–	–	–	–	–	F	–	–	–	–	–	+*	–	–
C. lambica	+*	+	–	+	–	+	–	–	–	–	–	+	–	–	–	–	–	–	–	–	–	–	–	–
C. lipolytica[c]	+	+	–	+	–	–	+	–	–	–	–	–	–	–	–	–	–	–	–	–	–	+	–	–
C. lusitaniae[d]	+	+	–	+	+	+	–	+	–	+	–	+	–	+	–	F	–	–	–	–	–	–	–	–
C. parapsilosis[e]	+	+	–	+	+	+	–	+	–	–	–	+	–	+	–	F	F	F	–	F	F	–	–	–
C. rugosa	+	+	–	+	–	–	–	+	–	–	–	+*	–	–	–	–	–	–	–	–	–	–	–	–

C. tropicalis[d,e]	+	+	+	−	+	+	+	−	+	−	+	+	+	−	F	F	F	F*	F*	−	−
C. zeylanoides	−	+	−	−	+	+	−	−	−	−	−	+	−	−	−	−	−	−	−	−	−
Cryptococcus neoformans	+	R	+	−	+	+	+	+	+	−	+	+	+	+	−	−	−	−	−	+	+
C. albidus	−*	−	−	−	+*	+*	+*	+*	+*	+*	+*	+*	+*	+	−	−	−	−	−	+	−
C. laurentii	+*	−	+	−	+	+	+	+	+	+	+	+	+	+	−	F*	−	−	−	+	+
C. luteolus	−	−	+	−	+	+	−	+	+	+	+	+	+	+	−	−	−	−	−	+	−
C. terreus	−*	−	+	−	+*	+*	+*	−	+*	+*	+*	+*	+	−	−	−	−	−	−	+	−
C. uniguttulatus	−	−	−	−	+	+	−	−*	−*	−	−*	−*	+	−*	−	−	−	−	−	+	−
R. glutinis	+	−	+	−	+	+	+	+	+	+	+	+	−	−	F	F	F	F	−	−	−
R. rubra	+	−	+	−	+	+	+	+*	+*	+*	+*	+*	+	−	F*	F	F*	F	F	−	−
S. cerevisiae	+	+	+	−	+	+	+	+	+	+	+	+	+	−	−	−	−	−	−	−	−
H. anomala	+*	−	+	−	+	+	+	+	+	+	+	+	+	+	−	−	−	−	−	+	+
G. candidum	−*	+	−	−	+	−	+	+	+	−	+	−	−	−	−	−	−	−	−	−	−
B. capitatus	+	+	+	+	−	−	−	+	−	+	+	+	−	−	−	−	−	−	−	−	−

[a]Adapted from P. R. Murray, E. J. Baron, J. H. Jorgensen, M. A. Pfaller, and R. H. Yolken (ed.), *Manual of Clinical Microbiology*, 8th ed., ASM Press, Washington, D.C., 2003.

[b]Symbols: +, growth greater than that of the negative control; −, negative reaction; *, some isolates may give the opposite reaction; R, rare; F, the sugar is fermented (i.e., gas is produced); W, weak fermentation.

[c]*C. lipolytica* assimilates erythritol; *C. krusei* does not. Maximum growth temperatures are 43 to 45°C for *C. krusei* and 33 to 37°C for *C. lipolytica*.

[d]*C. lusitaniae* assimilates rhamnose; *C. tropicalis* usually does not.

[e]*C. parapsilosis* assimilates L-arabinose; *C. tropicalis* usually does not.

Fungal Diagnosis

Fungal Diagnosis

Table 6.5 Characteristics of selected *Trichosporon* species[a]

Characteristic	T. asahii	T. asteroides	T. cutaneum	T. inkin	T. mucoides	T. ovoides
Assimilation of:						
L-Rhamnose	+	−	+	−	+	+
Melibiose	−	−	+	−	+	−
Raffinose	−	−	+	−	+	V
Ribitol	V	V	+	−	+	−
Xylitol	V	+	+	−	+	V
L-Arabinitol	+	+	+	−	+	−
Galactitol	−	−	−	−	+	−
Growth at 37°C	+	V	−	+	+	+
Urease	+	+	+	+	+	+
0.01% Cycloheximide	+	V	−	V	+	+
0.1% Cycloheximide	−	V	−	−	+	−
Appresoria	−	−	−	+	−	+

[a]Adapted from P. R. Murray, E. J. Baron, J. H. Jorgensen, M. A. Pfaller, and R. H. Yolken (ed.), *Manual of Clinical Microbiology*, 8th ed., ASM Press, Washington, D.C., 2003.

Table 6.6 Characteristics of *Aspergillus* species[a]

	Diagnostic characteristics	A. fumigatus	A. flavus	A. niger
	Colony morphology	Velvety-powdery, blue-green to gray, reverse white-tan	Velvety-powdery, yellow-dark yellowish green, reverse gold to red-brown	Velvety-powdery, yellow-black, reverse buff
	Seriation	Unseriate	Biseriate	Biseriate
	Conidiophore			
	Microscopic morphology	Smooth	Rough	Smooth, long, straight

conidia
vesicle
conidiophore

uniseriate
phialide
(no metula)

foot cell

[a]Illustrations from D. H. Larone, *Medically Important Fungi, a Guide to Identification,* 4th ed., ASM Press, Washington, D.C., 2002.

(continued)

Fungal Diagnosis

Fungal Diagnosis

Table 6.6 Characteristics of *Aspergillus* species[a] *(continued)*

Illustration	Diagnostic characteristics	A. nidulans	A. terreus	A. versicolor
	Colony morphology	Velvety, dark green to purplish-brown, reverse buff to deep red	Velvety, tan to cinnamon brown, reverse yellow to tan	Green to gray-green or tan with patches of pink or yellow, reverse variable
	Seriation	Biseriate	Biseriate	Biseriate
	Conidiophore	Smooth, short, brown	Smooth	Smooth
	Microscopic morphology			

conidia
vesicle
conidiophore

phialide ⎱ = biseriate
metula ⎰ phialide

foot cell

[a]Illustrations from D. H. Larone, *Medically Important Fungi, a Guide to Identification*, 4th ed., ASM Press, Washington, D.C., 2002.

Table 6.7 Opportunistic moniliaceous fungi[a]

Diagnostic characteristics	Penicillium	Paecilomyces	Scopulariopsis	Gliocladium	Trichoderma
Colony morphology	Velvet, green, reverse white to cream; if red diffusing pigment, rule out *P. marneffei*	Velvety, yellowish brown or mauve, never bright green or blue-green; off-white, pinkish, yellow or pale brown reverse	Powdery, cream-cinnamon or dark gray to brown-black; reverse usually tan, occasionally darker	Fluffy dark green, reverse white	Fluffy green, reverse colorless or yellow-orange
Microscopic morphology					

[a]Illustrations from D. H. Larone, *Medically Important Fungi, a Guide to Identification*, 4th ed., ASM Press, Washington, D.C., 2002. The *Paecilomyces* illustration is from the third edition.

(continued)

Fungal Diagnosis

Fungal Diagnosis

Table 6.7 Opportunistic moniliaceous fungi[a] (continued)

Diagnostic characteristics	Fusarium	Acremonium	Phialemonium	Lecythophora	Beauveria
Colony morphology	Cottony surface variable in color (white, cream, violet, or pink), reverse variable (white to dark pink); also consider *Cylindrocarpon*	Glabrous-feltlike, white, tan, light gray, or pale rose; reverse colorless, pale yellow, or pinkish; some species are dematiaceous	Flat, spready white-cream, yellow or green; reverse light with pale wine-buff or brown; some have green diffusing pigment	Moist-slimy, pink to salmon-orange; reverse pink or tan	Fluffy cream to pink; reverse white; also consider *Engyodontium*
Microscopic morphology					

[a]Illustrations from D. H. Larone, *Medically Important Fungi, a Guide to Identification*, 4th ed., ASM Press, Washington, D.C., 2002. The *Paecilomyces* illustration is from the third edition.

Table 6.8 Zygomycetes[a]

Diagnostic characteristics	Mucor	Rhizopus	Rhizomucor	Absidia	Syncephalastrum
Colony morphology	Fluffy gray to gray-brown, reverse white	Fluffy gray-brown, reverse white	Fluffy gray to dark-brown, reverse white	Fluffy gray, reverse white	Fluffy dark gray, reverse white
Microscopic morphology					
Maximum growth temp	37°C	45–50°C	54–58°C	45–50°C	40°C

[a]Illustrations from D. H. Larone, *Medically Important Fungi, a Guide to Identification*, 4th ed., ASM Press, Washington, D.C., 2002.

(continued)

Fungal Diagnosis

Fungal Diagnosis

Table 6.8 Zygomycetes[a] (continued)

Diagnostic characteristics	Cunninghamella	Saksenaea	Apophysomyces	Basidiobolus	Conidiobolus
Colony morphology	Fluffy gray, reverse white	Fluffy white, reverse white; use special media to enhance sporulation	Cream, yellow, or gray-brown; reverse white to pale-yellow; use special media to enhance sporulation	Flat, waxy, buff to gray-brown; satellite colonies formed by ejected conidia	Glabrous flat cream becoming covered with a white powdery mycelium, reverse white
Microscopic morphology					
Maximum growth temp	42°C	<37°C	42°C	37°C	35°C

[a] Illustrations from D. H. Larone, *Medically Important Fungi, a Guide to Identification*, 4th ed., ASM Press, Washington, D.C., 2002.

Table 6.9 Dimorphic moulds[a]

Diagnostic characteristics	*Blastomyces dermatitidis*	*Histoplasma capsulatum*	*Coccidioides* spp.	*Penicillium marneffei*	*Paracoccidioides brasiliensis*	*Sporothrix schenckii*
Direct exam						
Colony morphology at 25°C	Glabrous to velvety, white-gray, becoming tan; reverse cream-brown	Glabrous to velvety, white, becoming tan; reverse cream-brown	Glabrous to velvety, white-gray, becoming tan; reverse cream-brown	Green with gray-orange or purple-orange periphery; reverse buff, red diffusible pigment	Glabrous brown to wrinkled floccose, beige or white	Moist yeast-like texture, becoming wrinkled; surface reverse cream-brown

[a]Illustrations from D. H. Larone, *Medically Important Fungi, a Guide to Identification*, 4th ed., ASM Press, Washington, D.C., 2002.

(continued)

Fungal Diagnosis

Fungal Diagnosis

Table 6.9 Dimorphic moulds[a] *(continued)*

Diagnostic characteristics	*Blastomyces dermatitidis*	*Histoplasma capsulatum*	*Coccidioides* spp.	*Penicillium marneffei*	*Paracoccidioides brasiliensis*	*Sporothrix schenckii*
Microscopic exam						
Rule out	*Emmonsia, Chrysosporium, Scedosporium apiospermum*	*Emmonsia, Sepedonium*	*Arthrographis, Geotrichum, Malbranchea, Trichosporon*	Other *Penicillium* spp. producing red diffusible pigment	*Emmonsia*; on direct exam, *Blastomyces dermatitidis*	*Acrodontium* spp.

[a]Illustrations from D. H. Larone, *Medically Important Fungi, a Guide to Identification,* 4th ed., ASM Press, Washington, D.C., 2002.

Table 6.10 Characteristics of common *Trichophyton* species[a]

Diagnostic characteristics	T. mentagrophytes	T. rubrum	T. tonsurans	T. terrestre	T. verrucosum
Colony morphology	Variable cottony, velvety or granular, generally white; reverse white to pale yellow	Variable, cottony white; reverse deep red-brown	White to creamy yellow powdery or velvety surface, reverse lemon-yellow or red-brown	White to cream powdery to velvety surface, reverse pale, slightly yellow-gray	Very slow growing white to cream heaped colonies, reverse white to yellow-brown
Microscopic morphology					
Urease	+	–	+	+	
Trichophyton agars 1/4[b]	4+/4+	4+/4+	–/+	+/+	–/V
Growth at 37°C	+	+	+	–	+

[a] Illustrations from D. H. Larone, *Medically Important Fungi, a Guide to Identification*, 4th ed., ASM Press, Washington, D.C., 2002.

[b] –, no growth; +, restricted growth; 4+, maximum growth; V, variable.

Fungal Diagnosis

Fungal Diagnosis

Table 6.11 *Epidermophyton floccosum* and common *Microsporum* species[a]

Diagnostic characteristics	Epidermophyton floccosum	Microsporum canis var. canis	Microsporum gypseum complex
Colony morphology	Flat, slightly granular, sandy to olive-brown; reverse pale to yellow	Flat to velvety, pale to yellow; reverse yellow; also consider *M. praecox*	Granular, sandy color; reverse usually pale to brown
Microscopic morphology			

Diagnostic characteristics	*Microsporum audouinii*	*Microsporum cookei*	*Microsporum nanum*
Colony morphology	Flat to velvety; reverse pale salmon to pale brownish	Granular to velvety; reverse wine red	Powdery, sandy color; reverse reddish-brown
Microscopic morphology			

[a]Illustrations from D. H. Larone, *Medically Important Fungi, a Guide to Identification*, 4th ed., ASM Press, Washington, D.C., 2002.

Fungal Diagnosis

Fungal Diagnosis

Table 6.12 Dematiaceous fungi with macroconidia or other structures[a]

Diagnostic characteristics[b]	Bipolaris[c]	Dreschlera	Exserohilum	Helminthosporium
Microscopic morphology				

Diagnostic characteristics[b]	Alternaria	Curvularia	Chaetomium	Phoma
Microscopic morphology				

[a]Illustrations from D. H. Larone, *Medically Important Fungi, a Guide to Identification*, 4th ed., ASM Press, Washington, D.C., 2002.

[b]Colonies are woolly, rapidly growing, and shades of green and gray to black. Reverse is dark.

[c]In the past, most isolates of *Bipolaris* were mistakenly called *Dreschlera*; a germ tube test is needed for differentiation.

Fungal Diagnosis

Table 6.13 Dematiaceous fungi with small conidia[a]

Diagnostic characteristics[b]	Fonsecaea pedrosoi	Phialophora verrucosa	Rhinocladiella	Botrytis
Microscopic morphology			Also consider *Ramichloridium*	

Diagnostic characteristics[b]	Exophiala spp.	Wangiella	Phaeoannellomyces	Stachybotrys
Microscopic morphology				
Colony morphology and differential test	Nitrate positive; growth at 40°C variable	Nitrate negative; growth at 40°C positive	Nitrate positive; growth at 40°C variable	

[a] Illustrations from D. H. Larone, *Medically Important Fungi, a Guide to Identification*, 4th ed., ASM Press, Washington, D.C., 2002.

[b] Colonies are woolly, rapidly growing, and shades of green and gray to black. Reverse is dark. *Exophiala*, *Wangiella*, and *Phaeoannellomyces* are usually yeastlike when young.

Fungal Diagnosis

Fungal Diagnosis

Table 6.14 Differentiation of *Cladosporium* and *Cladophialophora* species[a]

Diagnostic characteristics[b]	Cladosporium spp.	Cladophialophora carrionii	Cladophialophora bantiana[c]
Microscopic morphology			
Gelatin hydrolysis	+	−	−
15% salt tolerance	+	−	−
Growth at 37°C	−	+	+
Growth at 42°C	−	−	Variable

[a] Illustrations from D. H. Larone, *Medically Important Fungi, a Guide to Identification*, 4th ed., ASM Press, Washington, D.C., 2002.

[b] Colonies rapidly growing, velvety or cottony, olive-gray to olive-brown or black. Reverse is black.

[c] *C. bantiana* now includes isolates previously classified as *Xylophypha emmonsii*. Isolates of *C. bantiana* from cerebral lesions exhibit growth at 40°C; some isolates (those previously classified as *X. emmonsii*) do not grow above 37°C.

Table 6.15 *Scedosporium* and *Dactylaria* species[a]

Diagnostic characteristics	*Scedosporium apiospermum* (asexual stage), *Pseudallescheria boydii* (sexual stage)	*Scedosporium prolificans*	*Dactylaria constricta* var. *gallopava*	*Dactylaria constricta* var. *constricta*
Colony morphology	Cottony white to gray or brown; reverse white, becoming gray or black	Cottony, light gray to black; reverse gray to black	Woolly and dark, olive-gray, reddish brown, or gray-black; reverse dark with a red to brown diffusible pigment	Woolly and dark, olive-gray, reddish brown, or gray-black; reverse dark with a red to brown diffusible pigment
Microscopic morphology	Graphium may be present Asexual Sexual			

[a]Illustrations from D. H. Larone, *Medically Important Fungi, a Guide to Identification*, 4th ed., ASM Press, Washington, D.C., 2002.

(continued)

Fungal Diagnosis

Table 6.15 *Scedosporium* and *Dactylaria* species[a] (continued)

Diagnostic characteristics	Scedosporium apiospermum (asexual stage), Pseudallescheria boydii (sexual stage)	Scedosporium prolificans	Dactylaria constricta var. gallopava	Dactylaria constricta var. constricta
Gelatin hydrolysis in <7 days	NA	NA	+	−
Cycloheximide tolerance	+ (the sexual stage may be inhibited by cycloheximide)	−	−	+
Growth at 37–45°C	37°C	45°C		

[a]Illustrations from D. H. Larone, *Medically Important Fungi, a Guide to Identification*, 4th ed., ASM Press, Washington, D.C., 2002.

Table 6.16 Dematiaceous fungi with hyphae[a]

Diagnostic characteristics	*Aureobasidium pullulans*	*Hormonema dematioides*	*Madurella grisea*	*Madurella mycetomatis*
Colony morphology	Smooth and moist; yellow, white, cream, light pink, or light brown, becoming black from development of arthroconidia	Smooth and moist; yellow, white, cream, light pink, or light brown, becoming black from development of arthroconidia	Slow-growing, velvety, dark gray to olive-brown; short tan or gray ariel hyphae; red-brown diffusible pigment may form in older cultures; sclerotia black	Slow-growing, smooth, folded and glabrous or powdery; white, yellowish-brown; reverse dark brown; a brown diffusible pigment usually formed; sclerotia reddish brown to black
Microscopic morphology	Conidia develop in a synchronous manner, each from its own locus	Conidia develop in a sequential manner from a single locus		
Assimilation of methyl α-ᴅ-glucoside (MDG)	Positive	Negative	NA	NA

[a]Illustrations from D. H. Larone, *Medically Important Fungi, a Guide to Identification*, 4th ed., ASM Press, Washington, D.C., 2002.

(continued)

Fungal Diagnosis

Fungal Diagnosis

Table 6.16 Dematiaceous fungi with hyphae[a] *(continued)*

Diagnostic characteristics	Piedraia hortae	Scytalidium	Nattrassia mangiferae
Colony morphology	Very slow growing, dark brown to black, heaped in the center with a flat periphery; some produce a reddish brown diffusible pigment; ascospores generally not found on routine mycological media	Rapidly growing, woolly, hyaline initially, becoming gray to brownish black; hyphae form one- or two-celled arthroconidia that are hyaline or pale brown	Rapidly growing, hyaline, becoming brown-black; pycnidia develop within 1–2 mo; the *S. dimidiatum* synanamorph is almost always present
Microscopic morphology			Pycnidia are variably shaped; conidia arise from phialides
Assimilation of methyl α-D-glucoside (MDG)	NA	NA	NA

[a]Illustrations from D. H. Larone, *Medically Important Fungi, a Guide to Identification*, 4th ed., ASM Press, Washington, D.C., 2002.

Parasitic Diagnosis

Diagnosis of most parasitic infections has traditionally been made by the microscopic examination of clinical material. This requires that highly trained technologists spend a significant amount of time examining individual specimens. In recent years, immunoassays have been developed to detect the more common parasites (e.g., *Entamoeba histolytica*, *Giardia lamblia*, and *Cryptosporidium parvum*). However, these tests are adjuncts to the microscopic examination of specimens for ova and parasites and can rarely replace microscopy. Likewise, a number of tests have been developed to detect parasite-specific nucleic acids. Although these amplification tests have been restricted primarily to research laboratories, it is anticipated that this will change in the future as the technology is simplified.

This section summarizes the tests currently available for the laboratory diagnosis of the most common parasitic infections. For additional information, the reader is referred to the *Manual of Clinical Microbiology*, 8th ed., 2003, and Garcia's *Diagnostic Medical Parasitology*, 4th ed., 2001.

Parasitic Diagnosis

Table 7.1 Detection methods for parasites[a]

Parasite	Culture	Microscopy	Antigen detection	Antibody detection	Molecular diagnostics
Free-living amebae					
Acanthamoeba	A	A	D	D	C
Naegleria	D	A	D	D	C
Intestinal and urogenital protozoa					
Balantidium coli	D	A	D	D	D
Blastocystis hominis	B	A	D	D	D
Cryptosporidium parvum	D	A	B	D	C
Cyclospora cayetanensis	D	A	D	D	C
Dientamoeba fragilis	D	A	D	D	D
Entamoeba histolytica/dispar	D	A	A	B	C
Giardia lamblia	D	A	A	D	C
Isospora belli	D	A	D	D	C
Trichomonas vaginalis	A	A	C	D	C
Blood and tissue protozoa					
Babesia	D	A	D	A	C
Leishmania	B	A	D	C	C

(continued)

Parasitic Diagnosis

Table 7.1 Detection methods for parasites[a] *(continued)*

Parasite	Culture	Microscopy	Antigen detection	Antibody detection	Molecular diagnostics
Plasmodium	C	A	B	C	C
Toxoplasma gondii	C	B	D	A	B
Trypanosoma	B	A	C	A	C
Microsporidia					
Many genera	D	A	D	D	C
Helminths—nematodes					
Ancylostoma duodenale	D	A	D	D	D
Ascaris lumbricoides	D	A	D	D	D
Brugia spp.	D	A	C	C	C
Capillaria philippinensis	D	A	D	D	D
Dracunculus medinensis	D	A	D	D	D
Enterobius vermicularis	D	A	D	D	D
Loa loa	D	A	C	C	C
Mansonella perstans	D	A	C	C	C
Necator americanus	D	A	D	D	D
Onchocerca volvulus	D	A	D	D	D
Strongyloides stercoralis	D	A	C	C	C
Toxocara canis	D	D	D	A	D

Trichinella spiralis	D	A	D	C
Trichuris trichiura	D	A	D	D
Wuchereria bancrofti	D	A	C	C
Helminths—trematodes				
Clonorchis sinensis	D	A	D	D
Fasciola hepatica	D	A	C	D
Fasciolopis buski	D	A	D	D
Paragonimus westermani	D	A	C	D
Schistosoma spp.	D	A	C	C
Helminths—cestodes				
Diphyllobothrium latum	D	A	D	D
Dipylidium caninum	D	A	D	D
Echinococcus granulosus	D	D	A	D
Echinococcus multilocularis	D	D	A	D
Hymenolepis diminuta	D	A	D	D
Hymenolepis nana	D	A	D	D
Taenia saginata	D	A	D	D
Taenia solium	D	A	A	D

[a] A, test is generally useful; B, test is useful under certain circumstances; C, test is seldom used for general diagnosis but may be available in reference laboratories; D, test is generally not used for laboratory diagnosis.

Parasitic Diagnosis

Microscopy

Acid-Fast Trichrome Chromotrope Stain

The acid-fast trichrome chromotrope stain is used to detected microsporidia, *Cryptosporidium*, *Cyclospora*, and *Isospora*. Specimens are stained with carbol fuchsin followed by Didier's trichrome solution (Chromotrope 2R, aniline blue, and phosphotungstic acid in acetic acid) and then washed with acid-alcohol followed by 95% ethanol. *Cryptosporidium*, *Cyclospora*, and *Isospora* stain bright pink or violet, and microsporidia appear pink.

Calcofluor White Stain

Calcofluor white binds to cellulose and chitin; it fluoresces best when exposed to long-wavelength UV light. Free-living amebae (i.e., *Acanthamoeba*, *Balamuthia*, and *Naegleria*) and larvae of *Dirofilaria* fluoresce.

Delafield's Hematoxylin Stain

Delafield's hematoxylin stain is used for thin and thick blood films for the detection of microfilaria. Structural detail (e.g., nuclei and sheaths) may show greater detail than with Giemsa or Wright's stains. This stain is not commercially available and so is typically used only in specialty laboratories.

Direct Fluorescent-Antibody Stain

A variety of organisms (e.g., *Cryptosporidium parvum* and *Giardia lamblia*) are detected directly in clinical specimens by using specific fluorescein-labeled antibodies. The labeled antibodies bind to the organisms and fluoresce green under UV light. The sensitivity and specificity of the stain are determined by the quality of the antibodies used in the reagents. Optimal detection of fluorescence requires the use of either a 420- to 490-nm (wide band) or 470- to 490-nm (narrow band) excitation filter and a 510- to 530-nm barrier filter.

Giemsa Stain

Giemsa stain and Wright's stain are modifications of Romanowsky stain, which combines methylene blue and eosin. Both stains are used for the detection of blood parasites (e.g., *Plasmodium, Babesia*, and *Leishmania*). A protozoan trophozoite has a red nucleus and gray-blue cytoplasm.

Parasitic Diagnosis

Iron Hematoxylin Stain

Iron hematoxylin stain is used for the detection and identification of fecal protozoa. Helminth eggs and larvae generally retain too much stain and are more easily identified with wet-mount preparations. Iron hematoxylin stain can be applied to either fresh stool specimens or ones preserved with polyvinyl alcohol or a similar preservative. Formalin-fixed specimens cannot be used.

Lugol's Iodine Stain

Iodine is added to "wet" preparations of parasitology specimens to enhance the contrast of the internal structures (e.g., nuclei and glycogen vacuoles). One disadvantage of this method is that protozoa are killed by the iodine and hence motility cannot be observed.

Modified Acid-Fast Stain

Acid-fast stains are used for detecting *Cryptosporidium*, *Cyclospora*, and *Isospora*. Because the protozoa can be readily decolorized, a weak acid-alcohol solution is used for removing the basic carbol fuchsin from non-acid-fast organisms. Organisms that retain this modified stain are referred to as being partially acid fast.

Modified Acid-Fast Stains (Weber Green, Ryan Blue)

The trichrome stain has been modified specifically for the detection of microsporidia. A higher concentration of dye and longer staining time are used to facilitate the staining of microsporidia. Weber Green stains the organisms pink with a green background, while the Ryan Blue also stains the organisms pink but with a blue background.

Trichrome Stain

The trichrome stain, like the iron hematoxylin stain, is a permanent stain that is used for the detection and identification of protozoa. The stain consists of a solution of three dyes (Chromotrope 2R, light green SF, and fast green FCF) in phosphotungstic acid and acetic acid. When staining is done properly, the specimen background is green and the protozoa have a blue-green to purple cytoplasm with red or purple-red nuclei, chromatoid bodies, erythrocytes, and bacteria. Parasite eggs and larvae usually stain red.

Parasitic Diagnosis

Wright's Stain

Wright's stain is a polychromatic stain that contains a mixture of methylene blue, azure B (from the oxidation of methylene blue), and eosin Y dissolved in methanol. The eosin ions are negatively charged and stain the basic components of cells orange to pink, while the other dyes stain the acidic cell structures various shades of blue to purple.

Specific Diagnostic Tests

Free-Living Amebae

Acanthamoeba. Chronic granulomatous amebic encephalitis, caused by several species of *Acanthamoeba*, can be diagnosed by microscopic examination of Giemsa- or trichrome-stained brain tissue and, rarely, cerebrospinal fluid (CSF). *Acanthamoeba* keratitis is diagnosed by direct microscopic examination of corneal scrapings or by culture of the specimen. Nucleic acid amplification (NAA) tests and serologic testing have been used only in research laboratories.

Naegleria. Primary meningoencephalitis, caused by *Naegleria fowleri*, is diagnosed by microscopic examination of Giemsa- or trichrome-stained brain tissue or detection of mobile trophozoites in CSF. Giemsa or trichrome staining can be performed on CSF, but Gram stains are unreliable (giving false-positive and false-negative results). NAA tests and serologic testing have been used only in research laboratories.

Intestinal and Urogenital Protozoa

Balantidium coli. *B. coli* is best detected by wet mount examination of stool specimens. The organism tends to overstain with trichrome stains and may be misidentified.

Blastocystis hominis. The role of *B. hominis* in human disease is controversial. The protozoa can be detected by microscopic examination (iodine wet mount, trichrome, or direct fluorescent-antibody [DFA] assay) or antigen tests (enzyme immunoassay [EIA]) of fecal specimens collected from symptomatic and asymptomatic individuals. Serologic testing is not useful because prolonged exposure is required before an antibody response is detected.

Cryptosporidium parvum. *C. parvum* infections are diagnosed by examining fecal specimens. This protozoon does not stain adequately with iodine or with permanent stains (trichrome or iron hematoxylin). It can be recognized by using a wet mount; however, modified acid-fast stains or the DFA test is more sensitive and specific. EIAs for the detection of *C. parvum* are also commercially available and have a sensitivity and specificity approaching 100%. PCR-based NAA tests have been developed but are restricted primarily to research laboratories. Serologic testing has not been used for diagnostic purposes.

Cyclospora cayetanensis. *C. cayetanensis* is detected by the microscopic examination of fecal specimens. The protozoon does not stain well with iodine, Giemsa, trichrome, or chromotrope stains. It is most commonly detected by using a modified acid-fast stain. It also autofluoresces under UV epifluorescence (green with 450- to 490-nm excitation filter; blue with 365-nm excitation filter). PCR-based NAA tests have been developed but are restricted to research laboratories. Serologic testing is not used for diagnostic purposes.

Dientamoeba fragilis. Microscopic examination of fecal specimens is the method used to diagnose *D. fragilis* infections. Because *D. fragilis* does not have a cyst stage, concentrated specimens should be examined with a permanent stain.

Entamoeba histolytica/dispar. Microscopy cannot reliably differentiate between *E. histolytica* (pathogenic) and *E. dispar* (nonpathogenic) unless erythrocytes are detected in the cytoplasm of *E. histolytica* trophozoites. These two protozoa are detected by examining clinical specimens (e.g., feces, tissue biopsy specimens, and abscess aspirates) using wet mount or permanent stains. A number of antigen detection tests (EIAs) can be used to identify *E. histolytica*. These tests are now more sensitive and specific than microscopy. PCR-based NAA tests are also available for the detection and identification of *E. histolytica*. The methods are as sensitive as antigen tests but are not yet widely available. Serologic testing is valuable for the diagnosis of extraintestinal infections because cysts or trophozoites may not be detected in stool specimens. Indirect hemagglutination (IHA) is the reference test. The Centers for Disease Control and Prevention (CDC) recommend the use of

≥1:256 as a criterion for a positive IHA serologic result. This level identifies 95% of patients with extraintestinal infections, 70% of patients with active disease localized to the intestines, and 10% of asymptomatic intestinal carriers. Positive titers may persist for years after successful therapy. EIA is a sensitive assay, which identifies significantly more patients with hepatic disease than does IHA. No cross-reactions with other amebas are observed. Detection of immunoglobulin M (IgM) antibodies is insensitive, even for patients with active invasive disease (positive in only 65% of these patients).

Giardia lamblia.   Microscopic examination of fecal specimens (wet mount, permanent stain, or DFA test [cyst specific]) for *G. lamblia* trophozoites and cysts is used to establish infection. EIAs are used extensively and are more sensitive and specific than microscopic methods. EIAs detect either cysts only or cysts and trophozoites (preferred test). PCR-based NAA methods have been developed and are at least as sensitive as microscopic methods.

Isospora belli.   As with *Cryptosporidium* and *Cyclospora*, the most common method used to detect *I. belli* in fecal specimens is the modified acid-fast stain. NAA tests are restricted to research laboratories, and serologic testing is not useful for diagnosis.

Trichomonas vaginalis.   *T. vaginalis* infections are most commonly diagnosed by microscopic examination (wet mount, DFA) of vaginal and urethral discharges, prostatic secretions, and urine sediments. The sensitivity of a microscopic examination is between 50 and 70%. Culture is more sensitive (>80%) and is considered the "gold standard." NAA and antigen tests have been developed but are not commercially available. Serologic testing is not useful.

Blood and Tissue Protozoa

Babesia spp.   *Babesia* infections are most commonly diagnosed by detecting parasitized erythrocytes in Giemsa-stained thin films of peripheral blood. For patients with low-grade parasitemia or inconclusive peripheral smears, serologic testing can be helpful. Antibody titers in the immunofluorescent-antibody (IFA) test rise rapidly during the first weeks of disease to 1:1,024 or higher and then gradually decline over the next 6 months. Low but detectable titers may persist for 1 year or more. Elevated antibody titers may be present in healthy individuals living in areas of endemic infection. Therefore, a positive serologic test result should be confirmed by detection of the parasite in blood smears. Cross-reactivity among *Babesia* species is variable; therefore, regional differences in serologic reactivity may be observed. A PCR-based NAA test has been developed but is restricted to research laboratories.

***Leishmania* spp.** Leishmaniasis is diagnosed by detection of amastigotes in clinical specimens or promastigotes in culture. Specimens should be collected from the margin of the lesion by aspiration, scraping, or punch biopsy. Tissue is used to make touch preparations and is submitted for histopathologic examination. Amastigotes are found in macrophages in Giemsa-stained preparations. PCR-based NAA tests have been developed to identify specific *Leishmania* species in tissue biopsy specimens. Specimens can also be cultured in NNN medium or Schneider's *Drosophila* medium supplemented with 30% fetal bovine serum. Although this is a sensitive procedure, cultures must be held for 4 weeks or longer. Serologic tests, including the IFA test, enzyme-linked immunosorbent assay (ELISA), and immunoblot (IB) test, have been developed for diagnosis but are available only in reference laboratories and at the CDC.

***Plasmodium* spp.** Malaria is most commonly diagnosed by detecting parasitized erythrocytes in Giemsa-stained thick and thin films of peripheral blood. If blood is collected with anticoagulant, EDTA but not heparin should be used. Examination of thick films is the most sensitive microscopic method, but identification of the *Plasmodium* species requires examination of thin films. Acidine orange has also been used to stain blood films. This method is sensitive, but species identification is difficult. PCR-based NAA tests have been developed and can identify *Plasmodium* at the species level. This test is at least as sensitive as examination of thick films but is currently restricted to reference laboratories. Antigen detection tests specific for *P. falciparum* histidine-rich protein 2 (HRP-2) and parasite lactate dehydrogenase (LDH) specific for *P. falciparum* and non-*P. falciparum* plasmodia have been developed. The HRP-2 assay has a sensitivity equivalent to that of microscopy; the LDH assays have not been adequately evaluated. None of these antigen tests are licensed in the United States. Although species-specific serologic tests have been developed, there is extensive cross-reactivity among *Plasmodium* species and these tests have not been used for diagnostic purposes.

Toxoplasma gondii. Microscopic examination of tissues and fluids is generally unrewarding, although tachyzoites and cysts may be observed in Giemsa-stained specimens. Additionally, parasites can be recovered by inoculating mice or cell cultures, but this also has a low yield. EIA antigen tests are insensitive and are not recommended. A PCR test has been developed and is useful for confirmation of congenital infections. This test is less useful for other forms of toxoplasmosis and is available only through reference laboratories. Serologic testing is the method of choice for the diagnosis of toxoplasmosis. A variety of commercial tests are available (IFA test, EIA, and agglutination) for measuring the IgM and IgG response to toxoplasma. Care must be used when tests using different assay methods are compared. For the diagnosis of an acute acquired infection, an IgG IFA test or EIA should be performed. If the test is negative in an immunocompetent person, the diagnosis is excluded. Detection of IgM antibodies or a fourfold or greater increase in the level of IgG antibodies (rarely observed) is consistent with an acute infection. Congenital infection can be diagnosed by demonstrating an acute infection in the mother and elevated antibodies in fetal blood. The presence of *Toxoplasma*-specific IgM or IgA antibodies in fetal serum confirms the diagnosis. Detection of parasite-specific DNA by PCR in amniotic fluid is also definitive evidence of disease. Ocular infections can be diagnosed by demonstrating local production of antibody or detection of parasite DNA. Most infections in immunocompromised patients represent reactivation disease. IgM antibody is usually not detected, and IgG antibody titers are consistent with chronic infections. Diagnosis is typically confirmed by detection of parasites or *Toxoplasma* DNA in tissue biopsy specimens or aspirated fluids.

Trypanosoma brucei. African trypanosomiasis is diagnosed by detection of trypanomastigotes in blood, lymph node aspirates, sternum bone marrow, or CSF. Parasites are present in the blood during febrile periods but are found in only small numbers when the patient is afebrile. Thick and thin films, as well as buffy coat cells, should be examined using the Giemsa stain. CSF should be concentrated before examination. ELISA has been used to detect parasitic antigens in serum and CSF.

PCR-based NAA tests have also been developed in reference laboratories. Serologic tests (IFA, ELISA, IHA, and agglutination) are used for epidemiologic studies but not for diagnosis.

Trypanosoma cruzi. American trypanosomiasis, caused by *T. cruzi*, is diagnosed during the acute phase of illness by detection of trypomastigotes in Giemsa-stained peripheral blood (thick film, thin film, or buffy coat cells). Blood smears are less reliable for detection of congenital infections and chronic disease. Immunoassays for parasitic antigens in sera and urine have been used for these infections. PCR-based NAA tests have been developed but are used primarily in research laboratories. Aspirates, blood, and tissues can be cultured in NNN medium with samples incubated for 4 weeks or longer. Serologic tests are available in reference laboratories and at the CDC. These tests include complement fixation (CF), IFA test, IHA, and ELISA. Most tests use an epimastigote antigen, and cross-reactions occur with other trypanosomes, *Leishmania*, and *Toxoplasma*. An elevated titer cannot be used to discriminate between active and past disease.

Microsporidia

As many as 140 genera have been described for the phylum Microsporidia, with at least 7 being implicated in human disease. Diagnosis is made most commonly by examination of fecal specimens or by cytologic or histopathologic testing. Fecal smears are prepared on glass slides (concentration of specimens results in a loss of organisms) and then stained with chromotrope-based stains or chemofluorescent agents (Calcofluor white). Immunofluorescent stains have been developed but are not widely used. Microsporidial spores have been detected by cytologic examination of concentrated fluids such as bronchoalveolar lavage fluid, biliary aspirates, duodenal aspirates, and CSF. Histologic examination of biopsy specimens has also been useful. NAA tests have been developed but are restricted to research laboratories. Serologic testing is not useful for the diagnosis of human infections.

Helminths: Nematodes

Ancylostoma duodenale. Hookworm infections are diagnosed by microscopic examination of fecal specimens with a direct smear for characteristic eggs. Heavy infections (e.g., >25 eggs per coverslip) are associated with anemia. Delays in examining the specimen should be avoided because eggs can hatch in nonpreserved specimens and release larval forms that can be misidentified as *Strongyloides*. Infection with other species of *Ancylostoma* (and other hookworms and *Strongyloides* species) can cause cutaneous larva migrans, where filariform larvae migrate through the skin layers and stimulate an inflammatory response. This disease is diagnosed on the basis of clinical presentation.

Ascaris lumbricoides. Roundworm infections are diagnosed by microscopic examination of fecal specimens for characteristic eggs (fertilized, decorticated, and unfertilized eggs). Fertilized eggs can be detected in a direct fecal smear or in concentrated specimens. Unfertilized eggs are not concentrated in floatation concentration methods. Adult worms may also be passed in feces or regurgitated.

***Brugia* spp.** Infections are detected by examining blood for the presence of microfilaria. Most infections consist of relatively few microfilaria in the blood, so that a large volume must be examined by either thick films or, more appropriately, concentration on a membrane filter (Knott technique). The worms are stained with Giemsa or hematoxylin. Identification of the specific microfilariae is based on their morphology (size, nuclear arrangement in the tail, and presence or absence of sheath). Antigen, antibody, and PCR-based NAA tests have also been developed for the detection of microfilarial infections. These tests are generally available through the CDC and research laboratories. Microfilariae circulate in blood in well-defined periodic cycles corresponding to the biting habits of the insect vector.

Capillaria philippinensis. Diagnosis is made on the basis of microscopic detection of characteristic eggs in fecal specimens. Larvae and adults are occasionally detected.

Dracunculus medinensis. Infections with the "Guinea worm" are diagnosed by recovery of the adult female worm when it migrates from the subcutaneous tissues to the skin surface. Adult male worms are small and are only rarely detected.

Enterobius vermicularis. Pinworm infections are diagnosed by microscopic examination of parasite eggs collected from the perianal folds. Eggs are collected with cellulose tape or a commercial paddle, transferred to a microscope slide, and examined directly or after exposure to 1 drop of toluene or xylene. Multiple specimens may have to be examined.

Loa loa. Refer to *Brugia*. *L. loa* has a diurnal periodicity. Adult worms may be detected when they migrate through the conjunctivae.

Mansonella perstans. Refer to *Brugia*. *M. perstans* has no periodicity.

Necator americanus. Refer to *Ancylostoma duodenale*.

Onchocerca volvulus. Adult worms live in subcutaneous tissues and deposit microfilaria in the skin tissue. Diagnosis is made by detecting the microfilaria in skin snips suspended in saline solutions. Skin snips should be collected from the scapular region or the iliac crest. Care must be used to not contaminate the specimen with blood.

Strongyloides stercoralis. Strongyloidiasis is diagnosed on the basis of microscopic examination of fecal specimens for characteristic larval forms. Eggs are rarely observed, and larvae may be scarce even in concentrated specimens, particularly in those from patients with chronic infections. Techniques developed to detect light infections include the Baermann procedure (fecal material is placed in a funnel with water, the larvae are allowed to migrate into the water, and the specimen is examined microscopically) and the agar plate method (fecal material is placed on an agar plate and then examined after 1 to 3 days for tracks of larvae migrating from the fecal mass). Multiple specimens may be needed to make the diagnosis. Adult worms, eggs, and larvae may be observed by histopathologic testing. Serologic tests (EIA and IB analysis) are available through the CDC. EIAs have a reported sensitivity between 84 and 92%. Cross-reactions can occur in patients with other nematode infections. Titers may persist, so serologic testing therefore cannot be used reliably to differentiate between current and past infections.

Toxocara canis. Human ingestion of *T. canis* eggs leads to visceral larva migrans, characterized by hypereosinophilia, hepatomegaly, fever, and pneumonitis. Diagnosis is based on clinical findings and serologic testing (EIA). The test sensitivity and specificity cannot be precisely assessed because alternative methods to demonstrate infection have not been developed.

However, the test sensitivity is estimated to vary from 70 to 80% and the specificity is estimated to be >90%.

Trichinella spiralis. Trichinosis is diagnosed by demonstration of encapsulated larvae in biopsy specimens of skeletal muscle, particularly deltoid and gastrocnemius muscles. Detection of larvae may be improved by digestion of muscle tissue with an acidic solution. Detectable antibodies do not develop until 3 to 5 weeks after infection (after the acute phase of disease); their levels peak in the second or third month and then decline slowly for several years. Antibodies are detected earlier by EIA than by other methods, but EIA is less specific. Positive EIA results can be confirmed by flocculation tests.

Trichuris trichiura. Diagnosis in patients with heavy infections is made by microscopic examination of a direct wet mount preparation of a fecal specimen. Concentration methods may be required to detect eggs in light infections.

Wuchereria bancrofti. Refer to *Brugia*. *W. bancrofti* has a nocturnal periodicity.

Helminths: Trematodes

Clonorchis sinensis. Infections with the Oriental liver fluke are diagnosed by microscopic examination of fecal specimens for characteristic eggs.

Fasciola hepatica. Infection with the intestinal fluke, *F. hepatica*, is diagnosed by microscopic examination of fecal specimens for characteristic eggs. Serologic tests (EIA and IB assay) are available through the CDC. EIA uses the excretory-secretory antigens. Specific antibodies appear within 2 to 4 weeks after infection. Sensitivity is excellent (95%); however, cross-reactivity with *Schistosoma* may occur. This can be resolved by using IB assays. Antibody titers fall rapidly following treatment and can be used to predict the response to therapy.

Fasciolopis buski. Infections with the liver fluke, *F. buski*, are diagnosed by microscopic examination of fecal specimens for characteristic eggs.

Paragonimus westermani. Infections with the lung fluke, *P. westermani*, are diagnosed by microscopic examination of fecal specimens and, less commonly, sputum for characteristic eggs. Serologic tests (EIA and IB assay) are available through the

CDC. EIA has a high sensitivity and specificity, and antibody titers can be monitored to assess the response to therapy.

***Schistosoma* spp.** The three most important blood flukes that infect humans are *S. mansoni*, *S. japonicum*, and *S. haematobium*. They produce morphologically characteristic eggs that can be detected in fecal specimens (*S. mansoni* and *S. japonicum*) or urine (*S. haematobium*). In chronic *S. mansoni* and *S. japonicum* infections, eggs accumulate in the walls of the intestine, rectum, and liver and may be scarce in fecal specimens. Biopsy of the rectum or cecum may be required to make a diagnosis. Likewise, biopsy of the bladder wall may be required to diagnose *S. haematobium* infection. Antigen (EIA) and antibody (EIA and IB assay) tests are available through the CDC. The tests have a high sensitivity for *S. mansoni* infections but a lower sensitivity for *S. japonicum* and *S. haematobium* infections. IB analysis is used to discriminate among the schistosome species.

Helminths: Cestodes

Diphyllobothrium latum. Fish tapeworm infections are diagnosed on the basis of detection of characteristic eggs or proglottids in fecal specimens.

Dipylidium caninum. Infections with the dog tapeworm, *D. caninum*, are diagnosed on the basis of detection of proglottids or egg packets in fecal specimens.

Echinococcus granulosus. Diagnosis of unilocular hydatid infection is difficult but is made by detecting cysts in tissues by using imaging techniques (e.g., X-ray analysis, ultrasonic scanning, and computed tomography). Aspiration of the cyst contents is not recommended. Serologic testing (IHA, IFA tests, and EIA) is also useful. The test sensitivity ranges from 60 to 90% and is improved when a combination of tests is used. Antibody reactivity in patients is influenced by the location and integrity of the cyst. Detectable antibodies are more common in patients with cysts in the bones and liver than in those with cysts in the lungs, brain, and spleen. Seroreactivity is always lower in patients with intact cysts. False-positive reactions may occur in persons with other helminthic infections, cancer, collagen vascular disease, and cirrhosis.

Echinococcus multilocularis. As with *E. granulosus*, infection with *E. multilocularis* (multilocular hydatid infection) is difficult. Definitive diagnosis is made by histologic examination of hepatic tissue. Serologic tests (EIA) have also been developed for diagnosis of infections with *E. multilocularis*. Purified antigens are used, which has improved the test sensitivity and specificity.

Hymenolepis diminuta. *H. diminuta* (mouse tapeworm) infections are diagnosed by finding characteristic eggs in fecal specimens. Proglottids are rarely observed.

Hymenolepis nana. *H. nana* (rat tapeworm) infections are diagnosed by finding characteristic eggs in fecal specimens. Proglottids are rarely observed.

Taenia saginata. Beef tapeworm infections are diagnosed by finding characteristic eggs or proglottids in fecal specimens.

Taenia solium. Infections with the pork tapeworm following ingestion of cysticerci are diagnosed by finding characteristic eggs or proglottids in fecal specimens. *T. solium* eggs are also infectious for humans. Ingestion of eggs leads to cysticercosis. Cysticerci can develop in any tissue, with diagnosis made on the basis of detection of the parasite in histologic preparations or on the basis of a serologic response (EIA and bentonite flocculation). Seropositivity is reported in 50 to 70% of patients with a single cyst, 80% of patients with multiple calcified lesions, and >90% of patients with multiple, noncalcified lesions. EIAs are less sensitive than the IB assay and cross-react with antibodies specific for other helminth infections. Current tests do not differentiate between active and inactive infections.

Parasitic Diagnosis

Table 7.2 Trophozoites of common intestinal amebae[a]

Organism	Size[b] (diam or length)	Motility	Nucleus (no. and visibility)	Appearance of stained: Peripheral chromatin	Appearance of stained: Karyosome	Appearance of stained: Cytoplasm	Appearance of stained: Inclusions
Entamoeba histolytica	5–60 μm; usual range, 15–20 μm; invasive forms may be >20 μm	Progressive, with hyaline, fingerlike pseudopodia; may be rapid	1; difficult to see in unstained preparations	Fine granules, uniform in size and usually evenly distributed; may appear beaded	Small, usually compact; centrally located but may also be eccentric	Finely granular, "ground glass"; clear differentiation of ectoplasm and endoplasm; if present, vacuoles are usually small	Noninvasive organism may contain bacteria; erythrocytes, if present, are diagnostic
Entamoeba hartmanni	5–12 μm; usual range, 8–10 μm	Usually nonprogressive	1; usually not seen in unstained preparations	Nucleus may stain more darkly than that of *E. histolytica*, although morphology is similar; chromatin may appear as solid ring rather than beaded	Usually small and compact; may be centrally located or eccentric	Finely granular	May contain bacteria; no erythrocytes
Entamoeba coli	15–50 μm; usual range, 20–25 μm	Sluggish, nondirectional, with blunt, granular pseudopodia	1; often visible in unstained preparations	May be clumped and unevenly arranged on membrane; may also appear as solid dark ring with no beads or clumps	Large, not compact; may or may not be eccentric; may be diffuse and darkly stained	Granular, with little differentiation into ectoplasm and endoplasm; usually vacuolated	Bacteria, yeast cells, other debris

(continued)

Parasitic Diagnosis

Parasitic Diagnosis

Table 7.2 Trophozoites of common intestinal amebae[a] *(continued)*

Organism	Size[b] (diam or length)	Motility	Nucleus (no. and visibility)	Appearance of stained:			
				Peripheral chromatin	Karyosome	Cytoplasm	Inclusions
Entamoeba polecki	10–12 μm	Usually nonprogressive, sluggish	1; occasionally seen on a wet preparation	Fine granules; may be interspersed with large granules; evenly arranged on membrane; chromatin may also be clumped at edge of membrane	Small, usually centrally located	Finely granular	May contain ingested bacteria
Endolimax nana	6–12 μm; usual range, 8–10 μm	Sluggish, usually nonprogressive	1; occasionally visible in unstained preparations	Usually no peripheral chromatin; nuclear chromatin may be quite variable	Large, irregularly shaped; may appear "blotlike"; many nuclear variations are common; may mimic *E. hartmanni* or *Dientamoeba fragilis*	Granular, vacuolated	Bacteria
Iodamoeba bütschlii	8–20 μm; usual range, 12–15 μm	Sluggish, usually nonprogressive	1; usually not visible in unstained preparations	Usually no peripheral chromatin	Large; may be surrounded by refractile granules that are difficult to see ("basket nucleus")	Coarsely granular; may be highly vacuolated	Bacteria, yeast cells, other debris

[a]Data from L. S. Garcia, *Diagnostic Medical Parasitology*, 4th ed., ASM Press, Washington, D.C., 2001.
[b]Wet-preparation measurements (in permanent stains, organisms usually measure 1 to 2 μm less).

Table 7.3 Cysts of common intestinal amebae[a]

				Appearance of stained:				
Organism	Size[b] (diam or length)	Shape	Nucleus (no. and visibility)	Peripheral chromatin	Karyosome	Cytoplasm, chromatoidal bodies	Glycogen[c]
Entamoeba histolytica	10–20 μm; usual range, 12–15 μm	Usually spherical	Mature cyst, 4; immature, 1 or 2; characteristics difficult to see on wet preparation	Fine, uniform granules, evenly distributed; nuclear characteristics may not be as clearly visible as in trophozoite	Small, compact, usually centrally located but occasionally eccentric	May be present; bodies usually elongate with blunt, rounded, smooth edges; may be round or oval	May be diffuse or absent in mature cyst; clumped chromatin mass may be present in early cysts
Entamoeba hartmanni	5–10 μm; usual range, 6–8 μm	Usually spherical	Mature cyst, 4; immature, 1 or 2; 2 nucleated cysts very common	Fine granules evenly distributed on membrane; nuclear characteristics may be difficult to see	Small, compact, usually centrally located	Usually present; bodies usually elongate with blunt, rounded, smooth edges; may be round or oval	May or may not be present, as in *E. histolytica*
Entamoeba coli	10–35 μm; usual range, 15–25 μm	Usually spherical; may be oval,	Mature cyst, 8; occasionally ≥16; immature cysts with ≥2	Coarsely granular; may be clumped and unevenly arranged on membrane; nuclear	Large, may or may not be compact and/or eccentric;	May be present (less frequently than in *E. histolytica*); splinter	May be diffuse or absent in mature cyst; clumped mass

(continued)

Parasitic Diagnosis

Table 7.3 Cysts of common intestinal amebae[a] *(continued)*

		Appearance of stained:				
Organism	Size[b] (diam or length)	Shape	Nucleus (no. and visibility)	Peripheral chromatin	Karyosome	Cytoplasm, chromatoidal bodies	Glycogen[c]
		triangular, or other; may be distorted on permanent stained slide owing to inadequate fixative penetration	nuclei occasionally seen	characteristics not as clearly defined as in trophozoite; may resemble *E. histolytica*	occasionally centrally located	shaped with rough, pointed ends	occasionally seen in mature cysts
Entamoeba polecki	5–11 μm	Usually spherical	Mature cyst, 1; may be visible in wet preparations; rarely 2 or 4 nuclei	Similar to trophozoite	Similar to trophozoite	Abundant, angular pointed ends; threadlike chromatoidal bodies may be present	May or may not be present

Endolimax nana	5–10 μm; usual range, 6–8 μm	Usually oval; may be round	Mature cyst, 4; immature cysts, 2, very rarely seen and may resemble cysts of *Enteromonas hominis*	Rarely present; small granules or inclusions are occasionally seen; fine linear chromatoidal bodies may be faintly visible on well-stained smears	Smaller than karyosome seen in trophozoites but generally larger than those of genus *Entamoeba*	No peripheral chromatin	Usually diffuse if present
Iodamoeba bütschlii	5–20 μm; usual range, 10–12 μm	May vary from oval to round; cyst may collapse owing to large glycogen vacuole space	Mature cyst, 1	No peripheral chromatin	Larger, usually eccentric refractile granules may be on one side of karyosome ("basket nucleus")	None; small granules are occasionally present	Large, compact, well-defined mass
Blastocystis hominis	6–40 μm	Usually spherical	Multiple nuclei surrounding a large central body	Not observed	Not observed	Large central body dominates internal structure	Not present

[a] Data from L. S. Garcia, *Diagnostic Medical Parasitology*, 4th ed., ASM Press, Washington, D.C., 2001.
[b] Wet-preparation measurements (in permanent stains, organisms usually measure 1 to 2 μm less).
[c] Stains reddish brown with iodine.

Parasitic Diagnosis

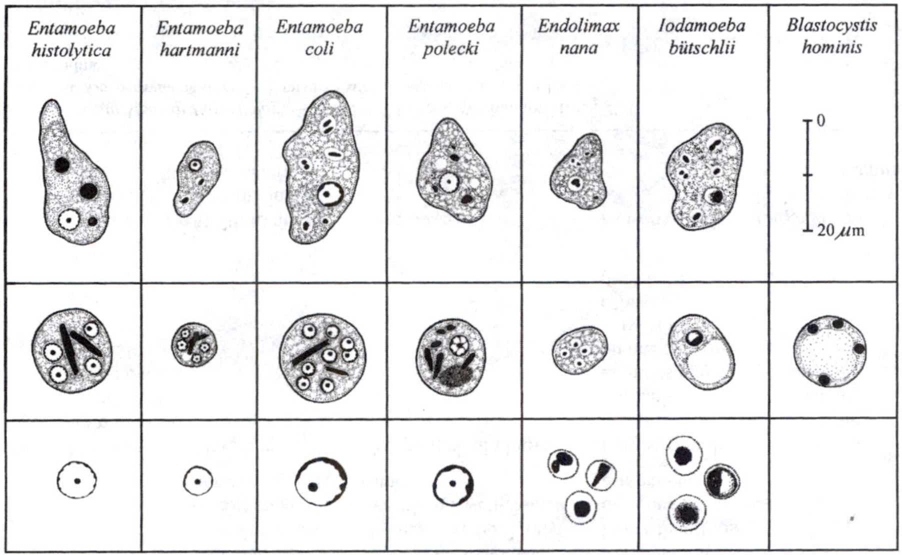

Parasitic Diagnosis

Figure 7.1 Intestinal amebae of humans. (Top row) Trophozoites. (Middle row) Cysts. (Bottom row) Trophozoite nuclei, shown in relative proportion. From P. R. Murray, E. J. Baron, J. H. Jorgensen, M. A. Pfaller, and R. H. Yolken (ed.), *Manual of Clinical Microbiology*, 8th ed., ASM Press, Washington, D.C., 2003.

Table 7.4 Trophozoites of flagellates[a]

Organism	Shape and size	Motility	Nucleus (no. and visibility)	No. of flagella[b]	Other features
Dientamoeba fragilis	Shaped like amebae; 5–15 μm (usual range, 9–12 μm)	Usually nonprogressive; pseudopodia are angular, serrated, or broad lobed and almost transparent	Percentage may vary, but 40% of organisms have 1 nucleus and 60% have 2 nuclei; not visible in unstained preparations; no peripheral chromatin; karyosome is cluster of 4–8 granules	No visible flagella	Cytoplasm finely granular and may be vacuolated with ingested bacteria, yeasts, and other debris; may be great variation in size and shape on single smear
Giardia lamblia	Pear shaped; 10–20 μm long; 5–15 μm wide	Falling-leaf motility may be difficult to see if organism is in mucus	2; not visible in unstained mounts	4 lateral, 2 ventral, 2 caudal	Sucking disk occupying 1/2–3/4 of ventral surface; pear shaped from front, spoon shaped from side
Chilomastix mesnili	Pear shaped; 6–24 μm long (usual range, 10–15 μm long), 4–8 μm wide	Stiff, rotary	1; not visible in unstained mounts	3 anterior, 1 in cytostome	Prominent cytostome extending 1/3–1/2 length of body; spiral groove across ventral surface

(continued)

Parasitic Diagnosis

Parasitic Diagnosis

Table 7.4 Trophozoites of flagellates[a] *(continued)*

Organism	Shape and size	Motility	Nucleus (no. and visibility)	No. of flagella[b]	Other features
Trichomonas hominis	Pear shaped; 5–15 μm long (usual range, 7–9 μm long), 7–10 μm wide	Jerky, rapid	1; not visible in unstained mounts	3–5 anterior; 1 posterior	Undulating membrane extends length of body; posterior flagellum extends free beyond end of body
Trichomonas vaginalis	Pear shaped; 7–23 μm long (usual range, 13 μm) 5–15 μm wide	Jerky, rapid	1; not visible in unstained mounts	3–5 anterior; 1 posterior	Undulating membrane extends 1/2 length of body; no free posterior flagellum; axostyle easily seen
Enteromonas hominis	Oval, 4–10 μm long (usual range, 8–9 μm long), 5–6 μm wide	Jerky	1; not visible in unstained mounts	3 anterior, 1 posterior	One side of body flattened; posterior flagellum extends free posteriorly or laterally
Retortamonas intestinalis	Pear shaped or oval; 4–9 μm long (usual range, 6–7 μm long), 3–4 μm wide	Jerky	1; not visible in unstained mounts	1 anterior, 1 posterior	Prominent cytostome extends approximately 1/2 length of body

[a]Data from L. S. Garcia, *Diagnostic Medical Parasitology*, 4th ed., ASM Press, Washington, D.C., 2001.
[b]Usually difficult to see.

Table 7.5 Cysts of flagellates[a]

Species	Size	Shape	Nuclei (no. and visibility)	Other features
Dientamoeba fragilis, *Trichomonas hominis*	No cyst stage	NA[b]	NA	NA
Giardia lamblia	8–19 μm long (usual range, 11–14 μm long), 7–10 μm wide	Oval, ellipsoidal, or round	4; not distinct in unstained preparations; usually located at one end	Longitudinal fibers in cysts may be visible in unstained preparations; deeply staining median bodies usually lie across longitudinal fibers; there is often shrinkage, and cytoplasm pulls away from cyst wall; may also be "halo" effect around outside of cyst wall due to shrinkage caused by dehydrating reagents
Chilomastix mesnili	6–10 μm long (usual range, 7–9 μm long), 4–6 μm wide	Lemon shaped with anterior hyaline knob	1; not distinct in unstained preparations	Cytostome with supporting fibrils, usually visible in stained preparation; curved fibril alongside of cytostome usually referred to as "shepherd's crook"

(continued)

Parasitic Diagnosis

Parasitic Diagnosis

Table 7.5 Cysts of flagellates[a] *(continued)*

Species	Size	Shape	Nuclei (no. and visibility)	Other features
Enteromonas hominis	4–10 µm long (usual range, 6–8 µm long), 4–6 µm wide	Elongate or oval	1–4; usually 2 lying at opposite ends of cyst; not visible in unstained mounts	Resembles *Endolimax nana* cyst; fibrils or flagella usually not seen
Retortamonas intestinalis	4–9 µm long (usual range, 4–7 µm long), 5 µm wide	Pear shaped or slightly lemon shaped	1; not visible in unstained mounts	Resembles *Chilomastix* cyst; shadow outline of cytostome with supporting fibrils extends above nucleus; bird beak fibril arrangement

[a] Data from L. S. Garcia, *Diagnostic Medical Parasitology*, 4th ed., ASM Press, Washington, D.C., 2001.
[b] NA, not applicable.

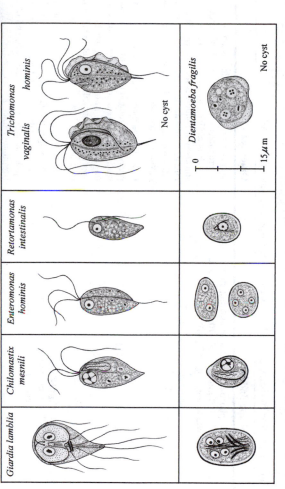

Figure 7.2 Intestinal and urogenital flagellates of humans. (Top row) Trophozoites. (Bottom row) Cysts. *D. fragilis* trophozoite is shown; no cyst stage. From P. R. Murray, E. J. Baron, J. H. Jorgensen, M. A. Pfaller, and R. H. Yolken (ed.), *Manual of Clinical Microbiology*, 8th ed., ASM Press, Washington, D.C., 2003.

Parasitic Diagnosis

Table 7.6 Morphological characteristics of ciliates, coccidia, microsporidia, and tissue protozoa[a]

Species	Shape and size	Other features[b]
Balantidium coli	Trophozoite: ovoid with tapering anterior; 50–100 µm long; 40–70 µm wide (usual width range, 40–50 µm) Cyst: spherical or oval; 50–70 µm in diam (usual range, 50–55 µm)	Trophozoite: 1 large, kidney-shaped macronucleus; 1 small, round micronucleus, which is difficult to see even in stained smears; macronucleus may be visible in unstained preparations; body is covered with cilia, which tend to be longer near cytostome; cytoplasm may be vacuolated Cyst: 1 large macronucleus visible in unstained preparations; micronucleus difficult to see; macronucleus and contractile vacuoles are visible in young cysts; in older cysts, internal structure appears granular; cilia difficult to see within cyst wall
Cryptosporidium parvum	Oocyst generally round, 4–5 µm in diam; each mature oocyst contains sporozoites, which may or may not be visible	Oocyst is the usual diagnostic stage in stool. Various other stages in life cycle can be seen in biopsy specimens taken from GI tract (brush borders of epithelial cells in intestinal tract) and other tissues (respiratory tract, biliary tract).

Cyclospora cayetanensis	Organisms generally round, 8–9 µm in diam; acid-fast like *Cryptosporidium* spp. but larger	Resemble nonrefractile spheres in wet-preparation smears; autofluoresce with epifluorescence; stain variably with acid-fast stains; appear clear, round, and somewhat wrinkled in trichrome stains
Isospora belli	Ellipsoidal oocyst; usual size, 20–30 µm long, 10–19 µm wide; sporocysts rarely seen out of oocysts but measure 9–11 µm	Mature oocyst contains 2 sporocysts with 4 sporozoites each; immature oocysts are usually seen in fecal specimens.
Microsporidia	Spores are extremely small and have been recovered from all body organs.	Histology results vary; acid-fast, trichrome, and Calcofluor white stains recommended for spores. Animal inoculation not recommended. Enteric infections in AIDS patients difficult to diagnose by examining stool specimens.
Toxoplasma gondii	Trophozoite (tachyzoite): crescent shaped; 4–6 µm long by 2–3 µm wide. Cyst (bradyzoite); generally spherical; 200 µm to 1 mm in diam	Diagnosis is most frequently based on clinical history and serologic evidence of infection.
Sarcocystis spp.	Oocyst with thin wall contains 2 mature sporocysts, each containing 4 sporozoites; oocyst frequently ruptures; ovoid sporocysts, each 9–16 µm long and 7.5–12 µm wide	Thin-walled oocyst or ovoid sporocysts occur in stool.

[a]Data from L. S. Garcia, *Diagnostic Medical Parasitology*, 4th ed., ASM Press, Washington, D.C., 2001.
[b]GI, gastrointestinal.

Parasitic Diagnosis

Parasitic Diagnosis

Table 7.7 Morphological characteristics of protozoa found in blood[a]

Organism	Diagnostic stage
Malaria parasites	
Plasmodium vivax (benign tertian malaria)	Ameboid rings; presence of Schüffner's dots; all stages seen in peripheral blood; mature schizont contains 16–18 merozoites; infects young RBCs[b]
Plasmodium ovale (ovale malaria)	Nonameboid rings; presence of Schüffner's dots; all stages seen in peripheral blood; mature schizont contains 8–10 merozoites; RBCs may be oval and have fimbriated edges; infects young RBCs
Plasmodium malariae (quartan malaria)	Rings are thick; no stippling; all stages seen in peripheral blood; presence of band forms and rosette-shaped mature schizont; lots of malarial pigment; infects mature RBCs
Plasmodium falciparum (malignant tertian malaria)	Multiple rings; appliqué/accolé forms; no stippling (rare Maurer's clefts); rings and crescent-shaped gametocytes seen in peripheral blood (no other developing stages, with rare exception of mature schizont); infects all RBCs
Babesia spp.	Ring forms only (resemble *P. falciparum* rings); seen in splenectomized patients; endemic in the United States (no travel history necessary); if present, "Maltese cross" configuration diagnostic

Trypanosoma brucei gambiense (West African sleeping sickness)	Trypomastigotes long and slender, with typical undulating membrane; lymph nodes and blood can be sampled; microhematocrit tube concentration helpful; examine spinal fluid in later stages of infection
Trypanosoma brucei rhodesiense (East African sleeping sickness)	Trypomastigotes long and slender, with typical undulating membrane; lymph nodes and blood can be sampled; microhematocrit tube concentration helpful; examine spinal fluid in later stages of infection
Trypanosoma cruzi (Chagas' disease, South American trypanosomiasis)	Trypomastigotes short and stumpy, often curved in C shape; blood sampled early in infection; trypomastigotes enter striated muscle (heart, GI[b] tract) and transform into amastigote form
Leishmania spp. (cutaneous; not actually a blood parasite but presented for comparison with *Leishmania donovani*)	Amastigotes found in macrophages of skin; presence of intracellular forms containing nucleus and kinetoplast diagnostic
Leishmania braziliensis (mucocutaneous; not actually a blood parasite but presented for comparison with *L. donovani*)	Amastigotes found in macrophages of skin and mucous membranes; presence of intracellular forms containing nucleus and kinetoplast diagnostic
Leishmania donovani (visceral)	Amastigotes found throughout reticuloendothelial system and in spleen, liver, bone marrow, etc.; presence of intracellular forms containing nucleus and kinetoplast diagnostic

[a]Data from L. S. Garcia, *Diagnostic Medical Parasitology*, 4th ed., ASM Press, Washington, D.C., 2001.
[b]GI, gastrointestinal; RBCs, erythrocytes.

Parasitic Diagnosis

Table 7.8 Morphological characteristics of blood and tissue nematodes

Parasite	Adult worm	Microfilaria
Brugia malayi	Threadlike; males 13–25 mm by 70–80 μm; females 43–55 mm by 130–170 μm	177–230 by 5–6 μm; sheathed; tail tapered; gap between subterminal and terminal nuclei
Loa loa	Males 30–35 mm by 350–430 μm; females 50–70 mm by 500 μm	230–250 by 6–8 μm; sheathed; tail tapered; nuclei extends to tip of tail
Mansonella perstans	Males 45 mm by 60 μm; females 70–80 mm by 120 μm	190–200 by 4 μm; unsheathed; tail tapered; nuclei extends to tip of tail
Mansonella ozzardi	Threadlike; males 24–28 mm by 70–80 μm; females 32–62 mm by 130–160 μm	163–203 by 3–4 μm; unsheathed; long, slender tail with nuclei at tip
Onchocerca volvulus	Males 19–42 mm by 130–210 μm; females 33–50 mm by 270–400 μm	304–315 by 5–9 μm; unsheathed; tail tapered; nuclei not at tip of tail
Wuchereria bancrofti	Threadlike; males 40 mm by 100 μm; females 80–100 mm by 250 μm	244–296 by 7–10 μm; sheathed; tail tapered; nuclei not at tip of tail

Table 7.9 Morphological characteristics of helminths[a]

Helminth	Diagnostic stage
Nematodes (roundworms)	
Ascaris lumbricoides	Egg: both fertilized (oval to round with thick, mammillated or tuberculate shell) and unfertilized (tend to be more oval or elongate, with bumpy shell exaggerated) eggs found in stool. Adult worms: 10–12 in. (ca. 25–30 cm), found in stool. Rarely (in severe infections), migrating larvae can be found in sputum.
Trichuris trichiura	Egg: barrel shaped with two clear, polar plugs. Adult worm: rarely seen. Eggs should be quantitated (rare, few, etc.), since light infections may not be treated.
Enterobius vermicularis	Egg: football shaped with one flattened side. Adult worm: about 3/8 in. (ca. 1 cm) long, white with pointed tail. Female migrates from anus and deposits eggs on perianal skin.
Ancylostoma duodenale, Necator americanus	Egg: eggs of two species identical; oval with broadly rounded ends, thin shell, and clear space between shell and developing embryo (8–16-cell stage). Adult worms: rarely seen in clinical specimens.
Strongyloides stercoralis	Rhabditiform larvae (noninfective) usually found in stool; short buccal cavity or capsule with large, genital primordial packet of cells ("short and sexy"). In very heavy infections, larvae are occasionally found in sputum and/or filariform (infective) larvae can be found in stool (slit in tail).
Ancylostoma braziliensis	Humans are accidental hosts. Larvae will wander through outer layer of skin, creating tracks (severe itching and eosinophilia). There are no practical microbiological diagnostic tests.

(continued)

Parasitic Diagnosis

Table 7.9 Morphological characteristics of helminths[a] *(continued)*

Helminth	Diagnostic stage
Toxocara cati or *Toxocara canis*	Humans are accidental hosts. Dog or cat ascarid eggs are ingested with contaminated soil; larvae wander through deep tissues (including eye); can be mistaken for cancer of eye; serologic tests helpful for confirmation; eosinophilia
Cestodes (tapeworms)	
Taenia saginata	Scolex (4 suckers, no hooklets) and gravid proglottid (>12 branches on single side) are diagnostic; eggs indicate *Taenia* spp. only (thick, striated shell, containing 6-hooked embryo or oncosphere); worm usually approx 12 ft (ca. 3.7 m) long
Taenia solium	Scolex (4 suckers with hooklets) and gravid proglottid (<12 branches on single side) are diagnostic; eggs indicate *Taenia* spp. only (thick, striated shell, containing 6-hooked embryo or oncosphere); worm usually approx 12 ft (ca. 3.7 m) long
Diphyllobothrium latum	Scolex (lateral sucking grooves) and gravid proglottid (wider than long, reproductive structures in center, "rosette"); eggs operculated
Hymenolepis nana	Adult worm not normally seen; egg round to oval with thin shell, containing 6-hooked embryo or oncosphere with polar filaments lying between embryo and egg shell
Hymenolepis diminuta	Adult worm not normally seen; egg round to oval with thin shell, containing 6-hooked embryo or oncosphere with no polar filaments lying between embryo and egg shell
Echinococcus granulosus	Adult worm found only in carnivores (dog); hydatid cysts develop (primarily in liver) when humans accidentally ingest eggs from dog tapeworms; cyst contains daughter cysts and many scolices. Laboratory should examine fluid aspirated from cyst at surgery.

Echinococcus multilocularis
Adult worm found only in carnivores (fox or wolf); hydatid cysts develop (primarily in liver) when humans accidentally ingest eggs from carnivore tapeworms. Cyst grows like metastatic cancer with no limiting membrane.

Trematodes (flukes)

Fasciolopsis buski
Eggs found in stool; very large and operculated (morphology like that of *F. hepatica* eggs)

Fasciola hepatica
Eggs found in stool; cannot be differentiated from those of *F. buski*

Clonorchis (Opisthorchis) sinensis
Eggs found in stool; very small (<35 μm); operculated, with shoulders into which operculum fits

Paragonimus westermani
Eggs coughed up in sputum (brownish "iron filing" = egg packets); can be recovered in sputum or stool (if swallowed); eggs operculated, with shoulders into which operculum fits

Schistosoma mansoni
Eggs recovered in stool (large lateral spine); specimens should be collected with no preservatives (to maintain egg viability); worms in veins of large intestine

Schistosoma haematobium
Eggs recovered in urine (large terminal spine); specimens should be collected with no preservatives (to maintain egg viability); worms in veins of bladder

Schistosoma japonicum
Eggs recovered in stool (very small lateral spine); specimens should be collected with no preservatives (to maintain egg viability); worms in veins of small intestine

[a]Data from L. S. Garcia, *Diagnostic Medical Parasitology*, 4th ed., ASM Press, Washington, D.C., 2001.

Parasitic Diagnosis

Parasitic Diagnosis

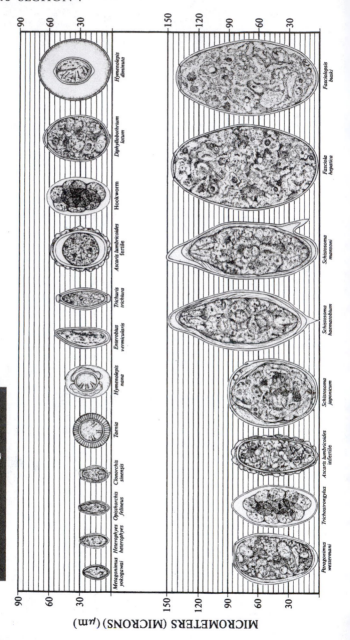

MICROMETERS (MICRONS) (μm)

Figure 7.3 Relative sizes of helminth eggs (from CDC). *Schistosoma mekongi* and *Schistosoma intercalatum* have been omitted. From M. Brooke and D. Melvin, *Morphology of Diagnostic Stages of Intestinal Parasites of Humans*, 2nd ed., U.S. Department of Health and Human Services publication (CDC) 84-8116, Centers for Disease Control and Prevention, Atlanta, Ga., 1984.

Table 7.10 Key to identification of common arthropods[a]

1. Three or four pairs of legs [2]
   Five or more pairs of legs [22]
2. Three pairs of legs with antennae (**insects: class Insecta**) [3]
   Four pairs of legs without antennae (**spiders, ticks, mites, scorpions: class Arachnida**) [20]
3. Wings present, well developed [4]
   Wings absent or rudimentary [12]
4. One pair of wings (**flies, mosquitos, midges: order Diptera**) [5]
   Two pairs of wings [6]
5. Wings with scales (**mosquitos: order Diptera**)
   Wings without scales (**other flies: order Diptera**)
6. Mouthparts adapted for sucking, with elongate proboscis [7]
   Mouthparts adapted for chewing, without elongate proboscis [8]
7. Wings densely covered with scales, proboscis coiled (**butterflies and moths: order Lepidoptera**)
   Wings not covered with scales; proboscis not coiled but directed backward (**bedbugs and kissing bugs: order Hemiptera**)
8. Both pairs of wings membranous, with similar structure, although size may vary [9]
   Front pair of wings leathery or shell-like, serving as covers for second pair [10]
9. Two pairs of wings similar in size (**termites: order Isoptera**)
   Hind wing much smaller than front wing (**wasps, hornets, and bees: order Hymenoptera**)
10. Front wings horny or leathery without distinct veins, meeting in a straight line down the middle [11]
    Front wings leathery or paperlike with distinct veins, usually overlapping in the middle (**cockroaches: order Dictyoptera**)
11. Abdomen with prominent cerci or forceps; wings shorter than abdomen (**earwigs: order Dermaptera**)
    Abdomen without prominent cerci or forceps; wings covering abdomen (**beetles: order Coleoptera**)
12. Abdomen with three long terminal tails (**silverfish and firebrats: order Thysanura**)
    Abdomen without three long terminal tails [13]
13. Abdomen with narrow waist (**ants: order Hymenoptera**)
    Abdomen without narrow waist [14]
14. Abdomen with prominent pair of cerci or forceps (**earwigs: order Dermaptera**)
    Abdomen without cerci or forceps [15]
15. Body flattened laterally; antennae small, fitting into grooves in side of head (**fleas: order Siphonaptera**)
    Body flattened dorsoventrally; antennae projecting from side of head, not fitting into grooves [16]
16. Antennae with nine or more segments [17]
    Antennae with three to five segments [18]
17. Pronotum covering head (**cockroaches: order Dictyoptera**)
    Pronotum not covering head (**termites: order Isoptera**)

(continued)

Table 7.10 Key to identification of common arthropods[a] (*continued*)

18. Mouthparts consisting of tubular jointed beak; three- to five-segment tarsi (**bedbugs: order Hemiptera**)
    Mouthparts retracted into head or of chewing type; one- or two-segment tarsi [19]
19. Mouthparts retracted into head, adapted for sucking blood (**sucking lice: order Anopleura**)
    Mouthparts of chewing type (**chewing lice: order Mallophaga**)
20. Body oval, consisting of single saclike region (**ticks and mites: subclass Acari**)
    Body divided into two distinct regions, a cephalothorax and an abdomen [21]
21. Abdomen joined to cephalothorax by slender waist; abdomen with segmentation indistinct or absent; stinger absent (**spiders: subclass Araneae**)
    Abdomen broadly joined to cephalothorax; abdomen distinctly segmented, ending with stinger (**scorpions: subclass Scorpiones**)
22. Five to nine pairs of legs or swimmerets; one or two pairs of antennae; principally aquatic organisms (**copepods, crabs, and crayfish: class Crustacea**)
    Ten or more pairs of legs; swimmerets absent; one pair of antennae; terrestrial organisms [23]
23. Only one pair of legs per body segment (**centipedes: class Chilopoda**)
    Two pairs of legs per body segment (**millipedes: class Diplopoda**)

[a] Data from J. Goddard, *Physician's Guide to Arthropods of Medical Importance*, CRC Press, Inc., Boca Raton, Fla., 1993, and National Communicable Disease Center, *Pictorial Keys: Arthropods, Reptiles, Birds, and Mammals of Public Health Significance*, Communicable Disease Center, Atlanta, Ga., 1969.

Vaccines, Susceptibility Testing Methods, and Susceptibility Patterns

Two important control measures for infectious diseases are vaccination to prevent infection and use of antimicrobial therapy to eradicate infections. This section provides information for both approaches. Tables 8.1 and 8.2 summarize immunization recommendations for pediatric and adult patients. These recommendations are published periodically in the *Morbidity and Mortality Weekly Report* and at the Centers for Disease Control and Prevention (CDC) website (hppt://www.cdc.gov/nip). The tables are a summary of the recommendations of the Advisory Committee on Immunization Practices (ACIP), the American Academy of Family Physicians (AAFP), the American College of Obstetricians and Gynecologists (ACOG), the American College of Physicians—American Society of Internal Medicine (ACP-ASIM), and the Infectious Diseases Society of America (IDSA).

Information regarding antimicrobial agents is subdivided into three sections: antimicrobial susceptibility testing methods, pharmacokinetic properties of antimicrobial agents, and antimicrobial susceptibility patterns. Tables 8.3 to 8.5 summarize the susceptibility testing guidelines provided by the National Committee for Clinical Laboratory Standards (NCCLS). The reader is referred to the NCCLS documents and website (www.nccls.org) for additional information. The pharmacokinetic properties of antimicrobial agents are summarized in Tables 8.6 to 8.10. These data should be used as a guide and are influenced by the dosing schedule, patient's underlying disease, and drug stability. The reader is referred to the infectious-disease and pharmacology texts cited in the Bibliography section for specific guidelines for therapeutic dosing. Antimicrobial susceptibility patterns are given in Tables 8.11 to 8.19, which summarize a number of well-controlled published reports of primarily U.S. isolates. Most data have been generated in selected national reference laboratories such as the Jones Group/JMI Laboratories, North Liberty, Iowa; Focus Technologies/MRL, Inc., Herndon, Va.; and the Clinical Microbiology Institute, Tualatin, Oreg. These data represent national trends. Because susceptibility patterns can vary regionally, it is important for each laboratory to determine the relevant antimicrobial susceptibility pattern for the patient population that it serves.

Vaccines, Susceptibility

Table 8.1 Recommended pediatric immunization schedule[a]

Vaccine	Recommended age for this dose	Minimum age for this dose	Recommended interval before next dose	Minimum interval before next dose
Hepatitis B				
First dose	Birth–2 mo	Birth	1–4 mo	4 wk
Second dose	1–4 mo	4 wk	2–17 mo	8 wk
Third dose	6–18 mo	6 mo		
Diphtheria-tetanus-pertussis				
First dose	2 mo	6 wk	2 mo	4 wk
Second dose	4 mo	10 wk	2 mo	4 wk
Third dose	6 mo	14 wk	6–12 mo	6 mo
Fourth dose	15–18 mo	12 mo	3 yr	6 mo
Fifth dose	4–6 yr	4 yr		
Haemophilus influenzae type b				
First dose	2 mo	6 wk	2 mo	4 wk
Second dose	4 mo	10 wk	2 mo	4 wk
Third dose	6 mo	14 wk	6–9 mo	8 wk
Fourth dose	12–15 mo	12 mo		

(continued)

Vaccines, Susceptibility

Vaccines, Susceptibility

Table 8.1 Recommended pediatric immunization schedule[a] *(continued)*

Vaccine	Recommended age for this dose	Minimum age for this dose	Recommended interval before next dose	Minimum interval before next dose
Inactivated poliovirus				
First dose	2 mo	6 wk	2 mo	4 wk
Second dose	4 mo	10 wk	2–14 mo	4 wk
Third dose	6–18 mo	14 wk	3.5 yr	4 wk
Fourth dose	4–6 yr	18 wk		
Pneumococcal conjugate				
First dose	2 mo	6 wk	2 mo	4 wk
Second dose	4 mo	10 wk	2 mo	4 wk
Third dose	6 mo	14 wk	6 mo	8 wk
Fourth dose	12–15 mo	18 wk		
Measles, mumps, rubella				
First dose	12–15 mo	12 mo	3–5 yr	4 wk
Second dose	4–6 yr	13 mo		

Varicella	12–15 mo	12 mo	4 wk	4 wk
Hepatitis A				
First dose	≥2 yr	2 yr	6–18 mo	6 mo
Second dose	≥30 mo	30 mo		
Influenza	6 mo	6 mo	1 mo	4 wk
Pneumococcal polysaccharide				
First dose	2 yr	2 yr	5 yr	5 yr
Second dose	7 yr	7 yr	5 yr	5 yr

[a]Data from Centers for Disease Control and Prevention, General recommendations on immunization: recommendations of the Advisory Committee on Immunization Practices and the American Academy of Family Physicians, *Morb. Mortal. Wkly. Rep.* **51**(RR-2):1–35, 2002.

Vaccines, Susceptibility

Vaccines, Susceptibility

Table 8.2 Recommended adult immunization schedule[a]

Vaccine	Age group (yr)		
	19–49	50–64	≥65
Tetanus/diphtheria	One booster dose every 10 yr	One booster dose every 10 yr	One booster dose every 10 yr
Influenza	One dose annually for persons with medical or occupational indications and their immediate contacts	One dose annually	One dose annually
Pneumococcal polysaccharide	One dose for persons with medical indications or one dose for persons with immunosuppressive conditions	One dose for persons with medical indications or one dose for persons with immunosuppressive conditions	One dose for persons unvaccinated or to revaccinate a person who has not received the vaccine in >5 yr
Hepatitis A	Two doses (6–12 mo apart) for persons with medical, behavioral, occupational, or other indications	Same as for 19–49-yr age group	Same as for 19–49-yr age group

Hepatitis B	Three doses (at 2–4 mo intervals) for persons with medical, behavioral, occupational, or other indications	Same as for 19–49-yr age group	Same as for 19–49-yr age group
Measles-mumps-rubella (MMR)	One dose if vaccination history is unreliable; two doses for persons with occupational, geographic, or other indications	Same as for 19–49-yr age group	Same as for 19–49-yr age group
Varicella	Two doses (1–2 mo apart) for susceptible persons (without a reliable history of natural disease, vaccination, or antibody response)	Same as for 19–49-yr age group	Same as for 19–49-yr age group
Meningococcal polysaccharide	One dose for persons with medical or other indications	Same as for 19–49-yr age group	Same as for 19–49-yr age group

[a]Data from Centers for Disease Control and Prevention, Recommended adult immunization schedule—United States, 2002–2003. *Morb. Mortal. Wkly. Rep.* **51**(40):904–908, 2002. Refer to this document and the CDC website (http://www.cdc.gov/nip) for detailed information about special considerations and contraindications for vaccinations.

Vaccines, Susceptibility

Table 8.3 National Committee for Clinical Laboratory Standards (NCCLS) documents related to antimicrobial susceptibility testing[a]

No.	Title
M2-A8	Performance Standards for Antimicrobial Disk Susceptibility Tests (2003)
M6-A	Protocols for Evaluating Dehydrated Mueller-Hinton Agar (1996)
M7-A6	Methods for Dilution Antimicrobial Susceptibility Tests for Bacteria That Grow Aerobically (2003)
M11-A5	Methods for Antimicrobial Susceptibility Testing of Anaerobic Bacteria (2001)
M21-A	Methodology for the Serum Bactericidal Test (1999)
M23-A2	Development of In Vitro Susceptibility Testing Criteria and Quality Control Parameters (2001)
M24-A	Antimycobacterial Susceptibility Testing of *Mycobacterium*, *Nocardia*, and Other Aerobic Actinomycetes (2003)
M26-A	Methods for Determining Bactericidal Activity of Antimicrobial Agents (1999)
M27-A2	Reference Method for Broth Dilution Antifungal Susceptibility Testing of Yeasts (2002)
M31-A2	Performance Standards for Antimicrobial Disk and Dilution Susceptibility Tests for Bacteria Isolated from Animals (2002)
M32-P	Evaluation of Lots of Mueller-Hinton Broth for Antimicrobial Susceptibility Testing (2001)
M33-P	Antiviral Susceptibility Testing (2000)
M37-A2	Development of In Vitro Susceptibility Testing Criteria and Quality Control Parameters for Veterinary Antimicrobial Agents (2002)
M38-A	Reference Method for Broth Dilution Antifungal Susceptibility Testing of Filamentous Fungi (2002)
M39-A	Analysis and Presentation of Cumulative Antimicrobial Susceptibility Test Data (2002)
M44-P	Method of Antifungal Disk Diffusion Susceptibility Testing of Yeasts (2003)
M100-S14	Performance Standards for Antimicrobial Susceptibility Testing (2004)
SC21-L	Susceptibility Testing (collection of documents: M2, M7, M11, M21, M24, M27, M31, and M100)

[a]Documents available from NCCLS (940 West Valley Road, Suite 1400, Wayne, PA 19087; telephone, 610-688-0100; FAX, 610-688-0700; E-mail, exoffice@nccls. org; Website, http://www.nccls.org).

Table 8.4 NCCLS quality control organisms for antimicrobial susceptibility tests

Quality control organism	Test(s)
Staphylococcus aureus ATCC 25923	Disk diffusion
Staphylococcus aureus ATCC 29213	Agar and broth dilution
Enterococcus faecalis ATCC 29212	Disk diffusion and agar and broth dilution
Enterococcus faecalis ATCC 51299	Agar and broth dilution
Escherichia coli ATCC 25922	Disk diffusion and broth dilution
Escherichia coli ATCC 35218	Disk diffusion and broth dilution
Pseudomonas aeruginosa ATCC 27853	Disk diffusion and broth dilution
Haemophilus influenzae ATCC 49247	Disk diffusion and broth dilution
Haemophilus influenzae ATCC 49766	Disk diffusion and broth dilution
Neisseria gonorrhoeae ATCC 49226	Disk diffusion and broth dilution
Streptococcus pneumoniae ATCC 49619	Disk diffusion and broth dilution
Helicobacter pylori ATCC 43504	Agar dilution
Campylobacter jejuni ATCC 33560	Agar dilution
Bacteroides fragilis ATCC 25285	Agar and broth dilution
Bacteroides thetaiotaomicron ATCC 29741	Agar and broth dilution
Eubacterium lentum ATCC 43055	Agar and broth dilution
Mycobacterium avium ATCC 700898	Agar or broth dilution
Mycobacterium peregrinum ATCC 700686	Broth dilution
Mycobacterium kansasii ATCC 12478	Agar or broth dilution
Mycobacterium marinum ATCC 927	Agar or broth dilution
Mycobacterium tuberculosis (H37Rv) ATCC 27294	Agar or broth dilution
Aspergillus flavus ATCC 204304	Broth dilution
Aspergillus fumigatus ATCC 204305	Broth dilution
Candida parapsilosis ATCC 22019 (QC strain)	Broth dilution
Candida krusei ATCC 6258 (QC strain)	Broth dilution
Candida parapsilosis ATCC 90018 (reference strain)	Broth dilution
Candida albicans ATCC 90028 (reference strain)	Broth dilution
Candida albicans ATCC 24433 (reference strain)	Broth dilution
Candida tropicalis ATCC 750 (reference strain)	Broth dilution

Vaccines, Susceptibility

Vaccines, Susceptibility

Table 8.5 Summary of NCCLS antimicrobial susceptibility test methods for bacteria, mycobacteria, and fungi[a]

Organism	Test method	Medium	Inoculum	Incubation conditions
Staphylococcus spp.	Disk diffusion	MHA	Direct	Air; 16–18 h (oxac, vanco: 24 h); 35°C
	Broth/agar dilution	CAMHB/MHA (oxac + 2% NaCl)	Direct	Air; 16–20 h (oxac, vanco: 24 h); 35°C
	Agar screen (S. aureus)	MHA + 4% NaCl + oxac (6 μg/ml)	Direct	Air; 24 h; 35°C
Streptococcus pneumoniae	Disk diffusion	MHA + 5% sheep blood	Direct	5% CO$_2$; 20–24 h; 35°C
	Broth dilution	CAMHB + 2–5% LHB	Direct	Air; 20–24 h; 35°C
Streptococcus, other spp.	Disk diffusion	MHA + 5% sheep blood	Direct	5% CO$_2$; 20–24 h; 35°C
	Broth/agar dilution	CAMHB + 2–5% LHB, or MHA + 5% sheep blood	Direct	5% CO$_2$ (agar) or air (broth); 20–24 h; 35°C
Enterococcus spp.	Disk diffusion	MHA	Direct; broth	Air; 16–18 h (vanco: 24 h); 35°C
	Broth/agar dilution	CAMHB/MHA	Direct; broth	Air; 16–20 h (vanco: 24 h); 35°C
	Agar screen	BHIA + gent (500 μg/ml)	Direct; broth	Air; 24 h; 35°C
		BHIA + strep (2,000 μg/ml)	Direct; broth	Air; 24–48 h; 35°C
		BHIA + vanco (6 μg/ml)	Direct; broth	Air; 24 h; 35°C

Listeria spp.	Broth dilution	CAMHB + 2–5% LHB	Direct; broth	Air; 16–20 h; 35°C
Neisseria gonorrhoeae	Disk diffusion	GCA + 1% supplement	Direct	5% CO$_2$; 20–24 h; 35°C
	Agar dilution	GCA + 1% supplement	Direct	5% CO$_2$; 20–24 h; 35°C
Neisseria meningitidis	Disk diffusion	CAMHB + 2–5% LHB	Direct	5% CO$_2$; 24 h; 35°C
	Broth/agar dilution	MHA + 5% sheep blood	Direct	5% CO$_2$; 24 h; 35°C
Haemophilus spp.	Disk diffusion	HTM agar	Direct	5% CO$_2$; 16–18 h; 35°C
	Broth dilution	HTM broth	Direct	Air; 20–24 h; 35°C
Enterobacteriaceae	Disk diffusion	MHA	Direct; broth	Air; 16–18 h; 35°C
	Broth/agar dilution	CAMHB/MHA	Direct; broth	Air; 16–20 h; *(Yersinia pestis,* 24 h); 35°C
Vibrio cholerae	Disk diffusion	MHA	Direct; broth	Air; 16–18 h; 35°C
	Broth/agar dilution	CAMHB/MHA	Direct; broth	Air; 16–20 h; 35°C
Pseudomonas aeruginosa	Disk diffusion	MHA	Direct; broth	Air; 16–18 h; 35°C
	Broth/agar dilution	CAMHB/MHA	Direct; broth	Air; 16–20 h; 35°C
Acinetobacter spp.	Disk diffusion	MHA	Direct; broth	Air; 16–18 h; 35°C
	Broth/agar dilution	CAMHB/MHA	Direct; broth	Air; 16–20 h; 35°C
Pseudomonas, other spp.	Broth/agar dilution	CAMHB/MHA	Direct	Air; 16–20 h; 35°C
Campylobacter spp.	Agar dilution	MHA + 5% sheep blood	Direct	Microaerophilic; 24 h; 42°C
Helicobacter pylori	Agar dilution	MHA + 5% aged sheep blood	Direct	Microaerophilic; 3 days; 35°C
Bacillus anthracis	Broth dilution	CAMHB	Direct	Air; 16–20 h; 35°C

(continued)

Vaccines, Susceptibility

Vaccines, Susceptibility

Table 8.5 Summary of NCCLS antimicrobial susceptibility test methods for bacteria, mycobacteria, and fungi[a] (continued)

Organism	Test method	Medium	Inoculum	Incubation conditions
Anaerobes	Broth/agar dilution	Brucella broth/agar + hemin (5 µg/ml), vitamin K_1 (1 µg/ml), 5% lysed sheep blood	Direct; broth	Anaerobic; 42–48 h; 35°C
Nocardia spp.	Broth dilution	CAMHB	Direct; broth	Air; 2–5 days; 35°C
Mycobacteria, rapid growers	Broth dilution	CAMHB + 0.02% Tween 80	Direct; broth	Air; 3–5 days; 30°C
	Agar disk elution	MHA + OADC	Direct; broth	Air; 3–5 days; 30°C
Mycobacteria, slow growers	Proportion agar dilution	7H10 agar + OADC	Direct; broth	5–10% CO_2; 3 wk; 37°C
Fungi (yeasts)	Broth dilution	Commercial broth systems	Direct; broth	5–14 days; 37°C
	Broth dilution	RPMI 1640 broth	Direct	Air; 46–50 h (Cryptococcus, 70–74 h); 35°C
Fungi (moulds)	Broth dilution	RPMI 1640 broth	Direct	Air; 46–50 h (Rhizopus spp., 21–26 h; Pseudallescheria boydii; 70–74 h); 35°C

[a]Inoculum can be prepared either directly with isolated colonies on an agar plate (direct) or after growth of the organism in a broth culture (broth).
Abbreviations: MHA, Mueller-Hinton agar; CAMHB, cation-adjusted Mueller-Hinton broth; NaCl, sodium chloride; LHB, lysed horse blood; BHIA, brain heart infusion agar; GCA, GC agar; HTM, Haemophilus test medium; OADC, oleic acid supplement; CNS, coagulase-negative staphylococci; oxac, oxacillin; gent, gentamicin; strep, streptomycin; vanco, vancomycin.

Table 8.6 Pharmacokinetic properties of antibacterial agents[a]

| Antimicrobial agent | Half-life in serum (h) | Unit dose | Avg peak level in serum (μg/ml)[b] | | |
			p.o.	i.m.	i.v.[c]
Amikacin	2–2.5	7.5 mg/kg		15–20	20–40
Amoxicillin	1	500 mg	6–8		
Amoxicillin-clavulanate	1.3/1.0	250/125 mg	3.3 (Amox) 1.5 (Clav)		
Ampicillin	1.1	500 mg 1 g	2.5–5	8–10	40
Ampicillin-sulbactam	1.1/1.0	3 g 1.5 g			120 (Amp) 60 (Sulb) 18 (Amp) 13 (Sulb)
Azithromycin	48	500 mg	0.4		3.5
Azlocillin	1	2 g			130
Aztreonam	1.7	1 g		45	90–160
Bacampicillin	1.1	800 mg	13		
Carbenicillin	1.1	1g		20–30	150
Carbenicillin indanyl sodium	1.1	764 mg	10		
Cefaclor	0.6	500 mg	16		
Cefadroxil	1.5	500 mg	10		
Cefamandole	0.5–1	1 g		20–36	90–140
Cefazolin	1.8	1 g		65	185

(continued)

Table 8.6 Pharmacokinetic properties of antibacterial agents[a] *(continued)*

Antimicrobial agent	Half-life in serum (h)	Unit dose	Avg peak level in serum (μg/ml)[b]		
			p.o.	i.m.	i.v.[c]
Cefepime	2	1 g		30	82
Cefdinir	1.7	300 mg	1.6		
Cefditoren	1.6	200 mg	3.1		
		400 mg	4.4		
Cefixine	3–4	400 mg	3.5		
Cefmetazole	1.5	1 g			70
Cefonicid	4	1 g		98	220
Cefoperazone	2	1 g		65–75	153
Ceforanide	3	1 g		70	125
Cefotaxime	1	1 g		20	40–45
Cefotetan	3–4.5	1 g		50–80	160
Cefoxitin	1	1 g		20–25	55–110
Cefpirome	2	1 g		45	85
Cefpodoxime	2.5	200 mg	2.3		
Cefprozil	1.5	500 mg	10.5		
Ceftazidime	2	1 g		40	70
Ceftibuten	2.5	400 mg	15		
Ceftizoxime	1.5	1 g		39	80–90
Ceftriaxone	6–9	500 mg		40–45	150
		1 g			

Cefuroxime	1.5	750 mg		27	50
Cefuroxime axetil	1.5	500 mg	9		
Cephalexin	0.9	500 mg	18		
Cephalothin	0.6	1 g			30–60
Cephapirin	0.6	1 g			40–70
Cephradine	0.8	500 mg	16		
Chloramphenicol	4	1 g	10–18		10–15
Chlortetracycline	6–9	500 mg	2–4	12	
Cinoxacin	1–1.5	500 mg	15		
Ciprofloxacin	3.5	400 mg	3.0		4.5
		500 mg	4.0		
		750 mg			
Clarithromycin	5–7	250 mg	1–2		
		500 mg	3–4		
		1,000 mg XL[d]	2–3		
Clinafloxacin	5.2	200 mg	1.5		
Clindamycin	2.5	300 mg	3		
		600 mg		6	
Cloxacillin	0.5	500 mg	10		10–12
Colistimethate sodium	2–4.5	150 mg		5–6	
Daptomycin	9	4 mg/kg			70
		6 mg/kg			82
Demeclocycline	12	300 mg	1–2		
Dicloxacillin	0.5–0.7	500 mg	15		

(continued)

Vaccines, Susceptibility

Vaccines, Susceptibility

Table 8.6 Pharmacokinetic properties of antibacterial agents[a] *(continued)*

Antimicrobial agent	Half-life in serum (h)	Unit dose	Avg peak level in serum (µg/ml)[b]		
			p.o.	i.m.	i.v.[c]
Dirithromycin	40	500 mg	0.5		
Doxycycline	18–22	100 mg	2.5		4
Enoxacin	4–6	400 mg	3–5		
Ertapenem	4	1 g		70	155
Erythromycin	1.5	500 mg	2–3		
		1 g			10
Fleroxacin	12	400 mg	5		7–8
Fosfomycin	5.7	3 g	25		
		50 mg/kg			275
Fusidic acid	13–19	500 mg	25–30		50
Gatifloxacin	7	400 mg	4		4.5
Gemifloxacin	7–8	800 mg	4		
Gentamicin	2–3	1.5 mg/kg	4–6		4–8
Imipenem	1	500 mg			25–35
Kanamycin	2.2–3	7.5 mg/kg		20–25	
Levofloxacin	6–8	500 mg	5.5		6.5
		750 mg	8.5		12
Lincomycin	5	500 mg	3.5	10	16–21
		600 mg			
Linezolid	5	600 mg	15		15

Lomefloxacin	6.5	400 mg	3		
Loracarbef	1	400 mg	14		
Meropenem	1	500 mg	15		25–35
Methicillin	0.5	1 g			60
Metronidazole	8	500 mg	12		20–25
Mezlocillin	1	1 g			15
		3 g			260
Minocycline	14–16	100 mg	1		4.5
Moxifloxacin	12	400 mg	4.5		
Nafcillin	0.5	500 mg			5–8
		1 g			20–40
Nalidixic acid	1.5	1 g	20–50		
Netilmicin	2.5	2 mg/kg		5–7	6–8
Nitrofurantoin	0.3	100 mg	<2		
Norfloxacin	3.3	400 mg	1.5		
Ofloxacin	5	400 mg	4		
Ornidazole	13	500 mg	10		20
Oxacillin	0.5	500 mg	4–6	14–16	40
		1 g			
Oxytetracycline	9	500 mg	1–2		
Pefloxacin	10	400 mg	3		5.5
Penicillin G	0.5	500 mg	1.5–2.5		
Aqueous		1×10^6 U		8–10	10
Benzathine		1.2×10^6 U		0.1–0.15	

(continued)

Vaccines, Susceptibility

Table 8.6 Pharmacokinetic properties of antibacterial agents[a] *(continued)*

Antimicrobial agent	Half-life in serum (h)	Unit dose	Avg peak level in serum (µg/ml)[b]		
			p.o.	i.m.	i.v.[c]
Procaine		1.2×10^6 U		3	
Penicillin V	0.3	500 mg	3–5		
Piperacillin	1.1	2 g			36
		4 g			240
Piperacillin-tazobactam	1.1/1.0	3.375 g			242 (Pip)
					24 (Tazo)
		4.5 g			298 (Pip)
					34 (Tazo)
Pivampicillin	0.5–1	350 mg	2		
Polymyxin B	6–7	2.5 mg/kg			5
Quinupristin-dalfopristin	1/0.75	7.5 mg/kg			3 (Q)
					7.5 (D)
Rifampin	2–5	600 mg	7–9		10
Sparfloxacin	20	200 mg	1.1		
Spectinomycin	1–2	2 g		100	
Spiramycin	3.8	2 g	3		
Streptomycin	2–3	1 g		25–50	
Sulfadiazine	17	2 g	100–150		
Sulfadoxine	150–200	1 g	50–75		

Drug		Dose			
Sulfamethizole	4–7	2 g	60		
Sulfamethoxazole	10–12	1 g	40		
Sulfisoxazole	5–7	2 g	170		
Teicoplanin	45	200 mg		7	
		400 mg			20–40
Telithromycin	9–10	800 mg	2		
Tetracycline	8	500 mg	4		8
Ticarcillin	1.2	1 g		20–30	
		3 g			190
Ticarcillin-clavulanate	1.2/1.0	3.1 g			330 (Ticar)
					8 (Clav)
Timidazole	12–14	2 g	40		40
Tobramycin	2–2.8	1.5 mg/kg		4–6	4–8
Trimethoprim	10–12	100 mg	1		
TMP-SMX		160/800 mg	3 (TMP)		9 (TMP)
			46 (SMX)		106 (SMX)
Trovafloxacin (alatrofloxacin i.v.)	11	300 mg			4.5
Vancomycin	6	500 mg			20–40

[a] Adapted from P. R. Murray, E. J. Baron, J. H. Jorgensen, M. A. Pfaller, and R. H. Yolken (ed.), *Manual of Clinical Microbiology*, 8th ed., ASM Press, Washington, D.C., 2003.

[b] p.o., oral; i.m., intramuscular; i.v., intravenous.

[c] At 30 min following intravenous infusion.

[d] Extended-release formulation.

Table 8.7 Pharmacokinetic properties of antimycobacterial agents

Antimicrobial agent	Half-life in serum (h)	Unit dose[a]	Avg peak level in serum (µg/ml)
p-Aminosalicylic acid	2	4 g p.o.	20
Cycloserine	3	250 mg p.o.	10
Clofazimine	70 days	300 mg p.o.	0.7–1.0
Dapsone	10–50 (avg 28)	200 mg p.o.	2.3
Ethambutol	4	25 mg/kg p.o.	2–5
Ethionamide	2	250 mg p.o.	2
Isoniazid	2.8	300 mg p.o.	7
		800 mg p.o.	10–15
Pyrazinamide	9–10	0.5 g p.o.	5
		3 g p.o.	30
Rifabutin	45	300 mg p.o.	0.3–0.5
Rifampin	2–3	600 mg p.o.	5–10

[a] p.o., oral; i.v., intravenous.

Table 8.8 Pharmacokinetic properties of antiviral agents

Antimicrobial agent	Half-life in serum (h)	Unit dose	Avg peak level in serum (μg/ml)
Abacavir	1.5	300 mg p.o.	2.9
Acyclovir	2.5–3.5	5 mg/kg i.v.	9.8
Adefovir	7.5	10 mg p.o.	0.02
Amantadine	14	200 mg p.o.	0.5
Amprenavir	7.1–10.6	1,200 mg p.o.	5.4
Cidofovir	2.5	3 mg/kg i.v.	9.8
Delavirdine	5.8	400 mg p.o.	19
Didanosine (ddi)	1.6	300 mg p.o.	1.6
Efavirenz	40–55	600 mg p.o.	4.1
Famciclovir	3.0	500 mg p.o.	3–4
Foscarnet	4.0	57 mg/kg i.v.	155
Ganciclovir	3.0	5 mg/kg i.v.	9
Indinavir	1.5–2.0	800 mg p.o.	12.6 μM
Lamivudine (3TC)	3–6	2 mg/kg p.o.	1.5
Lopinavir	5–6	400 mg/kg p.o.	9
Nelfinavir	3.5–5	750 mg p.o.	3–4
Nevirapine	25–30	200 mg p.o.	2
Oseltamivir	6–10	75 mg p.o.	0.3

(continued)

Vaccines, Susceptibility

Vaccines, Susceptibility

Table 8.8 Pharmacokinetic properties of antiviral agents *(continued)*

Antimicrobial agent	Half-life in serum (h)	Unit dose	Avg peak level in serum (µg/ml)
Ribavirin	9.5	400 mg p.o.	0.6
Rimantadine	36.5	100 mg p.o.	0.24
Ritonavir	3–5	300 mg p.o.	7.8
Saquinavir	1–2	1,200 mg p.o.	4.7
Stavudine	1.0	70 mg p.o.	1.4
Tenofovir	17	300 mg p.o.	0.12
Valacyclovir	2.5–3.5	1,000 mg p.o.	5.6
Zalcitabine	2.7	0.5 mg p.o.	7.6 ng/ml
Valganciclovir	3.0	900 mg p.o.	5.6
Zalcitabine (ddC)	1.2	200 mg p.o.	1.1
Zanamivir	2.5–5.1	5 mg inhalant	17–142 ng/ml
Zidovudine	1.1	200 mg p.o.	1.2

Table 8.9 Pharmacokinetic properties of antifungal agents[a]

Antimicrobial agent	Half-life in serum (h)	Unit dose	Avg peak level in serum (µg/ml)
Amphotericin B	15 days	0.4–0.7 mg/kg i.v.	0.5–3.5
Amphotericin B lipid complex		5 mg/kg i.v.	1.7
Liposomal amphotericin B		2.5 mg/kg i.v.	31
Flucytosine	3–6	2.5 g p.o.	30–45
Fluconazole	22–35	200 mg p.o.	10.2
		800 mg p.o.	40–60
Ketoconazole	7–10	200 mg p.o.	1.5–3.1
		400 mg p.o.	7
Itraconazole	24–42	200 mg p.o.	0.2–0.4
Voriconazole	6	200 mg p.o.	2.7–6
Caspofungin	8	70 mg i.v.	10

Vaccines, Susceptibility

Table 8.10 Pharmacokinetic properties of antiparasitic agents

Antimicrobial agent	Half-life in serum (h)	Unit dose	Avg peak level in serum (µg/ml)
Albendazole	9	400 mg p.o.	0.2–3.0
Mebendazole	2.5–5.5	100 mg p.o.	0.03–0.09
Dapsone	14–35	100 mg p.o.	1.8
Diethylcarbamazine	2–17	0.5 mg/kg p.o.	0.1–0.15
Ivermectin	10–16	12 mg p.o.	46
		1 g p.o.	0.5–1.2
Pentamidine	6.5–9.0	4 mg/kg i.v.	0.3–1.4
Praziquantel	1–3	40 mg/kg p.o.	1.0–1.6
Pyrimethamine	80–95	25 mg p.o.	0.1–0.3
Mefloquine	2–3 wk	250 mg p.o.	0.3

Table 8.11 Antibacterial agents for specific bacteria

Organism	Antibiotics	
	Generally active[a]	Unpredictable activity
Acinetobacter spp.	**Carbapenems**	β-Lactam – β-lactamase inhibitors
Actinobacillus spp.	**Cephalosporins**, rifampin, aminoglycosides, tetracyclines	Penicillins
Actinomyces spp.	**Penicillin**, doxycycline, broad-spectrum cephalosporins	Clindamycin, macrolides
Aeromonas hydrophila	**Broad-spectrum cephalosporins**, carbapenems, fluoroquinolones	Macrolides, aminoglycosides, tetracyclines
Anaplasma phagocytophila	**Doxycycline**	Chloramphenicol
Arcanobacterium haemolyticum	**Penicillin**, cephalosporins, carbapenems, vancomycin, macrolides, clindamycin, tetracyclines, fluoroquinolones	
Bacillus anthracis	**Penicillin**, ciprofloxacin	
Bacillus cereus	**Vancomycin**, carbapenems, macrolides, clindamycin, fluoroquinolones, gentamicin	Sulfonamides, tetracycline
Bacteroides fragilis group	**Metronidazole**	Clindamycin, carbapenems, cefoxitin, β-lactam – β-lactamase inhibitors

(continued)

Vaccines, Susceptibility

Vaccines, Susceptibility

Table 8.11 Antibacterial agents for specific bacteria *(continued)*

Organism	Antibiotics	
	Generally active[a]	Unpredictable activity
Bartonella henselae	**Erythromycin**, doxycycline	Penicillins, cephalosporins, carbapenems, aminoglycosides, fluoroquinolones, trimethoprim-sulfamethoxazole
Bordetella pertussis	**Macrolides**, trimethoprim-sulfamethoxazole, fluoroquinolones	
Borrelia burgdorferi	**Doxycycline or broad-spectrum cephalosporins,** penicillins, macrolides	Fluoroquinolones
Brucella spp.	**Doxycycline**, trimethoprim-sulfamethoxazole	Cephalosporins
Burkholderia cepacia	**Trimethoprim-sulfamethoxazole**	Fluoroquinolones
Burkholderia pseudomallei	**Carbapenems**, penicillins	Fluoroquinolones, broad-spectrum cephalosporins
Campylobacter jejuni	**Macrolides**, tetracyclines	Fluoroquinolones
Campylobacter fetus	**Carbapenem**, aminoglycosides	Ampicillin, macrolides
Capnocytophaga spp.	**Clindamycin**, β-lactam−β-lactamase inhibitors	Fluoroquinolones, carbapenems
Cardiobacterium hominis	**Penicillin**, cephalosporins, carbapenems, tetracycline	
Chlamydia trachomatis	**Doxycycline**, erythromycin	
Chlamydophila pneumoniae	**Doxycycline**, macrolides, fluoroquinolones	
Chlamydophila psittaci	**Doxycycline**, macrolides, fluoroquinolones	
Citrobacter freundi	**Broad-spectrum cephalosporins**, carbapenems, fluoroquinolones	Fluoroquinolones

Organism	Susceptibility	Alternatives
Citrobacter koseri	**Broad-spectrum cephalosporins**, carbapenems, fluoroquinolones	
Clostridium botulinum	**Penicillin**	
Clostridium difficile	**Metronidazole**, vancomycin	
Clostridium perfringens	**Penicillin**, cephalosporins, tetracyclines, clindamycin	
Clostridium tetani	**Penicillin**	
Corynebacterium diphtheriae	**Erythromycin**, penicillin, clindamycin, cephalosporins, vancomycin, fluoroquinolones, aminoglycosides	Trimethoprim-sulfamethoxazole
Corynebacterium jeikeium	**Vancomycin**	Fluoroquinolones
Corynebacterium urealyticum	**Vancomycin**	Fluoroquinolones, macrolides, tetracyclines
Coxiella burnetii	**Doxycycline**, macrolides, fluoroquinolones	
Ehrlichia chaffeensis	**Doxycycline**	Chloramphenicol
Ehrlichia ewingii	**Doxycycline**	Chloramphenicol
Eikenella corrodens	**Penicillin**, broad-spectrum cephalosporins, tetracyclines, fluoroquinolones	Aminoglycosides
Enterobacter aerogenes	**Carbapenems**	Broad-spectrum cephalosporins, fluoroquinolones
Enterobacter cloacae	**Carbapenems**	Broad-spectrum cephalosporins, fluoroquinolones
Enterococcus faecalis	**Penicillin, ampicillin, or vancomycin with gentamicin**	Imipenem, fluoroquinolones

(continued)

Vaccines, Susceptibility

Vaccines, Susceptibility

Table 8.11 Antibacterial agents for specific bacteria *(continued)*

	Antibiotics	
Organism	**Generally active**[a]	**Unpredictable activity**
Enterococcus faecium		**Penicillin,** ampicillin, or vancomycin with gentamicin
Erysipelothrix rhusiopathiae	**Penicillin,** cephalosporins, carbapenems, macrolides, clindamycin, fluoroquinolones	
Escherichia coli	β-Lactam–β-lactamase inhibitors, fluoroquinolones, broad-spectrum cephalosporins	
Francisella tularensis	**Streptomycin** or gentamicin, carbapenems, fluoroquinolones	Tetracyclines
Fusobacterium spp.	**Metronidazole,** carbapenems, penicillin, clindamycin	Broad-spectrum cephalosporins
Hafnia alvei	β-Lactam–β-lactamase inhibitors, fluoroquinolones, broad-spectrum cephalosporins	
Haemophilus aphrophilus	**Penicillin,** broad-spectrum cephalosporins	
Haemophilus ducreyi	**Broad-spectrum cephalosporins,** fluoroquinolones, macrolides	Penicillins, β-lactam–β-lactamase inhibitors, tetracyclines, trimethoprim-sulfamethoxazole
Haemophilus influenzae	Broad-spectrum cephalosporins, trimethoprim-sulfamethoxazole	Ampicillin
Kingella kingae	**Cephalosporins,** penicillins, carbapenems, aminoglycosides, macrolides	Clindamycin

Klebsiella granulomatis	**Tetracyclines**, macrolides, trimethoprim-sulfamethoxazole, aminoglycosides, fluoroquinolones
Klebsiella oxytoca	**Broad-spectrum cephalosporins**, fluoroquinolones, carbapenems
Klebsiella ozaenae	**Fluoroquinolones**, carbapenems
Klebsiella pneumoniae	**Broad-spectrum cephalosporins**, fluoroquinolones, carbapenems
Lactobacillus spp.	**Penicillin or ampicillin with aminoglycoside**
Legionella pneumophila	**Macrolides**, fluoroquinolones, rifampin
Leptospira interrogans	**Penicillin**, doxycycline, cephalosporins
Leuconostoc spp.	**Carbapenems**, aminoglycosides, tetracyclines
Listeria monocytogenes	**Penicillin or ampicillin with aminoglycoside**, vancomycin
Moraxella catarrhalis	**Cephalosporins**, fluoroquinolones, carbapenems, tetracyclines, macrolides
Morganella morganii	**Carbapenems**
Mycoplasma pneumoniae	**Macrolides**, tetracyclines
Neisseria gonorrhoeae	**Broad-spectrum cephalosporins**
Neisseria meningitidis	**Penicillin**, broad-spectrum cephalosporins
Nocardia spp.	**Sulfonamides**, carbapenems, amikacin, linezolid

	Penicillins, cephalosporins, aminoglycosides
	Penicillin, cephalosporins
	Fluoroquinolones, broad-spectrum cephalosporins
	Broad-spectrum cephalosporins
	Aminoglycosides, fluoroquinolones
	Penicillin, tetracyclines, macrolides, fluoroquinolones
	Fluoroquinolones, broad-spectrum cephalosporins

(continued)

Vaccines, Susceptibility

Vaccines, Susceptibility

Table 8.11 Antibacterial agents for specific bacteria *(continued)*

Organism	Antibiotics	
	Generally active[a]	Unpredictable activity
Pasteurella multocida	**Penicillin**, cephalosporins, carbapenems, fluoroquinolones, tetracyclines	Macrolides, clindamycin
Plesiomonas shigelloides	**Cephalosporins**, carbapenems, β-lactam–β-lactamase inhibitors, fluoroquinolones	
Porphyromonas spp.	**Metronidazole**, carbapenems, clindamycin	Broad-spectrum cephalosporins
Prevotella spp.	**Metronidazole**, carbapenems, clindamycin	Broad-spectrum cephalosporins
Proteus mirabilis	**Ampicillin**, broad-spectrum cephalosporins, carbapenems	
Proteus vulgaris	**Broad-spectrum cephalosporins**, carbapenems, fluoroquinolones	
Providencia spp.	**Broad-spectrum cephalosporins**, carbapenems, fluoroquinolones	
Pseudomonas aeruginosa	**Carbapenems**	Broad-spectrum cephalosporins, fluoroquinolones
Rhodococcus equi	**Carbapenems**, vancomycin, aminoglycosides, fluoroquinolones	Macrolides, clindamycin, tetracyclines
Rickettsia spp.	**Doxycycline**, fluoroquinolones	Erythromycin
Rothia mucilaginosa	**Penicillin**, cephalosporins, carbapenems, vancomycin	Aminoglycosides, clindamycin, macrolides
Salmonella enterica serovar Typhi	**Fluoroquinolones**, broad-spectrum cephalosporins	Chloramphenicol, amoxicillin, trimethoprim-sulfamethoxazole

Organism	Therapy of choice[a]	Alternative
Salmonella spp.	**Fluoroquinolones**, broad-spectrum cephalosporins	Chloramphenicol, amoxicillin, trimethoprim-sulfamethoxazole
Serratia marcescens	**Broad-spectrum cephalosporins**, carbapenems, fluoroquinolones	
Shigella spp.	**Fluoroquinolones**, azithromycin	Trimethoprim-sulfamethoxazole, ampicillin
Staphylococcus spp. (ox-susc.)	**Oxacillin**, vancomycin, cephalosporins, imipenem, macrolides, clindamycin, fluoroquinolones	
Staphylococcus spp. (ox-res.)	**Vancomycin**	Carbapenems, fluoroquinolones
Stenotrophomonas maltophilia	**Trimethoprim-sulfamethoxazole**	Fluoroquinolones
Streptobacillus moniliformis	**Penicillin**, tetracyclines	
Streptococcus agalactiae (group B)	**Penicillin**, cephalosporins, carbapenems, vancomycin	Penicillin (drug of choice if susc.)
Streptococcus, anginosus group	**Penicillin**, cephalosporins, carbapenems, vancomycin	Penicillin (drug of choice if susc.)
Streptococcus, mitis group	**Cephalosporins**, carbapenems, vancomycin	
Streptococcus pneumoniae	**Cephalosporins**, carbapenems, vancomycin	Macrolides
Streptococcus pyogenes (group A)	**Penicillin**, cephalosporins, carbapenems, vancomycin	
Treponema pallidum	**Penicillin**, broad-spectrum cephalosporins, tetracyclines	Tetracyclines, trimethoprim-sulfamethoxazole
Tsakamurella spp.	**Carbapenems**, aminoglycosides, fluoroquinolones	Trimethoprim-sulfamethoxazole
Vibrio cholerae	**Doxycycline**, fluoroquinolones	Aminoglycosides
Vibrio vulnificus	**Doxycycline with ceftazidime**	Broad-spectrum cephalosporins
Yersinia enterocolitica	**Fluoroquinolones**, trimethoprim-sulfamethoxazole	Chloramphenicol, ciprofloxacin, doxycycline
Yersinia pestis	**Streptomycin or gentamicin**	

[a]Therapy of choice in bold type.

Vaccines, Susceptibility

Vaccines, Susceptibility

Table 8.12 Antimicrobial activity of broad-spectrum agents against more than 3,000 clinical isolates[a]

Antibiotic	% of isolates susceptible								
	Escherichia coli	*Klebsiella* spp.	*Citrobacter* spp.	*Enterobacter* spp.	*Proteus mirabilis*	*Serratia* spp.	*Pseudomonas aeruginosa*	*Acinetobacter* spp.	*Staphylococcus aureus*
Imipenem	100	100	100	99.3	100	96.8	88.5	88.4	100
Meropenem	100	100	100	99.3	100	98.8	93.1	84.1	100
Ceftriaxone	99.4	98.4	88.2	83.1	100	96.3	14.3	34.8	99.4
Ceftazidime	99.4	98.0	87.1	82.2	100	96.3	85.7	58.0	90.7
Cefepime	100	100	98.8	98.0	100	98.8	87.9	53.6	100
Piperacillin-tazobactam	98.1	94.7	87.1	84.9	100	98.8	91.5	62.3	100
Gentamicin	95.4	96.0	91.8	94.7	93.9	95.1	87.9	59.4	98.7
Tobramycin	96.0	96.0	92.9	93.4	94.6	92.7	92.2	71.0	96.0
Ciprofloxacin	92.7	96.8	92.9	92.1	90.5	95.1	72.3	56.5	92.0

[a] Data from P. R. Rhomberg, R. N. Jones, and the MYSTIC Program Study Group, Antimicrobial spectrum of activity for meropenem and nine broad-spectrum antimicrobials: report from the MYSTIC Program (2002) in North America, *Diagn. Microbiol. Infect. Dis.* **47:**365–372, 2003.

Table 8.13 Susceptibility patterns for gram-negative bacteria associated with nosocomial bacteremia[a]

Antibiotic	% of isolates susceptible[b]					
	Escherichia coli	*Klebsiella pneumoniae*	*Enterobacter cloacae*	*Pseudomonas aeruginosa*	*Serratia marcescens*
Ampicillin	59	2	4	2	3
Ampicillin-sulbactam	62	60	16	2	11
Ticarcillin-clavulanate	79	67	59	85	85
Cefotaxime	98	88	63	22	93
Ceftriaxone	99	91	61	27	91
Ceftazidime	97	87	58	88	95
Imipenem	99	99	99	90	96
Ciprofloxacin	99	92	93	85	93
Gentamicin	97	87	88	81	92
Trimethoprim-sulfamethoxazole	86	83	85	13	96

[a] Data from M. B. Edmond, S. E. Wallace, D. K. McClish, M. A. Pfaller, R. N. Jones, and R. P. Wenzel, Nosocomial bloodstream infections in United States hospitals: a three-year analysis, *Clin. Infect. Dis.* **29:**239–244, 1999.

[b] Frequency of gram-negative rods responsible for nosocomial bacteremia: *E. coli*, 26.5%; *K. pneumoniae*, 25.1%; *E. cloacae*, 21.1%; *P. aeruginosa*, 20.6%; *S. marcescens*, 6.7%. Gram-positive cocci (coagulase-negative *Staphylococcus*, *S. aureus*, and *Enterococcus*) were responsible for 64.4% of infections; gram-negative rods were responsible for 27.0%, and yeasts were responsible for 8.4%.

Vaccines, Susceptibility

Table 8.14 Susceptibility patterns for bacteria associated with pneumonia in hospitalized patients[a]

Antibiotic	% of isolates susceptible[b]				
	Staphylococcus aureus	*Pseudomonas aeruginosa*	*Streptococcus pneumoniae*	*Klebsiella* spp.	*Haemophilus influenzae*
Ampicillin	9.5	0	90.7	5.4	71.4
Ticarcillin-clavulanate	NT[c]	74.4	NT	93.1	100
Piperacillin-tazobactam	NT	85.6	NT	97.5	100
Oxacillin	56.2	NT	NT	NT	NT
Cefuroxime	NT	0	NT	85.7	100
Ceftriaxone	56.2	13.6	97.2	99.5	100
Ceftazidime	56.2	78.3	NT	96.6	100
Cefepime	56.2	80.5	98.8	99.5	100
Imipenem	56.2	85.6	87.8	100	100
Meropenem	NT	89.1	NT	100	100

Ciprofloxacin	55.7	72.4	NT	97.5	100
Levofloxacin	57.0	71.5	98.8	97.5	100
Gatifloxacin	64.7	67.0	99.2	98.0	100
Erythromycin	44.7	NT	74.8	NT	NT
Clindamycin	60.3	NT	90.7	NT	NT
Quinupristin/dalfopristin	99.7	NT	100	NT	NT
Linezolid	100	NT	100	NT	NT
Tetracycline	91.4	3.9	80.5	85.2	100
Trimethoprim-sulfamethoxazole	89.9	0	74.0	94.6	82.4

[a]Data from D. J. Hoban, D. J. Biedenbach, A. H. Mutnick, and R. N. Jones, Pathogen of occurrence and susceptibility patterns associated with pneumonia in hospitalized patients in North America: results of the SENTRY Antimicrobial Surveillance Study (2000). *Diagn. Microbiol. Infect. Dis.* **45:**279–285, 2003.
[b]The five most frequent causes of pneumonia in hospitalized patients in this study were *S. aureus* (28.0%), *P. aeruginosa* (20.0%), *S. pneumoniae* (9.1%), *Klebsiella* spp. (7.5%), and *H. influenzae* (7.3%).
[c]NT, not tested.

Vaccines, Susceptibility

Vaccines, Susceptibility

Table 8.15 Susceptibility patterns for gram-negative bacteria associated with urinary tract infections in hospitalized patients[a]

Antibiotic	% of isolates susceptible[b]					
	Escherichia coli	*Klebsiella spp.*	*Pseudomonas aeruginosa*	*Proteus mirabilis*	*Enterobacter spp.*
Ampicillin	57.6	0.5	0.8	89.3	6.7
Amoxicillin-clavulanate	85.2	92.2	0.9	87.3	2.2
Imipenem	100	100	91.2	100	100
Piperacillin-tazobactam	95.8	95.2	95.6	100	73.3
Nalidixic acid	93.1	81.9	1.8	82.7	84.4
Ciprofloxacin	96.3	92.2	75.2	93.3	91.1
Levofloxacin	96.6	95.2	71.7	94.7	93.3
Nitrofurantoin	96.5	47.0	0	0	26.7
Trimethoprim-sulfamethoxazole	76.7	86.1	0	90.7	86.7

[a] Data from D. Mathai, R. N. Jones, M. A. Pfaller, and the SENTRY Participant Group North America, Epidemiology and frequency of resistance among pathogens causing urinary tract infections in 1,510 hospitalized patients: a report from the SENTRY Antimicrobial Surveillance Program (North America), *Diagn. Microbiol. Infect. Dis.* **40:**129–136, 2001.

[b] Frequency of gram-negative rods responsible for urinary tract infections in hospitalized patients: *E. coli*, 61.7%; *Klebsiella* spp., 14.5%; *P. aeruginosa*, 9.9%; *P. mirabilis*, 6.5%; *Enterobacter* spp., 3.9%. Gram-positive cocci (*Enterococcus*, coagulase-negative *Staphylococcus*, *S. aureus*, beta-hemolytic and *Streptococcus*) were responsible for 21.3% of infections, and gram-negative rods were responsible for 78.7%.

Table 8.16 Antimycobacterial agents for specific mycobacteria

Mycobacterium species	Antimycobacterial agents[a]		
	Primary or first choice	Secondary or second choice	Primary resistance likely
M. tuberculosis, M. bovis, M. africanum	INH, RMP, PZA, EMB	SM, ciprofloxacin, ofloxacin, sparfloxacin, rifapentine, ethionamide	*M. bovis* and *M. bovis* BCG are considered resistant to PZA
M. avium, M. intracellulare	Clarithromycin, EMB, azithromycin	Amikacin, ciprofloxacin, rifabutin	INH, PZA
M. leprae	Clarithromycin, dapsone, RMP	Ethionamide, prothionamide, minocycline, clofazimine	
M. haemophilum, M. malmoense, M. simiae, M. szulgai, M. xenopi, M. ulcerans	Clarithromycin, EMB, RMP	Amikacin, ciprofloxacin, rifabutin, INH, SM	PZA; primary drugs have proven clinical utility for some but not all species
M. scrofulaceum	Lymphadenitis (surgical excision without chemotherapy)	Clarithromycin, azithromycin	INH, PZA
M. kansasii	RMP	INH, EMB, clarithromycin	PZA
M. marinum	Doxycycline or minocycline, EMB, RMP, sulfonamides	Clarithromycin, azithromycin	INH, PZA
M. chelonae, M. fortuitum, M. abscessus, M. mucogenicum, M. smegmatis group	Amikacin, cefoxitin, ciprofloxacin, clarithromycin, doxycycline or minocycline, sulfonamides	Cefmetazole, ofloxacin, imipenem (*M. fortuitum* group, *M. smegmatis*, and *M. mucogenicum* only), tobramycin (*M. chelonae* only)	INH, PZA, RMP, SM, EMB, clofazimine

[a]INH, isoniazid; EMB, ethambutol; RMP, rifampin; PZA, pyrazinamide; SM, streptomycin; PAS, *p*-aminosalicylic acid.

Vaccines, Susceptibility

Table 8.17 Antiviral agents for specific viruses

Virus	Antiviral agents
Adenovirus	Cidofovir, ribavirin
Epstein-Barr virus	Foscarnet
Hepatitis B virus	Alpha interferon; lamivudine
Hepatitis C virus	Alpha interferon or ribavirin with alpha interferon (chronic disease)
Herpes simplex virus	Acyclovir, valacyclovir, penciclovir, famciclovir, foscarnet (for acyclovir-resistant virus)
Human cytomegalovirus	Ganciclovir, cidofovir, valganciclovir, foscarnet, fomivirsen
Human herpesvirus 6	Foscarnet, cidofovir, ganciclovir
Human immunodeficiency virus	Highly active antiretrovirus therapy (HAART)[a]: combination of two reverse transcriptase (RT) inhibitors (zidovudine, didanosine, zalcitabine, stavudine, lamivudine, abacavir, or tenofovir) with a protease inhibitor (indinavir, ritonavir, saquinavir, nelfinavir, amprenavir, or lopinavir) or nonnucleoside RT inhibitor (nevirapine, delavirdine, or efavirenz)
Human papillomavirus	Podofilox, alpha interferon, imiquimod
Influenza A virus	Amantadine, rimantadine, zanamivir, oseltamivir, ribavirin
Influenza B virus	Zanamivir, oseltamivir, ribavirin
Parainfluenza virus	Ribavirin
Respiratory syncytial virus	Ribavirin
Varicella-zoster virus	Acyclovir, valacyclovir, famciclovir, foscarnet

[a] For specific guidelines, refer to the CDC website (www.cdc.gov) or see Centers for Disease Control and Prevention, Guidelines for using antiretroviral agents among HIV-infected adults and adolescents: recommendations of the Panel on Clinical Practices for Treatment of HIV, *Morb. Mortal. Wkly. Rep.* **51**(RR-7):1–55, 2002.

Table 8.18 Antifungal agents for specific fungi

Organism	Antifungal agents		
	Generally active	Moderately active	Generally inactive
Yeasts			
Candida albicans	Amphotericin B, caspofungin, fluconazole, itraconazole	Ketoconazole	
C. glabrata	Caspofungin	Amphotericin B, fluconazole, itraconazole	Ketoconazole
C. guillermondii	Fluconazole, itraconazole	Amphotericin B, caspofungin	Ketoconazole
C. krusei	Caspofungin	Amphotericin B, itraconazole	Fluconazole, ketoconazole
C. lusitaniae	Caspofungin, fluconazole, itraconazole	Amphotericin B, ketoconazole	
C. parapsilosis	Amphotericin B, caspofungin, fluconazole, itraconazole	Ketoconazole	
C. tropicalis	Amphotericin B, caspofungin, fluconazole, itraconazole	Ketoconazole	
Cryptococcus neoformans	Amphotericin B plus flucytosine, fluconazole	Itraconazole	Caspofungin, ketoconazole

(continued)

Vaccines, Susceptibility

Vaccines, Susceptibility

Table 8.18 Antifungal agents for specific fungi *(continued)*

Organism	Antifungal agents		
	Generally active	Moderately active	Generally inactive
Malassezia spp.	Selenium sulfide, ketoconazole, itraconazole, amphotericin B, terbinafine		
Trichosporon spp.	Amphotericin B plus flucytosine, terbinafine	Caspofungin	
Dimorphic fungi			
Blastomyces dermatitidis	Amphotericin B, itraconazole	Ketoconazole, caspofungin	Fluconazole, flucytosine
Coccidioides immitis	Amphotericin B, fluconazole, itraconazole	Ketoconazole, caspofungin	Flucytosine
Histoplasma capsulatum	Amphotericin B, itraconazole	Fluconazole, ketoconazole, caspofungin	Flucytosine
Paracoccidioides brasiliensis	Amphotericin B, itraconazole, ketoconazole	Caspofungin, fluconazole	Flucytosine
Penicillium marneffei	Amphotericin B, itraconazole, terbinfine	Fluconazole	
Sporothrix schenckii	Potassium iodide, itraconazole, terbinafine, amphotericin B		Flucytosine, ketoconazole, fluconazole

Other moulds			
Aspergillus spp.	Amphotericin B (except for *A. terreus*), itraconazole	Caspofungin	Ketoconazole, fluconazole
Chromoblastomycosis agents[a]	Itraconazole, flucytosine		Amphotericin B
Dematiaceous fungi	Itraconazole, voriconazole	Ketoconazole	*Scedosporium prolificans:* all drugs
Dermatophytes[b]	Miconazole, itraconazole, ketoconazole, clotrimazole, fluconazole, terbinafine, nystatin, griseofulvin		
Eumycetoma agents[c]		Amphotericin, voriconazole, ketoconazole, itraconazole	Fluconazole
Zygomycetes[d]	Amphotericin B		Caspofungin, fluconazole, itraconazole, ketoconazole, flucytosine
Other fungi			
Pneumocystis jiroveci	Trimethoprim-sulfamethoxazole, pentamidine isethionate	Atovaquone, clindamycin-primaquine	

[a] Chromoblastomycosis agents include *Phialophora* and *Cladophialophora* spp.
[b] Dermatophytes include *Epidermophyton, Microsporum,* and *Trichophyton* spp.
[c] Eumycetoma agents include *Madurella, Pseudallescheria, Acremonium,* and *Fusarium* spp.
[d] Zygomycetes include *Mucor, Rhizopus,* and *Absidia* spp.

Vaccines, Susceptibility

Table 8.19 Antiparasitic agents for specific parasites

Parasite	Antiparasitic agents
Protozoa	
Acanthamoeba spp.	Pentamidine(?)
Babesia microti	Atovaquone plus azithromycin, clindamycin plus quinine
Balantidium coli	Tetracycline, metronidazole
Cryptosporidium parvum	Nitazoxanide(?), paromomycin plus azithromycin(?)
Cyclospora cayetanensis	Trimethoprim-sulfamethoxazole
Entamoeba histolytica	Metronidazole, paromomycin, iodoquinol
Giardia lamblia	Metronidazole, furazolidone, paromomycin
Isospora belli	Trimethoprim-sulfamethoxazole, pyrimethamine plus folinic acid
Leishmania spp.	Sodium stibogluconate or meglumine antimonite, amphotericin B, fluconazole
Naegleria fowleri	Amphotericin B
Plasmodium falciparum	
Chloroquine susceptible	Chloroquine
Chloroquine resistant	Mefloquine, doxycycline, atovaquone-proquanil
Plasmodium, other spp.	Chloroquine plus primaquine
Toxoplasma gondii	Pymethamine plus sulfadiazine plus leucovorin; spiramycin (during pregnancy)
Trichomonas vaginalis	Metronidazole
Trypanosoma cruzi	Nifurtimox
Trypanosoma brucei	Pentamidine, melarsoprof, eflornithine
Microsporidia	Albendazole
Nematodes	
Dracunculus medinensis	Metronidazole
Enterobius vermicularis	Albendazole, mebendazole
Hookworm	Albendazole, mebendazole
Onchocerca volvulus	Ivermectin
Other filarial nematodes	Ivermectin, diethylcarbamazine
Strongyloides stercoralis	Ivermectin
Toxocara spp.	Albendazole, mebendazole
Trichinella spiralis	Albendazole, mebendazole
Trichuris trichiura	Albendazole, mebendazole
Trematodes	
Clonorchis sinensis	Praziquantel, albendazole
Fasciola hepatica	Triciabendazole
Schistosoma spp.	Praziquantel
Other trematodes	Praziquantel
Cestodes	
Cysticercus cellulosae	Albendazole, praziquantel
Echinococcus spp.	Albendazole
Intestinal tapeworms	Praziquantel, niclosamide

Vaccines, Susceptibility

Bibliography

For additional information regarding the subjects discussed in this pocket guide, please refer to the following general texts.

Ash, L. R., and T. C. Orihel. 1997. *Atlas of Human Parasitology*, *4th* ed. American Society of Clinical Pathologists, Chicago, Ill.

Atlas, R., and L. Parks. 1993. *Handbook of Microbiological Media.* CRC Press, Inc., Boca Raton, Fla.

Collier, L., A. Balows, and M. Sussman. 1998. *Topley & Wilson's Microbiology and Microbial Infections*, *9th* ed. Edward Arnold, London, United Kingdom. (Note: The *10th* edition will be published in 2004.)

de Hoog, G. S., J. Guarro, J. Gene, and M. J. Figueras. 2000. *Atlas of Clinical Fungi*, *2nd* ed. Universitat Rovira i Virgili, Reus, Spain.

Difco Laboratories. 1998. *Difco Manual*, *11th* ed., Difco Laboratories, Division of Becton Dickinson and Co., Sparks, Md.

Dismukes, W. E., P. G. Pappas, and J. D. Sobel. 2003. *Clinical Mycology.* Oxford University Press, Oxford, United Kingdom.

Garcia, L. S. 2001. *Diagnostic Medical Parasitology*, *4th* ed. ASM Press, Washington, D.C.

Holt, J., N. Krieg, P. Sneath, J. Staley, and S. Williams. 1994. *Bergey's Manual of Determinative Bacteriology*, *9th* ed. The Williams & Wilkins Co., Baltimore, Md.

Kucers, A., S. Crowe, M. L. Grayson, and J. Hoy. 1997. *The Use of Antibiotics: a Clinical Review of Antibacterial, Antifungal and Antiviral Drugs*, *5th* ed. Butterworth Heinemann, Oxford, United Kingdom.

Larone, D. H. 2002. *Medically Important Fungi, a Guide to Identification*, *4th* ed. ASM Press, Washington, D.C.

Mandell, G. L., J. E. Bennett, and R. Dolin. 2000. *Principles and Practice of Infectious Diseases*, *5th* ed. Churchill Livingstone, Philadelphia, Pa. (Note: The sixth edition will be published in 2005.)

Miller, J. M. 1998. *A Guide to Specimen Management in Clinical Microbiology*, 2nd ed. ASM Press, Washington, D.C.

Murray, P. R., E. J. Baron, J. H. Jorgensen, M. A. Pfaller, and R. H. Yolken. 2003. *Manual of Clinical Microbiology*, 8th ed. ASM Press, Washington, D.C.

Murray, P. R., K. Rosenthal, G. Kobayashi, and M. Pfaller. 2002. *Medical Microbiology*, 4th ed. Mosby, St. Louis, Mo.

Richman, D. D., R. J. Whitley, and F. G. Hayden. 2002. *Clinical Virology*, 2nd ed. ASM Press, Washington, D.C.

Rose, N. R., R. G. Hamilton, and B. Detrick. 2002. *Manual of Clinical Laboratory Immunology*, 6th ed. ASM Press, Washington, D.C.

Weyant, R. S., C. W. Moss, R. E. Weaver, D. G. Hollis, J. G. Jordan, E. C. Cook, and M. I. Daneshvar. 1996. *Identification of Unusual Pathogenic Gram-Negative Aerobic and Facultatively Anaerobic Bacteria*, 2nd ed. The Williams & Wilkins Co., Baltimore, Md.

Index

NOTES

NOTES

NOTES

NOTES